Best of Five MCQs for the MRCP Part 1

Volume 2

Best of Five MCQs for the MRCP Part 1

Volume 2

Edited by

Iqbal Khan

Consultant Gastroenterologist and Associate Director of Undergraduate Education, Northampton General Hospital, Northampton, UK

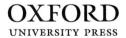

OXFORD
UNIVERSITY PRESS

Great Clarendon Street, Oxford, OX2 6DP,
United Kingdom

Oxford University Press is a department of the University of Oxford.
It furthers the University's objective of excellence in research, scholarship,
and education by publishing worldwide. Oxford is a registered trade mark of
Oxford University Press in the UK and in certain other countries

First Edition published in 2017

Impression: 5

Published in the United States of America by Oxford University Press
198 Madison Avenue, New York, NY 10016, United States of America

British Library Cataloguing in Publication Data
Data available

Library of Congress Control Number: 2016945122

Set ISBN 978–0–19–878792–1
Volume 1 978–0–19–874672–0
Volume 2 978–0–19–874716–1
Volume 3 978–0–19–874717–8

Printed in Great Britain by
Clays Ltd, Elcograf S.p.A.

PREFACE

The Membership of the Royal College of Physicians (MRCP) is a mandatory exam for trainees in the UK intending to enter a career in a medical speciality. The MRCP exam has three parts: MRCP Part 1 (written paper); MRCP Part 2 (written paper); and MRCP Part 2 Clinical Examination (PACES).

The MRCP (UK) Part 1 Examination is designed to assess a candidate's knowledge and understanding of the clinical sciences relevant to medical practice and of common or important disorders to a level appropriate for entry to specialist training. Candidates must sit two papers, each of which is three hours in duration and contains 100 multiple choice questions in 'best of five' format. These are designed to test candidates' core knowledge, the ability to interpret information, and clinical problem solving. The MRCP Part 1 requires a huge breadth of information to be revised.

Whilst books and resources are available, there is a huge variation in the number and quality of practice questions available. Online revision websites can be very expensive and impractical for busy junior doctors in clinical posts. These three volumes have been written with these busy junior doctors in mind and are designed to be studied one volume at a time. The three volumes together cover the full syllabus of the MRCP part 1 exam, and the number of questions per speciality is proportional to that seen in the exam. It is suggested that doctors preparing for the exam should carry one of the books into work each day and use every opportunity to study, even if it is for brief intervals. When time permits a more detailed review of the subject should take place to ensure full understanding of each topic.

The questions have been written and reviewed by experts in their respective fields and I would like to use this opportunity to thank each and every one of the for their excellent contributions.

Iqbal Khan

CONTENTS

ABBREVIATIONS

µmol/L	micromoles per litre
A&E	Accident and Emergency
ABG	arterial blood gas
ACE	angiotensin-converting enzyme
ACTH	adrenocorticotropic hormone
ADH	alcohol dehydrogenase
ADP	aminolaevulinic acid dehydratase porphyria
AGA	antigliadin antibody
AHO	Albright's hereditary osteodystrophy
AIDS	acquired immune deficiency syndrome
AIP	acute intermittent porphyria
Alb	albumin
ALP	alkaline phosphatase
ALT	alanine aminotransferase
AMA	anti-mitochondrial antibody
anti-HBc	anti-hepatitis B core
anti-HBe	anti-E antigen
anti-HBs	anti-hepatitis B surface
AST	aspartate aminotransferase
BCG	bacille Calmette–Guérin
BD	bis in die
Beta-HCG	Beta-human chorionic gonadotropin
BHH	benign hypocalciuric hypercalcemia
BHIVA	British HIV Association
BM	blood glucose monitoring
BMI	body mass index
BNF	British National Formulary
BNP	B-type natriuretic peptide
BP	blood pressure; bullous pemphigoid

bpm	beats per minute
Ca_2	calcium
CDAD	Clostridium difficile-associated diarrhoea
CDI	Clostridium difficile-associated infection
CEP	congenital erythropoietic porphyria
CIN	cervical intraepithelial neoplasia
CL	cutaneous leishmaniasis
CNS	central nervous system
CO_2	carbon dioxide
COPD	chronic obstructive pulmonary disease
Cr	creatinine
CRA	central retinal artery
CRP	C-Reactive Protein
CSF	cerebrospinal fluid
CT	computed tomography
CTPA	CT pulmonary angiography
CXR	chest X-ray
DCL	diffuse cutaneous leishmaniasis
DCCT	Diabetes Control and Complications Trial
DDAVP	desmopressin acetate (1-deamino-8-D-arginine vasopressin)
DEXA	dual energy X-ray absorptiometry
DI	diabetes insipidus
DIDMOAD	diabetes insipidus, diabetes mellitus, optic atrophy, and deafness
DKA	diabetic ketoacidosis
DNA	deoxyribonucleic acid
DRESS	drug rash, eosinophilia, and systemic symptoms
DVT	deep vein thrombosis
ECCO	European Crohn's and Colitis Organisation
ELISA	enzyme-linked immunosorbent assay
EM	erythema multiforme
EMA	endomysial antibody
ERCP	endoscopic retrograde cholangiopancreatogram
ESR	erythrocyte sedimentation rate
ETEC	enterotoxigenic E. coli
FAP	familial adenomatous polyposis
FBC	full blood count

FDA	Food and Drug Administration
FHH	familial hyocalciuric hypocalcaemia
FNA	fine-needle aspiration
FNA	fine-needle aspiration biopsy
FSH	follicle stimulating hormone
FVC	forced vital capacity
GBS	Guillain–Barré syndrome
GCS	Glasgow Coma Scale
g/dL	grammes per decilitre
GFD	gluten-free diet
GFR	glomerular filtration rate
GI	gastrointestinal
g/l	gramme per litre
GGT	gamma-glutamyl transferase
GORD	gastro-oesophageal reflux disease
GP	general practitioner
GVHD	graft versus host disease
HAART	highly active anti-retroviral therapy
HACEK	Haemophilus, Aggregatibacter (previously Actinobacillus), Cardiobacterium, Eikenella, Kingella
Hb	haemoglobin
HBeAg	hepatitis B E antigen
HBIg	hepatitis B immune globulin
HBsAg	hepatitis B surface antigen
HBV	hepatitis B virus
HCC	hepatocellular carcinoma
hCG	human chorionic gonadotropin
HH	hereditary haemochromatosis
HHT	hereditary haemorrhagic telangiectasia
HIV	human immunodeficiency virus
HLA	human leukocyte antigen
HNPCC	hereditary non-polyposis colon cancer
HPV	human papilloma virus
HR	heart rate
HRS	hepatorenal syndrome
HTN	hypertension
HUS	haemolytic uremic syndrome

IBD	inflammatory bowel disease
IBS	irritable bowel syndrome
IE	infective endocarditis
IgA	immunoglobulin A
IgD	immunoglobulin D
IgG	Immunoglobulin class G
IgM	immunoglobulin M
IM	intramuscular
INR	international normalized ratio
ITP	idiopathic thrombocytopenic purpura
ITU	intensive treatment unit
IU/L	international unites per litre
IU/ml	international units per millimetre
IV	intravenous
IVIg	intravenous immunoglobulin
JVP	jugular venous pressure
K	potassium
kg	kilogramme
KPa	kilo Pascal
LAD	left anterior descending coronary artery
LDH	lactate dehydrogenase
LFT	liver function test
LH	luteinizing hormone
LKM	liver-kidney microsomal antibody
LP	lichen planus
mcg/l	microgram per litre
MCA	middle cerebral artery
MCL	mucocutaneous leishmaniasis
MCV	mean corpuscular volume
MEN-1	multiple endocrine neoplasia type 1
MEN-2	multiple endocrine neoplasia type 2
mg	milligramme
MI	myocardial infarction
micromole/l	micromoles per litre
mmHg	millimetres of mercury (torr)
mmol/l	millimoles per litre

mOsm/kg	milliosmole per kilogram
MRCP	magnetic resonance cholangiopancreatography
MRI	magnetic resonance imaging
MRSA	methicillin-resistant Staphylococcus aureus
ms	milliseconds
MSU	midstream urine sample
MU	million units
MU/l	million units per litre
NA	sodium
NAFLD	non-alcoholic fatty liver disease
NASH	non-alcoholic steatohepatitis
NF-1	neurofibromatosis type 1
ng/ml	nanogrammes per millilitre
NMDA	N-methyl-d-aspartate
nml/l	nanomole per litre
NNRTI	non-nucleoside reverse transcriptase inhibitor
NRTI	nucleoside reverse transcriptase
NSAID	nonsteroidal anti-inflammatory drug
O_2	oxygen
od	omni die
OGD	oesophago-gastro- duodenoscopy
PA	plasma aldosterone
PaO_2	potential oxygen
PAS	periodic acid-Schiff
PBC	primary biliary cirrhosis
PCR	polymerase chain reaction
PCT	porphyria cutanea tarda
PDGFR	platelet derived growth factor receptor
PE	pulmonary embolism
PET	positron emission tomography
PG	pyoderma gangrenosum
pg/l	picogramme per litre
pH	potential hydrogen
PI	protease inhibitor
PITS	parietal inferior, temporal superior
PLT	primed lymphocyte test

PML	progressive multifocal leukoencephalopathy
pmol/l	picomole per litre
pO$_2$	potential oxygen
PPI	proton pump inhibitor
PR	by rectum
PSC	primary sclerosing cholangitis
PT	prothrombin time
PTH	parathyroid hormone
PV	pemphigus vulgaris
PVL	Panton–Valentine Leukocidin
QDS	quater die sumendum
RNA	ribonucleic acid
RPR	rapid plasma reagin
RT	Riedel's thyroiditis
SAA	serum amyloid A
SCC	squamous cell carcinoma
SeHCAT	selenium-homocholic acid taurine
SIADH	syndrome of inappropriate antidiuretic hormone
SIRS	systemic inflammatory response syndrome
SLE	systemic lupus erythematosus
SST	short synacthen test
TB	tuberculosis
TDS	ter die sumendum
TEN	toxic epidermal necrolysis
TIPSS	transjugular intrahepatic portosystemic shunt insertion
TNF	tumour necrosis factor
TNM	tumor-node-metastasis
TPHA	treponema pallidum haemagglutination assay
TPMT	thiopurine methyltransferase
TSH	thyroid stimulating hormone
tTG	tissue tranglutaminase
U&E	urea and electrolytes
U/l	units per litre
UC	ulcerative colitis
USS	ultrasound scan
VAP	ventilator-associated pneumonia

VDRL	Venereal Disease Research Laboratory
VHL	Von Hippel–Lindau disease
VLCFA	very long chain fatty acids
WBC	white blood cell count
WCC	white cell count
XLDPP	X-linked dominant protoporphyria
ZE	Zollinger–Ellison

1. **A 52-year-old man presents to the clinic for review some six weeks after starting phenytoin for complex partial seizures. He is very concerned as he has a rash which began on his face but quickly spread over the upper body. It begins as large, painful macules, but the top layer of skin sheds to reveal very moist raw skin underneath. He has a temperature of 37.8°C, and a BP of 135/70 mmHg; the remainder of his examination is normal. Investigations: Hb 13.2, WCC 8.2 (Eosinophilia), PLT 181, Na 138, K 4.2, Cr 130. Which of the following is the most appropriate treatment?**

    A. Topical steroids
    B. Systemic corticosteroids
    C. Stop phenytoin
    D. Oral flucloxacillin
    E. Topical fucidin

2. **A 62-year-old woman presents to the clinic with painful eyes and blurring of vision. She has also been suffering from increasing mouth ulcers over the past few months. On examination she has multiple mouth ulcers and evidence of gingivitis. Slit lamp examination reveals evidence of corneal scarring. There are no significant skin rashes. Investigations: Hb 13.0, WCC 8.1, PLT 191, Na 137, K 4.2, Cr 124. Which of the following is the most likely diagnosis?**

    A. Pemphigus
    B. Bullous pemphigoid
    C. Behcet's syndrome
    D. Occular ciccatrical pemphigoid
    E. Anterior uveitis

3. **Koebner phenomenon is encountered in which of the following conditions?**

   A. Lupus vulgaris
   B. Pitryasis rosea
   C. Lichen planus
   D. Erythema nodosum
   E. Squamous cell carcinoma of the skin

4. **A 39-year-old woman presents to the clinic with an erythematous rash below her umbilicus and around her left wrist. She admits to wearing a cheap fashion watch and wearing a belt with a metal buckle. You suspect nickel allergy. Which of the following hypersensitivity reactions is likely to have occurred?**

   A. Type 1
   B. Type 2
   C. Type 3
   D. Type 4
   E. Type 5

5. **A 26-year-old woman comes to the clinic with her partner. They both have mild inherited ichthyosis vulgaris, they met via patient support group, and want to start a family. Which of the following is factually correct with regards to inheritance of the condition?**

   A. There is a 75% chance any offspring will have clinically significant disease
   B. There is a 25% chance that any offspring will not be affected by the disease and will not be a carrier of the mutation
   C. There is a 50% chance that any offspring will not have clinically significant disease
   D. There is a 100% chance that any offspring will be free of the disease
   E. There is a 100% chance that any offspring will be affected by the disease

6. **A 60-year-old lady feels that her nails have not grown over the last six months. Her hands are shown in Figure 1.1. She gets mildly breathless on exertion, but is otherwise well. Examination of the cardiorespiratory system and abdomen reveals bilateral ankle oedema, but no other abnormalities. Select the most appropriate initial investigation.**

   A. Abdominal ultrasound scan
   B. Chest radiograph
   C. Computed tomography scan of thorax, abdomen, and pelvis
   D. Electrocardiogram
   E. Transthoracic ECHO

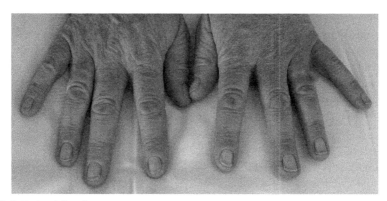

Figure 1.1 Patient's hands

7. **You notice a solitary pigmented lesion on the back of a 68-year-old man, whilst examining his respiratory system (see Figure 1.2). He has been admitted for a suspected exacerbation of chronic obstructive pulmonary disease, but is otherwise well. What is the most appropriate initial management?**
    A. Computed tomography staging scan
    B. Punch biopsy
    C. Reassure him that it is harmless
    D. Urgent referral to oncology to consider radiotherapy
    E. Urgent excision

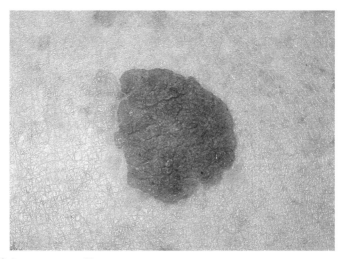

Figure 1.2 Solitary pigmented lesion

8. **An 80-year-old lady is admitted following a fall. She is febrile at 38.1°C. Examination of the cardiorespiratory and nervous systems reveals no gross abnormality. An enlarged spleen is detected on abdominal examination. She is also noted to have several plum-coloured plaques scattered on the trunk and limbs. Her initial bloods show anaemia and thrombocytopenia, but a mild neutrophilia. Select the likeliest diagnosis.**

   A. Acute Epstein–Barr virus infection
   B. Pyoderma gangrenosum
   C. Sarcoidosis
   D. Sweet's syndrome
   E. Urinary tract infection with exanthem

9. **A 43-year-old lady presents with a 4-week history of a non-itchy rash on the face. She has been systemically well and denies other symptoms. She has mild asthma which is well controlled on treatment. She describes Raynaud's phenomenon which occurs occasionally in winter. Examination reveals a symmetrical eruption on the central face, involving the nose, medial cheeks, with a few lesions on the forehead and chin. The eruption is comprised of erythematous papules, with a few pustules and some macular erythema. There Is no scaling. Select the likeliest diagnosis.**

   A. Acne vulgaris
   B. Chronic cutaneous (discoid) lupus erythematosus
   C. Malar rash of systemic lupus erythematosus
   D. Rosacea
   E. Seborrhoeic dermatitis

10. **A 24-year-old woman who works as a hairdresser is referred with a six-month history of a rash on the hands. Examination reveals dryness, scaling, and vesicles, worse on the palmar surfaces. Select the most appropriate investigation.**

    A. Bacterial and viral swabs
    B. Patch tests
    C. Prick tests
    D. Skin biopsy
    E. Specific IgE tests

11. **A 33-year-old man is concerned by the development of some mildly itchy, warty papules on the central chest and behind the ears. He is also noted to have nail dystrophy. He says that his father has similar problems. Select the likeliest diagnosis.**

    A. Darier's disease
    B. Hailey–Hailey disease
    C. Lichen planus
    D. Seborrhoeic keratoses
    E. Viral warts

12. **A 16-year-old boy presents with a red, scaly rash. The differential diagnosis is thought to lie between eczema and psoriasis. Which one of the following would favour the diagnosis of eczema?**

    A. Genital involvement
    B. Hyperlinear palms
    C. Koebner phenomenon
    D. Onycholysis
    E. Well-demarcated areas of involvement

13. **A 30-year-old woman is referred with an eruption confined to the ankles and wrists. Which of the following features would most support a diagnosis of lichen planus?**

    A. Raynaud's phenomenon
    B. Scaly plaques
    C. Scarring
    D. Soreness rather than pruritus
    E. Violaceous papules

14. **A 70-year-old man is seen with a three-day history of suspected maculopapular drug exanthem. He remains well in himself, though he was recently discharged from the rehabilitation ward following a stroke. During his admission, he suffered from two seizures and a urinary tract infection. He has a previous history of gout. His drug history is as follows: allopurinol for five years; amlodipine for three years; aspirin for five weeks; simvastatin for five weeks; perindopril for five weeks; phenytoin for four weeks; seven-day course of trimethoprim which ended seven days ago. Select the likeliest culprit drug.**

A. Allopurinol
B. Aspirin
C. Perindopril
D. Phenytoin
E. Trimethoprim

15. **A 58-year-old man presents with a five-day history of a rapidly extending eruption, characterized by scaling and erythema. He complains of feeling cold although his temperature is 37.1°C. Examination confirms that almost his entire skin surface is affected. He is tachycardic at 116 bpm; BP is 105/62. Which one of the following statements about erythroderma is correct?**

A. A skin biopsy should be taken to exclude toxic epidermal necrolysis
B. Erythroderma means a rash covering the majority of the skin surface area
C. Erythrodermic patients should receive prophylactic antibiotics
D. High output cardiac failure is a potential complication
E. The commonest cause is mycosis fungoides

16. **You are reviewing a patient with Crohn's disease in the clinic. He has had multiple flare-ups over the last year, requiring several courses of steroids, despite taking asacol (5-ASA) continuously. You wish to start him on azathioprine therapy. Which single blood test is essential prior to starting azathioprine?**

A. Iron studies
B. TPMT level (thiopurine methyltransferase)
C. Folic acid levels
D. G6PD level (glucose-6-phosphate dehydrogenase)
E. High density lipoprotein level

17. **Which of the following skin lesions is not associated with diabetes mellitus?**

    A. Acanthosis nigricans
    B. Necrobiosis lipoidica
    C. Lipohypertrophy
    D. Eruptive xanthomata
    E. Erythema nodosum

18. **Which of the following statements regarding bullous pemphigoid is correct?**

    A. Bullae are intra-epidermal
    B. Direct immunofluoresence demonstrates linear deposits of IgG along the epidermal basement membrane zone
    C. It is usually precipitated by alcohol
    D. Extensor surfaces of the limbs are usually involved
    E. Neutrophilia is usually seen

19. **A 35-year-old woman is referred with a necrotic ulcer displaying a purple border on the lower leg. Which of the following conditions is most likely to be associated with the likely skin condition?**

    A. Type 2 diabetes mellitus
    B. Ulcerative colitis
    C. SLE
    D. Rheumatoid arthritis
    E. Pernicious anaemia

20. **A 23-year-old woman presents to the clinic with diarrhoea suggestive of malabsorption, and weight loss of some 6 kg during the past three months. Her GP has checked some routine bloods and found her to be anaemic with a low albumin. In addition, she is anti-TTG antibody postiive. Which of the following skin changes is most likely to be seen?**

    A. Erythematous plaques with associated bullous lesions
    B. Painful erythematous nodules on the lower leg
    C. Vesicobullous eruption on the buttocks
    D. Deep inflammatory fissures in the inguinal folds
    E. Large ulcerated lesion with a violaceous border on the lower leg

21. **A 64-year-old lady sustained a dog bite to the right hand four hours earlier. An empirical prophylaxis cover with antibiotic was deemed necessary as the wound was deep and required extensive toileting in the emergency room. Which of the following antibiotics is regarded most appropriate?**

    A. Flucloxacillin
    B. Erythromycin
    C. Penicillin
    D. Co-amoxiclav
    E. Tetracycline

22. **A 63-year-old man presents with a three-month history of blistering on his face and hands. He feels that the skin on his hands has become thinner and is more easily traumatized than usual. He reports no systemic symptoms and has no significant past medical history. Examination reveals several erosions, scars from previous bullae, and milia formation. There is no mucous membrane involvement. Select the likeliest diagnosis.**

    A. Bullous impetigo
    B. Bullous pemphigoid
    C. Dermatitis herpetiformis
    D. Pemphigus vulgaris
    E. Porphyria cutanea tarda

23. **A 32-year-old lady is referred with an eruption on the hands. Apart from a cold sore on the lip, she has otherwise been well. Examination reveals discrete erythematous lesions on the palms, each with central blistering and two surrounding concentric rings of different hues. Select the most likely diagnosis.**

    A. Bullous pemphigoid
    B. Erythema multiforme
    C. Nodular vasculitis
    D. Pemphigus vulgaris
    E. Secondary syphilis

24. **A 35-year-old delivery driver attends the emergency department with an exacerbation of itching. He has been suffering from urticaria on most days for the last three months, for which his general practitioner has prescribed chlorphenamine 4 mg twice daily. He takes no other regular medication. He denies facial swelling, respiratory symptoms, and light-headedness. Examination reveals widespread weals. Select the most appropriate management plan.**

    A. Cetirizine 20 mg once daily
    B. Chlorphenamine increased to 4 mg four to six times per day
    C. Intramuscular adrenaline and intravenous chlorphenamine
    D. Intravenous hydrocortisone
    E. Prednisolone 30 mg once daily for five days

25. **A 17-year-old girl presents to her GP with a generalized skin rash. She had been prescribed pencillin two weeks earlier for a streptococcal throat infection, but is concerned as she has begun a relationship with a new sexual partner a short while ago. On examination she is apyrexial and her throat looks normal now. She has multiple erythematous scaly plaques on her skin, however, ranging from a few mm to up to 10–15 mm in diameter. Which of the following is the most likely diagnosis?**

    A. Reiter's syndrome
    B. Antibiotic allergy
    C. Guttate psoriasis
    D. Stevens Johnson syndrome
    E. Rheumatic fever

26. **A 25-year-old woman who has received a liver transplant after a paracetamol overdose comes to the clinic for review some two weeks after her transplant. She has begun to develop a painful maculopapular rash over both the palms of her hands and the soles of her feet and has been suffering from increasing diarrhoea. Investigations: haemoglobin 10.2 g/dl (11.5–16.5), white cells 5.1 x 10^9/l (4–11), platelets 149 x 10^9/l (150–400), sodium 138 mmol/l (135–146), potassium 3.9 mmol/l (3.5–5), creatinine 103 micromol/l (79–118), ALT 225 U/l (5–40), albumin 27 g/l (35–50). Which of the following is the most likely diagnosis?**

    A. Acute graft versus host disease
    B. Chronic graft versus host disease
    C. Sirolimus toxicity
    D. Drug-induced psoriasis
    E. Cyclosporin-related dermatitis

27. **Which of the following is not seen in a patient with hereditary haemorrhagic telangiectasia?**
    A. Pale conjunctiva
    B. Hepatic bruit
    C. Hyperpigmentation of the lips
    D. Clubbing
    E. Cyanosis

28. **A 35-year-old man is noted to have bilateral lesions on the shins. Closer examination reveals yellow, atrophic plaques with prominent telangiectasia and an erythematous, annular border. Select the most appropriate management plan.**
    A. Chest radiography and pulmonary function tests for possible sarcoidosis
    B. Computed tomography scan of the thorax and abdomen to search for occult malignancy
    C. Fasting glucose to exclude diabetes mellitus
    D. Skin biopsy to confirm the diagnosis of basal cell carcinoma
    E. Skin scraping should be obtained, prior to treating with a topical antifungal

29. **A 41-year-old woman with coeliac disease is seen regarding an asymptomatic eruption on the legs. Examination reveals palpable purpura. Which one of the following statements is correct?**
    A. A strict gluten-free diet will lead to resolution of the rash
    B. Blood pressure and urinalysis should be checked
    C. Coagulation screen should be performed
    D. She should be admitted for treatment with systemic steroids
    E. The diagnosis is lichen planus and topical steroids should be commenced

30. **A 67-year-old man presents with an enlarging ulcer on the leg. He has a history of ischaemic heart disease and type 2 diabetes mellitus. Examination reveals a 3 cm ulcer with an irregular, undermined, violaceous border which you think may be pyoderma gangrenosum. Which one of the following statements about pyoderma gangrenosum is correct?**
    A. Associated with myeloproliferative disorders
    B. Heals without scarring
    C. Histopathological changes are diagnostic
    D. Requires treatment with broad spectrum antibiotics
    E. Typically asymptomatic

31. **A 22-year-old woman is concerned about an enlarging mole on her leg. Concerning melanoma, which one of the following statements is?**

A. If a melanoma in situ is fully excised, the patient can be deemed cured
B. Lentigo maligna is a particularly aggressive form of the disease
C. Melanoma is the commonest type of skin cancer seen in the black population
D. Most melanomas respond well to chemotherapy
E. The diameter of the tumour at diagnosis is the most accurate prognostic indicator

32. **An 85-year-old retired postman presents with an enlarging lesion on the right temple (see Figure 1.3). Select the likeliest diagnosis.**

A. Amelanotic melanoma
B. Basal cell carcinoma
C. Giant molluscum contagiosum
D. Seborrhoeic keratosis
E. Squamous cell carcinoma

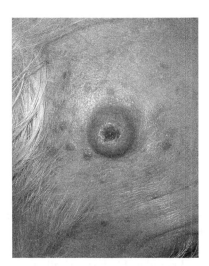

Figure 1.3 Enlarging lesion

33. **A 24-year-old woman with a history of type 1 diabetes presents to the clinic with a collapse. On examination in the emergency department she is heavily pigmented. Her BP is 100/60, pulse is 95 and regular. She claims that her insulin dose has remained the same, but has been suffering more hypos over the past few weeks. Of note in her blood tests is that her sodium is low at 128, and a TSH is elevated at 9.2. Which of the following is the most likely diagnosis?**

   A. Addison's disease
   B. Cushing's syndrome
   C. Hypothyroidism
   D. Dehydration
   E. Haemochromatosis

34. **What percentage of the UK population is affected by psoriasis?**

   A. 0.5%
   B. 2%
   C. 5%
   D. 5%
   E. 12%

35. **Which of the following is associated with autosomal recessive inheritance?**

   A. Peutz–Jeghers syndrome
   B. Cowden's disease
   C. LEOPARD syndrome.
   D. Hereditary haemorrhagic telangiectasia
   E. Xeroderma pigmentosum

36. **A 62-year-old man with a history of type 1 diabetes comes to the foot clinic for review. There is a dry, shallow wound on the plantar aspect of his left foot. He has a history of microalbuminuria and peripheral neuropathy and takes ramipril and amlodipine in addition to his insulin. His BP is 132/70, pulse is 75 and regular. He has a shallow wound on the plantar aspect of his left foot. His ankle brachial pressure index (ABPI) is 0.85. Which of the following is the most appropriate dressing for his wound?**

   A. Alginate
   B. Jelonet
   C. Elastoplast
   D. Foam
   E. Silver

37. **A 36-year-old man with a history of HIV is commenced on abacavir but then presents to the emergency department with an acute hypersensitivity reaction. You are aware that abacavir hypersensitivity is associated with a certain HLA subtype. Which of the following subtypes is most likely to be associated abacavir hypersensitivity?**

A. B1502

B. B1508

C. B5701

D. DQ602

E. DR3

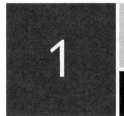

DERMATOLOGY

ANSWERS

1. C. Stop phenytoin

Phenytoin is recognized as a cause of toxic epidermal necrolysis, a dangerous condition resulting in a severe erythematous rash leading to epidermal necrolysis. Withdrawal of the offending agent is the key intervention. Use of systemic corticosteroids is somewhat controversial as they may be associated with increased mortality. Other drugs which cause the condition include allopurinol, non-steroidals, lamotrigine, and penicillins.

Ramrakha PS et al., *Oxford Handbook of Acute Medicine*, Third Edition, Oxford University Press, 2010, Chapter 12, Dermatological emergencies, Toxic epidermal necrolysis (TEN) 1.

2. D. Occular ciccatrical pemphigoid

This picture is consistent with occular ciccatrical pemphigoid, which results in mouth ulcers, and subepithelial conjunctival fibrosis, which untreated can lead to corneal scarring and fibrosis, eventually blindness. Topical therapy is rarely effective, and oral corticosteroids +/− cyclophosphamide are required. Potential antigens identified include epiligrin, and an unidentified 45 kDa protein.

Spickett G, *Oxford Handbook of Clinical Immunology and Allergy*, Second Edition, 2006, Oxford University Press, Chapter 11, Autoimmune eye disease, Ocular cicatricial pemphigoid.

3. C. Lichen planus

Koebner phenomenon occurs when new skin lesions erupt at the site of traumatic injuries in areas of apparently normal skin. Lichen planus, pemphigus vulgaris, molluscum contagiosum, and vitiligo are associated with this phenomena. Other causes include psoriasis and warts.

Crissey JT, Parish LC, Holubar KH, *Historical Atlas of Dermatology and Dermatologists*, Parthenon Publishing Group, 2002.

4. D. Type 4

Nickel allergy is a type 4 hypersensitivity reaction, and occurs when nickel (in metals such as a belt buckle or watch strap) reacts with keratin in the skin to drive an immune reaction. The antigen is presented to T cells by macrophages, which then leads to expansion of T-cell clones which specifically react with nickel. These help to drive production of cytokines leading to infiltration of activated neutrophils at the site of nickel deposition. Type 1 hypersensitivity is immediate and is IgE-mediated, occurring in response to an allergen. Examples include urticaria and hayfever. Type 2 hypersensitivity includes sensitivity to self, in other words autoimmunity. Examples include Grave's disease and Goodpasture's. Type 3 hypersensitivity is immune complex-mediated disease, examples include serum sickness and post-streptococcal glomerulonephritis. Type 5 hypersensitivity is used in some circles to describe a subset of type 2 hypersensitivity where antibodies bind to cell surface receptors, for example in Grave's.

Wilkins R et al., Oxford Handbook of Medical Sciences, Second Edition, Oxford University Press, 2011, Chapter 12, Infection and immunity, Hypersensitivity

5. B. There is a 25% chance that any offspring will not be affected by the disease and will not be a carrier of the mutation

This question is tricky as inherited ichthyosis is an autosomal dominant condition with incomplete penetrance. It is caused by mutations in the genes coding for filaggrin, and at least two mutations, including p.R501X and c.2282del4, are recognized in affected patients. Hence those carrying one mutation usually have only mild clinical disease, although those who are homozygotes or compound heterozygotes may be severely affected. The condition is not responsive to corticosteroids, although some patients may respond to retinoids. The main aim of therapy is to achieve adequate skin hydration.

Burge S, Wallis D, Oxford Handbook of Medical Dermatology, Oxford University Press, 2011, Chapter 31, Skin in infancy and childhood, Red scaly skin in neonates and infants

6. B. Chest radiograph

This patient has yellow discoloration of all of the fingernails. There is mild onycholysis at the lateral borders of a few nails. The cuticles are absent. These features, along with the history of markedly slowed growth indicates yellow nail syndrome. This is a rare disorder which usually begins in middle age and is difficult to treat. The nail changes may be associated with lymphoedema, as in this case. There may be lung abnormalities, particularly effusions (in around one-third of patients). Other associations include bronchiectasis, recurrent lower respiratory tract infection, and sinusitis. Lymphatic impairment is thought to be responsible for the condition, but the aetiology is poorly understood. There are sparse reports suggesting that yellow nail syndrome can be paraneoplastic, but in the absence of other suspicious findings, whole body computed tomography is not indicated as an initial investigation.

Ngan V, Yellow nail syndrome, Dermnet, 2009. http://dermnetnz.org/hair-nails-sweat/yellow-nails.html

7. C. Reassure him that it is harmless

This lesion is a typical seborrhoeic keratosis. It is sharply demarcated with a matt surface and has a 'stuck on' appearance. The surface is warty, with numerous fissures. It is mainly mid-brown, with some ill-defined darker areas; there is also a skin-coloured component adjacent to the main part of lesion. Seborrhoeic keratoses can range in colour from pink, through skin coloured to various shades of brown and virtually black. They become more numerous with advancing age and are extremely common. They have no malignant potential. Atypical lesions can often be mistaken for skin cancer. The lesion shown here, however, can confidently be diagnosed clinically, so no intervention is indicated (symptomatic lesions can be treated with cryotherapy or curettage). When melanoma is suspected, excision by an individual experienced in dealing with pigmented lesions is the management of choice. In practice, this is usually a dermatologist or plastic surgeon and an urgent referral is warranted.

Balin AK, Seborrheic keratosis, Emedicine, 2009. http://emedicine.medscape.com/article/1059477-overview

8. D. Sweet's syndrome

Sweet's syndrome or acute febrile neutrophilic dermatosis typically presents with fever and the abrupt onset of tender, red to purple papules, nodules or plaques. The lesions may blister. Peripheral neutrophilia is common. Although many cases are idiopathic, others are precipitated by underlying infection or drugs. There is also a well recognized association with malignancy, particularly myeloproliferative disease, as in the case described. The diagnosis should be confirmed on skin biopsy. The rash usually responds very well to systemic corticosteroids, but investigations are required to exclude an underlying cause. Acute Epstein–Barr virus infection or infectious mononucleosis usually presents in a much younger age group. If a rash is present, it would be expected to be maculopapular or morbilliform in morphology. Pyoderma gangrenosum has clinical and histological similarities with Sweet's disease, but causes rapidly enlarging, painful ulcers with an undermined, violaceous border. It is usually treated with systemic corticosteroids or immunosuppression. The cutaneous manifestations of sarcoidosis are protean, but the description here is classical for Sweet's syndrome. Erythema nodosum, which can be associated with sarcoidosis, typically gives rise to tender, subcutaneous nodules on the legs. The presentation with fall, pyrexia, and neutrophilia might initially suggest urinary tract infection with exanthem, but this would not explain the eruption.

Bae-Harboe Y-SC et al., Acute febrile neutrophilic dermatoses, *Emedicine*, 2010. http://emedicine. medscape.com/article/1122152-overview

9. D. Rosacea

The distribution and age of onset of this acneiform eruption are highly suggestive of rosacea, which also can lead to prominent telangiectasia. The pathogenesis is poorly understood. The condition usually begins in middle age and is often persistent. Treatment options include topical metronidazole or azelaic acid and oral tetracycline antibiotics. Chronic rosacea can lead to sebaceous hypertrophy usually on the nose, known as rhinophyma. Manifestations of ocular rosacea include blepharitis, conjunctivitis, and keratitis. The description is acneiform, with papules and pustules. However, acne vulgaris mostly occurs in a younger age group and lesions are not usually confined to the central face. Discoid lupus erythematosus gives rise to erythematous, scaly plaques, particularly on sun-exposed sites. It is a cause of scarring alopecia. Systemic lupus erythematosus is also a photosensitive condition; its classical malar rash may comprise macular erythema or a plaque, but pustules are not seen. The patient described is systemically well, making this diagnosis very much less likely. Seborrhoeic dermatitis may co-exist with rosacea but manifests as mildly erythematous, superficial plaques, with overlying waxy scale. It tends to be prominent in the nasolabial folds and can also cause scaling in the eyebrows and on the scalp.

Randleman JB, Loft ES, Song CD, Ocular rosacea, *Emedicine*, 2009. http://emedicine.medscape.com/ article/1197341-overview

10. B. Patch tests

The description is suggestive of eczema. Vesicles are more common in allergic than irritant dermatitis. In the context of chronic, bilateral findings confined to the hands, eczema herpeticum is unlikely; weeping or crusts might suggest bacterial infection, but these are not described in this case. Hairdressers are routinely exposed to numerous irritants and potentially sensitizing chemicals and hand eczema is a common result. Patch tests are required to identify allergic contact dermatitis (ACD). These assess for type 4 (delayed) allergy and involve application of multiple chemicals to the back. These stay in place for two days and definitive readings are taken after a further two days. Prick tests and specific IgE tests both check for type 1 (immediate) allergy and are not relevant to ACD. Hand eczema is a clinical diagnosis and a biopsy is not required.

Guidelines on the managemnet of contact dermatitis: an update, British Association of Dermatologists, *British Journal of Dermatology* 2009;160:946–954.

11. A. Darier's disease

Darier's disease is an autosomal dominantly inherited condition which is characterized by warty, greasy papules. These tend to predominate in seborrhoeic areas, including the central chest and back, the scalp and on the ears. Nail changes are common: a central V-shaped nick is typical. Palmar pits are found in the majority of patients. The diagnosis can be confirmed on skin biopsy. Some patients develop problems with superadded infection, either with bacteria or herpes simplex virus. Hailey–Hailey disease is another autosomal dominantly inherited condition, also known as benign familial pemphigus. It typically gives rise to erosions in flexural areas. Lichen planus is an inflammatory condition, characterized by intensely pruritic violaceous papules. Seborrhoeic keratoses are extremely common, acquired, benign lesions, but are unusual before the age of around 40. Viral warts are commonest in children and immunosuppressed individuals. The latter three conditions do not have a hereditary component.

Kwok P-Y et al., Keratosis follicularis (Darier disease), *Emedicine*, 2010. http://emedicine.medscape.com/article/1107340-overview

12. B. Hyperlinear palms

Typical features of eczema include prominent pruritus, skin dryness, fine scaling, and ill-defined erythema. Childhood eczema tends to affect the flexures and hands, though this pattern may be lost in adulthood. Psoriasis is characterized by well-defined plaques with a variable degree of overlying, adherent scale. It tends to predominate on the extensor surfaces, though other common sites include the scalp, umbilicus, natal cleft, and genitalia. The Koebner phenomenon is seen typically in psoriasis. Onycholysis is a key feature of psoriatic nail disease, though may arise from other causes. Eczema can also be associated with nail changes, most commonly horizontal ridging. Hyperlinearity of the palms is associated with mutations of the filaggrin gene. This gives rise to altered skin barrier function and predisposes to atopic eczema. Hyperlinear palms are also seen in ichthyosis vulgaris.

Brown SJ et al., Filaggrin null mutations and childhood atopic eczema: a population-based case-control study, *Journal of Allergy and Clinical Immunology* 2008;121:940–946.

13. E. Violaceous papules

Lichen planus (LP) is a disorder of unknown aetiology. Many clinical subtypes have been described. The commonest form, classical LP, gives rise to intensely itchy, violaceous polygonal papules which coalesce into plaques. Overlying fine white scale, known as Wickham's striae, is typically seen on the surface. As the lesions subside, they leave prominent post-inflammatory hyperpigmentation, but not scarring. LP tends to demonstrate the isomorphic response or Koebner phenomenon, whereby the eruption 'colonizes' sites of even minor trauma, usually after a delay of a few days. Nail changes such as tracheonychia (sandpapered nails) can be seen. Intra-oral changes, which may be asymptomatic, are common in LP. Classical LP usually responds well to application of a very potent topical steroid. Raynaud's phenomenon is associated with various connective tissue diseases, but not with LP.

Chuang T-Y, Stitle L, Lichen planus, *Emedicine*, 2010. http://emedicine.medscape.com/article/1123213-overview

14. E. Trimethoprim

Virtually any drug can cause an exanthem. The commonest culprits include allopurinol, antibiotics— especially sulfonamides and penicillins—anti-convulsants, and non-steroidal anti-inflammatory drugs. An accurate drug history, with timings, is essential when trying to tease out the cause of a drug exanthem. Unless the patient has previously been sensitized (when the rash usually appears after one or two doses), a lag of 1–2 weeks is typically seen between commencement of the drug and the onset of the eruption. Even if the drug has been stopped, the rash may still occur. Thus in this case, trimethoprim, a likely causative drug, has been taken in the likely time window. It should be avoided by this patient in future. It should be noted that certain more serious drug eruptions, such as Stevens–Johnson syndrome, toxic epidermal necrolysis, and DRESS (drug rash, eosinophilia, and systemic symptoms) may occur after a longer lag phase of around a month.

Blume JE et al., Drug eruptions, *Emedicine*, 2010. http://emedicine.medscape.com/article/1049474-overview

15. D. High output cardiac failure is a potential complication

Erythroderma is defined as redness and scaling covering at least 90% of body surface area. The commonest cause is eczema, followed by psoriasis, then drug eruption, then cutaneous T-cell lymphoma (including mycosis fungoides). Possible complications include dehydration, renal failure, electrolyte disturbance, temperature dysregulation, infection, hypoalbuminaemia, and high output cardiac failure. Toxic epidermal necrolysis (TEN) is a specific eruption, which is almost always attributable to drugs. It is characterized by fever, skin pain, and macular erythema, with blistering and denudation of the epidermis, and mucosal involvement. TEN does not usually enter the differential diagnosis of erythroderma.

Umar SH, Kelly AP, Erythroderma (Generalized Exfoliative Dermatitis), *Emedicine*, 2009. http://emedicine.medscape.com/article/1106906-overview

16. B. TPMT level (thiopurine methyltransferase)

Azathioprine is metabolized into 6-MP which is further metabolized into the active and cytotoxic components. TPMT is the enzyme that inactivates 6-MP through methylating thiopurine compounds. Patients with low or absent activity are at an increased risk of drug-induced bone marrow toxicity. TPMT level is determined genetically (11% of population have reduced levels and 3% have absent TPMT levels). Hence, it is essential to measure the TPMT levels prior to starting azathioprine or 6-MP medication, as this reading will guide you to give reduced dosage to those with reduced TPMT levels, thus reducing the risk of toxic side effects. Procollagen 3 is used to monitor hepatic fibrosis in patients on methotrexate.

Torkamani A et al., Azathioprine metabolism and role of TPMT, *Emedicine*. http://emedicine.medscape.com/article/1829596-overview

17. E. Erythema nodosum

Diabetes is associated with many skin disorders. Acanthosis nigricans is associated with insulin-resistant diabetes mellitus. Lipoatrophy and lipohypertrophy are both related to diabetes mellitus. Lipohypertrophy occurs secondary to the pharmacological effects of insulin repeatedly deposited at the same location. Eruptive xanthomata occurs secondary to hyperglycaemia associated with poor glycaemic control.

Mert A et al., Erythema nodosum: an experience of 10 years, *Journal of Infectious Diseases* 2004;36:424–427.

18. B. Direct immunofluoresence demonstrates linear deposits of IgG along the epidermal basement membrane zone

Bullous pemphigoid is an acute or chronic autoimmune disease involving the formation of bullae. It mainly affects the elderly population; involvement of the trunk, limbs, and flexures is common. The eruption can start with pruritus and urticated, erythematous lesions. Later tense blisters develop both on normal and erythematous skin. There may be mucosal involvement with blisters and erosions. The blisters are subepidermal and intact epidermis forms the roof. Autoantibodies, especially IgG, to the epidermal basement membrane zone are found in skin and blood. It may be precipitated by exposure to drugs including loop diuretics, ACE inhibitors, and penicillamine.

Langan SM et al., Bullous pemphigoid and pemphigus vulgaris—incidence and mortality in the UK, *British Medical Journal* 2008;337:a180.

19. B. Ulcerative colitis

Pyoderma gangrenosum is a rare non-infectious neutrophilic dermatosis commonly associated with underlying systemic disease. It can have a wide variety of presentations but the classical finding is that of a necrotic ulcer with characteristic violaceous undermined edges. Systemic associations include: ulcerative colitis and Crohn's disease, multiple myeloma, acute and chronic myeloid leukaemia, arthritis, and chronic active hepatitis. Out of the options listed above it is most likely to be associated with ulcerative colitis. Management may include intra-lesional triamcinalone, systemic corticosteroids, and second-line immunosuppressive agents.

Powell FC et al., Pyoderma gangrenosum: classification and management, *J Am Acad Dermatol* 1996;34(3):395–409.

20. C. Vesicobullous eruption on the buttocks

Inflammatory bowel disease (IBD) is associated with many extra-intestinal manifestations including the skin. Answer A refers to Sweet's syndrome. Sweet's syndrome is a neutrophilic dermatoses which is associated with underlying disease in 50% of cases. It is seen in association with inflammatory bowel disease, malignancy, commonly haematological malignancy, infection, and pregnancy. Answer B describes the clinical picture seen in erythema nodosum. Causes include systemic disease (IBD, sarcoid, Bechet's and Hodgkin's disease) infections, drugs (oral contraceptive pill, aspirin, dapsone and sulphonamides) and pregnancy. Answer D relates to the clinical manifestation of cutaneous Crohn's disease. Answer E describes the clinical picture of pyoderma gangrenosum. Systemic associations include: IBD, multiple myeloma, acute and chronic myeloid leukaemia, arthritis and chronic active hepatitis. Answer C relates to dermatitis herpetiformis. This is associated with coeliac disease.

Rook A et al., *Textbook of Dermatology*, Fourth Edition, Blackwell Scientific Publications, 2013.

21. E. Tetracycline

Dog-bite-related infections are polymicrobial, predominantly *Pasteurella multocida* and *Bacteroides spp*. Infected bites presenting less than 12 hours after injury are particularly likely to be infected with *Pasteurella spp.*, whereas those presenting more than 24 hours after the event are likely to be predominantly infected with staphylococci or anaerobes. The major basis for recommending co-amoxiclav is in-vitro sensitivity data. Co-amoxiclav covers *P. multocida*, the penicillin-resistant *S. aureus* and anaerobes. *Pasteurella multocida* is resistant to flucloxacillin and erythromycin. Penicillin and tetracycline are not effective against *P. multocida*.

Centers for Disease Control and Prevention, Nonfatal dog bite-related injuries treated in hospital emergency departments—United States, 2001, *Morbidity and Mortality Weekly Report* 2003;52(26):605–610.

22. E. Porphyria cutanea tarda

Features of porphyria cutanea tarda (PCT) include skin fragility, blistering, milia (tiny inclusion cysts which tend to occur after blistering), scarring, hypertrichosis, and (rarely) sclerodermoid changes. These occur on sun-exposed sites. The condition is caused by a defect in the haem biosynthetic pathway. Most PCT is acquired secondary to chronic liver disease, which leads to reduced activity of the enzyme uroporphyrinogen decarboxylase. The diagnosis should be confirmed by checking urinary, faecal, and red blood cell porphyrin levels. Work-up should include a non-invasive liver screen. Skin biopsies for histology and immunofluorescence can be helpful to rule out differential diagnoses. Treatment includes sun protection, venesection if iron overload is present, low-dose chloroquine, and management of any other underlying liver disease. Bullous impetigo is common in children: usually a golden crust is seen in addition to fragile bullae. Bullous pemphigoid gives rise to tense bullae, but skin fragility and a photo-distribution are not seen. Dermatitis herpetiformis is associated with friable, pruritic vesicles, classically at extensor sites. Pemphigus vulgaris is always associated with mucosal involvement.

Poh-Fitzpatrick MB, Porphyria cutanea tarda, *Emedicine*, 2010. http://emedicine.medscape.com/article/1103643-overview

23. B. Erythema multiforme

The description is of target lesions at an acral site, which is typical of erythema multiforme (EM). Central blistering occurs in some cases. There may also be mucosal involvement. EM is a reactive dermatosis. It is most commonly precipitated by *Herpes simplex* infection, as in this case. Other triggers include various infections, notably Mycoplasma, and occasionally drugs. The condition is self-limiting with resolution usually occurring within 10–14 days. Bullous pemphigoid (BP) and pemphigus vulgaris (PV) are immunobullous diseases caused by circulating antibodies. BP tends to present in elderly individuals with generalized, tense blisters. PV often begins in middle age; mucosal involvement is prominent and blisters are very friable with resultant superficial erosions. Nodular vasculitis leads to purpuric lumps, but not target lesions. Secondary syphilis has many possible manifestations. One of the classical findings is discrete scaly lesions on the palmoplantar surfaces, but not target lesions.

Plaza JA, Prieto VG, Erythema multiforme, *Emedicine*, 2010. http://emedicine.medscape.com/article/1122915-overview

24. A. Cetirizine 20 mg once daily

This patient has chronic urticaria. The mainstay of treatment is antihistamines. For a driver, it is important that these be non-sedating, so chlorphenamine is not the best choice. Unlicensed doses of antihistamines are often required to gain control of the condition, which may be highly symptomatic. This patient lacks features of anaphylaxis, so parenteral treatment with adrenaline, chlorphenamine, or hydrocortisone is not required. Systemic steroids may have a role in acute urticaria, or possibly in acute exacerbations, but should be reserved for the most refractory cases. Antihistaminic treatment has not been optimized in this case and therefore this approach should take precedence. Chronic urticaria (conventionally of greater than six weeks' duration) is usually idiopathic and allergy is rarely of relevance (in contrast to acute urticaria where not infrequently there is an obvious precipitant). The disease is characterized by pruritic weals; individual lesions are expected to resolve within 24 hours (though new ones may appear, such that the rash is always present). Weals of longer duration should raise the possibility of urticarial vasculitis. High doses of antihistamines may be required to control chronic urticaria. Occasionally, immunosuppression is required, but corticosteroids are not favoured for this chronic condition, in view of their poor long-term safety profile.

Urticaria and angioedema, British Association of Dermatologists, 2009. http://www.bad.org.uk/site/740/default.aspx

25. C. Guttate psoriasis

Guttate psoriasis is recognized to occur post-streptococcal infection, accounting for up to 60% of cases. The rash occurs around 14 days after infection and resolves spontaneously over the course of a few weeks, requiring little treatment apart from simple emollients. Very rarely are topical steroids or UV treatment actually required.

Collier J et al., *Oxford Handbook of Clinical Specialties*, Eighth Edition, Oxford University Press, 2009, Chapter 8, Dermatology, Psoriasis.

26. A. Acute graft versus host disease

This patient's symptoms are consistent with graft versus host disease, as evidenced by the typical rash, and diarrhoea which is consistent with mucus membrane and gut lining inflammation. Whilst the initial development of the condition is thought to be T-cell-mediated, other inflammatory cells are recruited as the condition worsens. Often the rash may extend to form confluent areas of erythema or even erythroderma in severe cases. Acute GVHD occurs within the first 100 days, and is primarily T-cell-mediated, with pre-formed clones existing to the donor tissue. Chronic GVHD is said to occur after 100 days, and both T-cell-mediated mechanisms and changes in humoral immunity are thought to drive the development of GVHD.

Ferrara JLM et al., Graft-versus-host disease, *Lancet* 2009;373:1550–1561. http://www.sciencedirect.com/science/article/pii/S0140673609602373

27. C. Hyperpigmentation of the lips

Hereditary haemorrhagic telangiectasia (HHT) is an autosomal dominant disorder due to mutations in ENG and ACVRL1 genes. This leads to abnormal blood vessel formation in the skin, mucous membranes, lungs, liver, and brain. This manifests as epistaxis, cutaneous telangiectasia, and visceral arteriovenous malformations. Patients often give a family history and present with symptoms of iron-deficient anaemia, telangiectasia of the nail beds and face (commonly lips and tongue), pallor, and spontaneous epistaxis. Furthermore, visceral arteriovenous malformations can lead to hepatic and pulmonary bruits, signs of cardiac failure, and subarachnoid haemorrhage. Hyperpigmentation of the lips is seen in Peutz–Jeghers syndrome.

HTT Foundation International. http://curehht.org/

28. C. Fasting glucose to exclude diabetes mellitus

This is a classical description of necrobiosis lipoidica. This is a condition of unknown aetiology. It occurs in 0.3% of patients with diabetes mellitus. It may occur in those without diabetes and sometimes precedes this diagnosis. It does not appear to be related to glycaemic control. The alternative answers all describe appropriate investigation of other problems. Dermatophyte infection also causes annular lesions, with a scaly edge. Various eruptions can be paraneoplastic, such as dermatomyositis or acanthosis nigricans. Basal cell carcinoma does not cause atrophy and bilateral lesions would be atypical. Sarcoidosis can be associated with erythema nodosum, which does typically affect the shins, but this manifests as firm, tender, subcutaneous nodules.

Barnes CJ, Davis L, Necrobiosis lipoidica, *Emedicine*, 2010. http://emedicine.medscape.com/article/1103467-overview

29. B. Blood pressure and urinalysis should be checked

Palpable purpura indicates the presence of vasculitis. Possible causes include connective tissue disease, Henoch–Schönlein purpura, hepatitis B or C infection, and drugs, though idiopathic cutaneous vasculitis is not uncommon. It is vital to exclude systemic involvement. Initial investigations should include blood pressure and urinalysis to screen for early renal involvement. Bloods should be taken for blood count, urea and electrolytes, liver enzymes, inflammatory markers, auto-antibodies (e.g. anti-nuclear and anti-neutrophil cytoplasmic antibodies), and anti-streptolysin O titre. If no systemic involvement is found, the rash may be managed conservatively with rest and/or compression. Oral steroids or other drugs (e.g. dapsone or colchicine) are sometimes used if the rash is causing symptoms such as pain, oedema, or ulceration. Otherwise, treatment should be directed at the underlying cause. Unless there are significant complications, admission is unnecessary. Lichen planus is very itchy and gives rise to violaceous, but not purpuric, papules. Coeliac disease is not associated with vasculitis, but dermatitis herpetiformis, which would be expected to settle with a strict gluten-free diet. Coagulation defects do not lead to palpable purpura.

Cohen SN, English JSC, Skin, nails and hair. In: *Chamberlain's Symptoms and Signs in Clinical Medicine*, Houghton A, Gray D (eds), Thirteenth Edition, Hodder Arnold, 2010.

30. A. Associated with myeloproliferative disorders

Pyoderma gangrenosum (PG) is an uncommon inflammatory condition of unknown aetiology. It has been reported in association with many diseases, but relatively common associations include myeloproliferative disorders, inflammatory bowel disease, rheumatoid arthritis, and diabetes mellitus. PG begins as a pustule or papulonodule, which breaks down to form an ulcer. This is usually very painful and can extend rapidly. Ulceration may be multifocal and is commonest on the legs. The condition sometimes demonstrates pathergy, with new lesions arising at sites of trauma. The ulcer edges are violaceous or gun-metal coloured and undermined; there is often pus in the base. The diagnosis is primarily clinical. Histology can be corroborative, but the dense neutrophil infiltrate is not specific for the condition. Treatment is with immunosuppressives, such as corticosteroids or cyclosporin. If not apparent, underlying associations should be sought. Ulcers tend to heal with cribriform scarring.

Jackson JM, Callen JP, Pyoderma gangrenosum, *Emedicine*, 2010. http://emedicine.medscape.com/article/1123821-overview

31. A. If a melanoma in situ is fully excised, the patient can be deemed cured

Melanoma in situ refers to a melanoma that is confined to the upper layer of skin, the epidermis. When melanoma cells breach into the dermis, the tumour is classed as invasive and it is only at this point that metastasis becomes possible. Melanoma is the type of cancer responsible for the greatest number of deaths in young people. It is much more common in Caucasians but may occur in darker skin types. However, the most common type of skin cancer in black people is squamous cell carcinoma. The most accurate prognostic indicator at diagnosis is the depth of the tumour, measured as the Breslow thickness. The primary treatment of melanoma is excision. Chemotherapy can be used for metastatic disease, but the response rate to standard treatment with dacarbazine is only around 10%. Lentigo maligna is a subtype of melanoma in situ which tends to occur in elderly individuals with chronically sun-damaged skin. It has a more indolent behaviour than other melanomas in situ, though it may become invasive in which case it is termed lentigo maligna melanoma.

Swetter SM, Malignant melanoma, *Emedicine*, 2010. http://emedicine.medscape.com/article/1100753-overview

32. E. Squamous cell carcinoma

The image shows a red, crateriform nodule with a central keratotic plug. This is the classical appearance of squamous cell carcinoma (SCC). The clinical differential diagnosis includes keratoacanthoma, a benign mimic of SCC which grows rapidly, demonstrates a plateau phase, and then regresses spontaneously. Amelanotic melanoma does not show keratinization. Basal cell carcinoma is usually skin coloured or pink, with a rolled, pearly edge, surface telangiectasia, and central ulceration or crust. Molluscum contagiosum is a self-limiting infection caused by a pox virus. It classically gives rise to umbilicated papules. Giant mollusca can occur, particularly in the immunosuppressed. Some can easily be mistaken for skin cancer, but the lesion in the picture, occurring on a sun-exposed site, is typical for SCC. Seborrhoeic keratosis is a very common benign lesion, manifesting as a skin-coloured or pigmented warty lesion, with a 'stuck on' appearance. Risk factors for SCC include lighter skin type, age, chronic sun exposure, and long-term immunosuppression. SCC is usually treated by excision, though radiotherapy is an alternative. Around 5% of cutaneous SCCs metastasize, usually to draining lymph nodes.

Jennings L, Schmults CD, Squamous cell carcinoma, *Emedicine*, 2010. http://emedicine.medscape.com/article/1101535-overview

33. A. Addison's disease

Although the TSH is elevated in this case, the pigmentation, low sodium, and frequent hypoglycaemia fit much better with a diagnosis of Addison's. Rehydration and corticosteroid replacement are the initial mainstays of therapy. Replacement of thyroid hormone can actually precipitate a worsening of the adrenal crisis. Cushing's leads to hyperglycaemia and weight gain. Haemochromatosis is associated with type 2 diabetes and not type 1 diabetes.

Longmore M et al., *Oxford Handbook of Clinical Medicine*, Nineth Edition, Oxford University Press, 2014, Chapter 5, Endocrinology.

34. B. 2%

The incidence of psoriasis varies greatly across the world, but approximately 2–3% of Caucasians suffer from the condition. The prevalence of psoriasis is around 50% less in individuals of African origin. The median age of onset is 28, although 15% of cases of psoriasis begin under the age of ten years. Alcohol is well recognized as an aetiological factor as are drugs such as beta-blockers and lithium. Skin trauma and infections including staphylococcus, streptococcus, and HIV are also recognized to precipitate episodes.

Fairhurst DA et al., Optimal management of severe plaque form of psoriasis, *American Journal of Clinical Dermatology* 2005;6(5):283–294.

35. E. Xeroderma pigmentosum

Xeroderma pigmentosum is an autosomal recessive disease characterized by photosensitivity, pageantry changes, premature ageing, and neoclassic and abnormal DNA repair. Some patients have neurological complications. Peutz–Jeghers syndrome is autosomal donminant and is characterized by the development of benign hamartomatous polyps in the gastrointestinal tract and hyperpigmented macules on the lips and oral mucosa. Cowden's disease is a rare autosomal dominant disorder. It is characterized by multiple hamartomatous lesions of ectodermal, endodermal, and mesodermal origin. There is a predisposition to malignant tumours, particularly of the breast. LEOPARD syndrome is a rare autosomal dominant disorder. Multiple lentigines are associated with a wide range of developmental defects. Hereditary haemorrhagic telangiectasia is an autosomal dominant dosease characterized by epistaxis, cutaneous telangiectasia, and arteriovenous malformations. Multiple telangiectasia occur at various characteristic sites: lips, oral cavity, fingers, and nose.

Ber Rahman S, Bhawan J, Lentigo, *International Journal of Dermatology* 1996;35:229–239.

36. B. Jelonet

Management of wounds in patients with diabetes is dependent upon the depth of the wound, the amount of exudate, presence or absence of infection, and arterial supply. In this case the arterial supply to the lower limbs is excellent, and there are no signs of infection. Given that there is only a small amount of exudate, jelonet is therefore the dressing of choice. Silver dressings are used when infection is suspected. Hydrocolloid and alginate are used for wounds when a large amount of exudate is present, and foam dressings are used when exudate needs to be contained.

Lesley K. Bowker, James D. Price, and Sarah C. Smith, *Oxford Handbook of Geriatric Medicine*, Second Edition, Oxford University Press, 2012, Chapter 18, Pressure injuries

37. C. B5701

B5701 was recognized in 2008/2009 to be associated with abacavir hypersensitivity, and a genetic test was developed to screen out high-risk individuals prior to starting abacavir anti-retroviral therapy. B1502 and B1508 are both associated with hypersensitivity to carbamazepine and increased risk of the development of Stevens–Johnson syndrome. DQ602 is a protective allele for autoimmune diabetes, and DR3 is a risk allele for autoimmune diabetes and rheumatoid arthritis.

Warrell DA et al., *Oxford Textbook of Medicine,* Fifth Edition, Oxford University Press, 2010, Section 23, 23.16, Cutaneous reactions to drug

1. **A 24-year-old woman with a history of congenital adrenal hyperplasia comes to the clinic for review. She is currently taking prednisolone and tells you that she thinks she is six weeks pregnant. Which of the following is a key feature of her pregnancy care?**

   A. Dexamethasone 20 mg should be started before week 10
   B. Her prednisolone should be increased immediately by 10 mg
   C. She should be given oestrogen during the pregnancy
   D. She should be given progesterone during the pregnancy
   E. A female child will usually require reconstructive therapy after birth

2. **Which of the following is about calcitonin?**

   A. A decline in Ca^{2+} level stimulates its release
   B. It has an analgesic effect
   C. It is secreted by special cells in the parathyroid gland
   D. It can be given by mouth
   E. It stimulates osteoblast activities

3. **A 32-year-old woman is treated with block–replace carbimazole/ thyroxine for Grave's disease. She presents to the clinic complaining of increasingly blurred vision. On examination she has lid retraction and proptosis. There is decreased visual acuity affecting both eyes. Her TSH is suppressed and her T4 is in the normal range. Which of the following is the most appropriate initial treatment?**

   A. Prednisolone 60 mg
   B. Methotrexate 10 mg
   C. Ciclosporin 10 mg
   D. Cyclophosphamide 100 mg
   E. Orbital radiotherapy

4. **A 43-year-old man is brought to the hospital with a hip fracture following a minor fall. Bone density measurement of the patient's spine and hip reveals osteoporosis. Which of the following should be measured in this patient?**

A. Serum B12 level

B. Serum testosterone

C. Calcitonin levels

D. Lipid profile

E. Vitamin E levels

5. **A 67-year-old man was referred with a calcium level of 2.91 mmol/l and parathormone hormone level (PTH) at 10 pg/l (normal value 2–2 pg/l). This patient's hypercalcaemia is most likely due to which of the following conditions?**

A. Sarcoidosis

B. Primary hyperparathyroidism

C. Hypervitaminosis D

D. Multiple myeloma

E. Malignancy with bone metastases

6. **A woman who is 31 weeks pregnant comes to the clinic. She is currently taking 10 mg of carbimazole for thyrotoxicosis, but is complaining of further palpitations and anxiety. Repeat thyroid function tests confirm that her TSH is <0.05. T3 and T4 are also above the upper limit of normal. Which of the following is the correct course of action?**

A. Increase her carbimazole

B. Switch to propylthiouracil

C. Partial thyroidectomy

D. Radioiodine

E. Deliver the baby by caesarean

7. **A 34-year-old woman is referred to the clinic with symptoms of thirst, tiredness, and indigestion. She is unaware of her past family medical history because she tells you she was adopted by a travelling family. On examination her blood pressure is 132/72, pulse is 75 and regular. Her BMI is 22 and general physical examination is unremarkable. Investigations: Hb 11.4 g/dl, WCC 8.4 x10^9/l, PLT 237 x10^9/l, Na$^+$ 137 mmol/l, K$^+$ 4.0 mmol/l, creatinine 103 micromol/l, glucose 3.5 mmol/l, gastrin 290 pmol/l (<55), calcium 2.91 mmol/l. Which of the following additional findings/diagnoses is most likely?**

   A. Hypercortisolaemia
   B. Medullary thyroid carcinoma
   C. VIPoma
   D. Phaeochromocytoma
   E. Insulinoma

8. **A 22-year-old woman is referred by her GP to the clinic because she has not had a period for some five months. She admits to enjoying long-distance running and tells you that she has lost a considerable amount of weight whilst training for a marathon. On examination her BMI is 18.5, pulse is 57 and regular; physical examination is normal apart from her low BMI. Investigations: Hb 12.1, WCC 7.9, PLT 169, Na 137, K 4.3, Cr 90, TSH 2.6, FSH and LH both well above the normal range. What is the most likely diagnosis?**

   A. Primary ovarian failure
   B. Autoimmune ovarian failure
   C. Ovarian failure due to low BMI
   D. Pregnancy
   E. Turner's syndrome

9. **A 22-year-old diabetic patient attends hospital with a week's history of feeling unwell. Over the last two days they have been vomiting and have not taken their normal insulin. The nurse takes their blood sugar which just reads 'high' on the glucometer. They look dehydrated and unwell. Which of the following statements is correct?**

   A. Total body potassium will be elevated
   B. Rehydration and insulin should always commence immediately concurrently
   C. Low molecular weight heparin should be administered
   D. Intravenous sodium bicarbonate should be considered
   E. Arterial blood gases would reveal a reduced anion gap

10. **What is the commonest cause of primary hyperaldosteronism in the UK?**

    A. Bilateral adrenal hyperplasia
    B. Conn's syndrome
    C. Cushing's syndrome
    D. Addison's disease
    E. Genetic enzyme defects

11. **You see a 45-year-old patient who has just had a myocardial infarct and has significant coronary artery disease. He has tested positive for familial hypercholesterolaemia. Which of these statements most closely reflects the pathophysiology of this condition?**

    A. Autosomal dominant LDL receptor mutation which reduces cholesterol clearance
    B. Autosomal recessive HDL receptor mutation which reduces cholesterol clearance
    C. Apolipoprotein B mutation
    D. Autosomal dominant with elevated VLDL
    E. Lipoprotein lipase deficiency

12. **A 24-year-old woman with type 1 diabetes comes to the clinic for review. She has been well controlled on a basal bolus insulin regime with an HbA1c of 7.3%, but most recently has begun to lose weight. She has also complained of stress, for which her GP recommended anti-depressants. Her BP is 112/70, her pulse is 90 and regular. There is a fine tremor on examination of her hands. Investigations: Hb 12.9, WCC 6.9, PLT 191, Na 137, K 4.2, Cr 105, HbA1c 7.3%. Which of the following is the most likely diagnosis?**

    A. Graves' disease
    B. Coeliac disease
    C. SLE
    D. Crohn's disease
    E. Addison's disease

13. **You are asked to review a 54-year-old woman who has suffered a Colles' fracture. She is found to have a T score of −2.8 and is confirmed to have osteoporosis. Which of the following conditions predisposes to reduced bone mineral density?**

A. Hypothyroidism
B. Obesity
C. Smoking
D. Late menopause
E. Early menarche

14. **A 17-year-old man with short stature comes to the clinic for review. He has struggled at school and finds sport particularly difficult because of muscle weakness and frequent cramps. Investigations: Hb 12.1, WCC 8.2, PLT 201, Na 137, K 4.3, Cr 122, Ca 2.05, PO4 1.8, PTH 22.1. Which of the following is the most likely finding on physical examination?**

A. Shortened first metacarpal
B. Shortened second and third metacarpals
C. Shortened fourth and fifth metacarpals
D. Shortened first phalanx
E. Shortened radius

15. **A 49-year-old man complains of profuse diarrhoea, frequently associated with facial flushing. The symptoms are often precipitated by alcohol. On examination a pansystolic murmur is heard over the praecordium, loudest at the lower left sternal edge. Transaminases are elevated with an ALT of 320 U/l and he is anaemic with an Hb of 10.2 g/dl. His symptoms are the result of over-production of which of the following hormones?**

A. Cholecystokinin
B. Serotonin
C. Vasoactive intestinal polypeptide
D. Gastrin
E. Somatostatin

16. **A 42-year-old woman presents to the oncology clinic for follow-up. She has recently undergone a thyroidectomy for medullary carcinoma of the thyroid. There is no history in the family of multiple endocrine neoplasia or familial medullary thyroid cancer. Which of the following is the percentage chance that she has a RET oncogene mutation?**

    A. 10%
    B. 20%
    C. 50%
    D. 75%
    E. 100%

17. **A 25-year-old woman comes to the clinic for review. It is four weeks since she has received radioiodine for Grave's thyrotoxicosis. She is in a stable relationship and she and her partner want to start a family. She is now euthyroid and wants to know how soon she may start a family. What does the guidance state on this matter?**

    A. One month post radioiodine
    B. Three months post radioiodine
    C. Six months post radioiodine
    D. Nine months post radioiodine
    E. Twelve months post radioiodine

18. **A 32-year-old woman is referred with difficult-to-manage hypertension. She is already managed with three anti-hypertensives: ramipril, bendroflumethiazide, and lacidipine. Her BP is still 155/95, clinical examination is otherwise normal. Blood testing reveals a potassium of 3.2, creatinine of 90. Her spot aldosterone:renin ratio is 845. Which of the following is the most appropriate next step in her management?**

    A. MRI abdomen
    B. Add doxazosin
    C. Add atenolol
    D. Echocardiogram
    E. Intravenous pyelogram

19. **A 66-year-old man presents to the emergency room complaining of severe thirst and polyuria. He has a long history of COPD and his GP has prescribed him a three-week course of doxycycline in an attempt to reduce his number of exacerbations. On examination his BP is 140/90, with a postural drop of 20/10. His sodium is 145 mmol/l, his glucose is mildly elevated at 7.2 mmol/l. Which of the following is the most appropriate way to manage him?**

   A. Stop his doxycycline
   B. Fluid restrict him
   C. Tell him to drink at least 4 litres of water per day
   D. BD vasopressin
   E. High dose bendroflumethiazide

20. **A 39-year-old woman presents as a new patient with hypertension. She has not started any treatment. Investigations reveal: serum sodium 136 mmol/l, serum potassium 2.7 mmol/l, urea 6.7 mmol/l, serum creatinine 98 micromol/l. Which of the following further investigations might be expected in this patient?**

   A. Low renin, low aldosterone
   B. Low renin, high aldosterone
   C. High renin, high aldosterone
   D. High renin, low aldosterone
   E. None of the above

21. **A 52-year-old woman presents with diarrhoea and flushing. She is on no medication. Her past history includes a cholecystectomy fours years previously and an appendicectomy last year. What is the likely cause for her symptoms?**

   A. Carcinoid tumour
   B. Menopause
   C. Phaeochromocytoma
   D. Thyrotoxicosis
   E. Whipple's disease

22. **An 18-year-old girl is being investigated for short stature, and a pituitary cause is suspected. What is the most appropriate investigation to detect growth hormone deficiency?**

    A. Clonidine test
    B. Growth hormone estimation pre- and post-exercise
    C. Growth hormone estimation during glucose tolerance test
    D. Growth hormone estimation following an insulin stress test
    E. Midnight and morning growth hormone estimation

23. **A 33-year-old woman complains of increased skin pigmentation. Six months previously she had undergone bilateral adrenalectomy for Cushing's syndrome. She is on fludrocortisone 100 micrograms daily and hydrocortisone 20 mg morning and 10 mg evening. What is the cause for her pigmentation?**

    A. Addison's disease
    B. Amyloidosis
    C. Haemochromatosis
    D. Nelson's syndrome
    E. Sarcoidosis

24. **A 25-year-old woman in the second trimester of her second pregnancy—the first pregnancy was normal and resulted in a live boy three years previously weighing 3.1 kg—presents with headaches, palpitations, and sweating. Her blood pressure is found to be 220/110 mmHg. What is the likely cause of her hypertension?**

    A. Carcinoid tumour
    B. Coarctation of the aorta
    C. Phaeochromocytoma
    D. Pre-eclampsia
    E. Thyrotoxicosis

25. **A 21-year-old woman with a history of type 1 diabetes comes to the clinic for review. She has begun losing weight over the past few months, despite feeling hungry most of the time. She has also had to take time off work because of anxiety. On examination her BMI is 19, her BP is 135/75, and she has a resting pulse of 92. Her chest is clear and she has a smooth goitre. A recent HbA1c demonstrates good glycaemic control at 7.1%. TSH is <0.05 and thyroid antibodies are positive. What appearance would you expect on thyroid isotope scan?**

    A. A focal hot spot of increased uptake
    B. Multiple areas of increased uptake
    C. Normal scan
    D. Globally decreased uptake
    E. Globally increased uptake

26. **Deficiency of which vitamin may result in Wernicke–Korsakoff syndrome?**

    A. Vitamin A
    B. Vitamin B1
    C. Vitamin B3
    D. Vitamin B6
    E. Vitamin B12

27. **A 42-year-old man presents with headache, thirst, and urinary frequency. His only past history was erythema nodosum. He is on no medication. Investigations reveal: Serum sodium 146 mmol/l, urea 12.2 mmol/l, serum creatinine 105 micromol/l, serum potassium 3.9 mmol/l, serum calcium (corrected) 2.46 mmol/l. What is the likely cause for his symptoms?**

    A. Cerebral sarcoidosis
    B. Craniopharyngioma
    C. Diabetes mellitus
    D. Hypopituitarism
    E. Retroperitoneal fibrosis

28. **You are asked to see a 43-year-old woman who has had a partial thyroidectomy a few hours previously. She is confused, agitated, threatening to take her own discharge, and has been noted to be in rapid atrial fibrillation. What is the likely cause for her symptoms?**

    A. Acute alcohol withdrawal
    B. Bipolar disorder
    C. Mitral stenosis
    D. Reaction to anaesthetic
    E. Thyroid storm

29. **A 70-year-old woman with a past history of heart disease and epilepsy complained of tiredness. Her thyroid function was found to be abnormal, though she was clinically euthyroid. Which of her following medications is the least likely to be the culprit for the biochemical abnormality?**

    A. Aspirin
    B. Amiodarone
    C. Carbamazepine
    D. Atenolol
    E. Phenytoin

30. **The 43-year-old sister of a woman who has emigrated to the UK from central Africa comes to visit. She is taken for a private visit to the local endocrinologist because she feels tired and lethargic. She admits to eating mainly local specialities at home. On examination her BP is 138/82, pulse is 80 and regular and BMI is 29. She has an obvious diffuse nodular goitre on examination of her neck. Her TSH is slightly elevated at 5.4 mU/l (0.5–4.5). What is the most likely diagnosis?**

    A. Hashimoto's disease
    B. Iodine deficiency
    C. Graves' disease
    D. Non-toxic multinodular goitre
    E. Toxic multinodular goitre

31. **A 28-year-old woman comes to the clinic complaining of a slowly enlarging hard mass on the right-hand side of her neck. There are no other associated symptoms and she is otherwise well; the only medication of note is the oral contraceptive pill. On examination she has a 3–4 cm mass on the right-hand side of her neck. Thyroid function testing reveals a TSH of 3.4 mU/l (0.5–4.5), her calcium is normal at 2.43 mmol/l (2.20–2.67). Which of the following is the most likely underlying cause?**

    A. Papillary carcinoma
    B. Follicular carcinoma
    C. Medullary carcinoma
    D. Anaplastic carcinoma
    E. Multinodular goitre

32. **A 78-year-old woman presents to the clinic for review after a second Colles' fracture. On further questioning she admits to being very poorly compliant with her bisphosphonate because of severe indigestion. Other past medical history of note includes a pulmonary embolus for which she was treated with warfarin for a period of six months. A T score is measured at –4.5. Which of the following is the most appropriate treatment?**

    A. Strontium
    B. Monthly risedronate
    C. Monthly ibandronate
    D. Calcium and vitamin D
    E. Denosumab

33. **A 32-year-old man who has had type 1 diabetes for 20 years comes to the clinic for review. His HbA1c has drifted higher over the past few months and has now reached 8.3% (67 mmol/mol). He has tried increasing his basal insulin, but is suffering from increased nocturnal hypoglycaemia. According to NICE guidelines, which is the most appropriate basal insulin for him?**

    A. NPH insulin
    B. Insulin glargine
    C. Insulin glulisine
    D. Insulin aspart
    E. Insulin lispro

34. **A 79-year-old man is brought to the emergency department by ambulance from his nursing home. He is known to take a number of medications for type 2 diabetes and the staff were unable to wake him from sleep in the morning. He has recently been investigated for chronic renal impairment and has been ill with diarrhoea and vomiting. On admission to the department his finger prick blood glucose is measured at 1.9 mmol/l. Which of the following medications is most likely to have been responsible?**

    A. Glibenclamide
    B. Acarbose
    C. Pioglitazone
    D. Gliclazide
    E. Glipizide

35. **A 30-year-old woman is seen (for the fourth time in two years) in accident and emergency with abdominal pain and vomiting. Clinical examination reveals a thin young woman with widespread skin pigmentation. Blood tests demonstrate hyponatraemia (Na 120 mmol/l). A pregnancy test is negative and abdominal X-ray is unremarkable. Due to persistent vomiting, she is admitted to the ward by the Endocrine registrar on call who considers a diagnosis of Addison's disease. A random cortisol level is sent and the laboratory subsequently phones through to inform you that this is undetectable. Which of the following is most in keeping with a diagnosis of primary (autoimmune) adrenal insufficiency?**

    A. A low plasma renin level
    B. A low 9 am ACTH level
    C. Elevated VLCFA (very long chain fatty acid) levels
    D. Eosinophilia
    E. Adrenal gland calcification

36. **A 32-year-old male lawyer presents with weight loss, agitation, and diarrhoea. On examination, he is noted to have warm skin and a sinus tachycardia. Blood tests confirm thyrotoxicosis (with a strongly positive TSH receptor antibody) and he is treated accordingly. Several months later, he presents with dry, gritty eyes. Having done some research on the internet, he is very concerned and would like to ask you some questions about Graves' opthalmopathy. Which of the following statements he presents to you is correct?**

    A. It is less common in cigarette smokers
    B. It is more common in women
    C. It occurs in 75% of patients with Graves' disease
    D. Loss of vision is common
    E. Proptosis is always symmetrical

37. **A 78-year-old female presents to her GP with general malaise, confusion, and abdominal pain. Her past medical history consists of hypertension for which she was treated with an ACE inhibitor. She gave up smoking two years ago, having previously smoked 20 cigarettes a day for 30 years. Investigations showed: normal full blood count, thyroid function, renal function; cCa: 2.89 mmol/l (2.2–2.65 mmol/l); PTH: 7.0 (1.6–9.3 pmol/l); ACE: 88 IU/l (10–70); 24-hour urinary Ca excretion: elevated. What is the most likely diagnosis?**

    A. Benign hypocalcuric hypercalcaemia (BHH)
    B. Hypercalcaemia related to ACE inhibitor treatment
    C. Hypercalcaemia related to malignancy
    D. Primary hyperparathyroidism
    E. Sarcoidosis

38. **A 23-year-old woman is brought into A&E drowsy and confused; she is unable to give a history. GCS is 9 and there is some vomit around her mouth. On examination the pulse rate is 102 bpm, BP 78/35 mmHg, SpO_2 is 98% on air and temperature is 37.5°C. On auscultation of her chest there are a few crackles at the right base. Her BM is 3.2 mmol/l. Blood tests reveal that the sodium is 123 mmol/l, potassium 5.9 mmol/l, urea 7.9 mmol/l, and creatinine 118 micromol/l. Which of the following treatments is most urgent?**

    A. Intravenous 50% dextrose with actrapid insulin
    B. Hypostop gel
    C. Hypertonic saline
    D. Intravenous hydrocortisone
    E. Intravenous co-amoxiclav

39. **A 38-year-old woman with a 30-year history of type 1 diabetes attends the clinic for review. She is currently managed with a basal bolus insulin glargine and actrapid regime. Her BP is 112/72, she has microalbuminuria, and a recent creatinine was 95 micromol/l. HbA1c is 7.1%. Which of the following is the most appropriate course of action?**

    A. Do nothing
    B. Move her to a basal bolus insulin regime
    C. Add enalapril titrated to maximal tolerated dose
    D. Add amlodipine titrated to maximal tolerated dose
    E. Add aspirin

40. **A 30-year-old woman complains of being thirsty more than usual and notes that she has been visiting the toilet more frequently to pass urine. No complaints about dysuria or foul-smelling urine. Her urea and electrolytes are as follows: Na 125 mmol/l (137–144), K 4.5 mmol/l (3.5–4.9), U 7.0 mmol/l (2.5–7.5), Cr 120 micromol/l (60–110), corrected Ca 2.40 mmol/l (2.12–2.65). Which would be the next appropriate investigation?**

    A. Serum Glucose
    B. Water Deprivation Test
    C. Synachten Test
    D. Liver Fuction Test
    E. Paired urine and serum osmolality.

41. **A 70-year-old man fell off a ladder and was knocked out. He had a CT head scan which revealed a 1.3 cm macroadenoma not encroaching the optic chiasm. He recovered well from the fall and examination, including visual fields, was entirely normal. His thyroid function tests, synacthen test, and testosterone levels were all normal. The prolactin level was 550 mU/l (50–450). Which is the most appropriate treatment?**

    A. Pituitary radiotherapy
    B. Transphenoidal hypophysectomy
    C. Monitor with serial imaging
    D. No further investigation/treatment required
    E. Commence cabergoline treatment

42. **An 80-year-old woman comes into hospital with confusion, and is unable to give a full history. On examination, she is underweight with a fine tremor of the fingers. She has lid lag and pretibial myxoedema. Her blood tests are as follows: TSH: 0.001 mu/l (0.5– 5 mu/l), total T4: 250 mmol/l (70–140 mmol/l), total T3: 3.5 nmol/l (1.2–2.6 nmol/l). What is the cause?**
    A. De Quervain's thyroiditis
    B. Graves' disease
    C. Excess thyroxine treatment
    D. Toxic nodule
    E. Unable to tell at this stage

43. **A 25-year-old woman with a history of Addison's disease comes to the clinic for review. She is currently taking 20 mg of hydrocortisone in the morning and 10 mg in the evening. Happily, she is eight weeks pregnant with her first child. Which of the following is the correct advice with respect to her corticosteroids?**
    A. Decrease dose by 5 mg/day
    B. Increase dose by 10 mg/day in the first trimester
    C. Increase dose by 10 mg/day in the third trimester
    D. Increase steroid dose in the first trimester by 10 mg/day until three months post-partum
    E. Give hydrocortisone 20 mg PO when labour begins

44. **With regard to multiple endocrine neoplasia type 1 (MEN-1), which is the most appropriate answer?**
    A. It is characterized by pancreatic, parathyroid, and thyroid tumours
    B. It is inherited in an autosomal recessive pattern
    C. Measurement of serum calcium is a useful screening test for suspected cases
    D. The gene for MEN-1 has been mapped to chromosome 13q11.
    E. It is associated with Marfanoid habitus

45. **A 63-year-old man, weighing 75 kg, presented in the A&E department after a car accident in which he pulled out into a main road and was hit by a passing car. He was not on any drugs. He complains of numbness in his fingers and blames the accident on this. He is found to be hypertensive (190/110 mmHg), with a pulse of 84 sinus rhythm, and routine blood tests reveal: urea 5.8 mmol/l, serum creatinine 100 micromol/l, serum potassium 4.5 mmol/l, random glucose 10.8 mmol/l, TSH less than 0.05 mIU/l. What is the cause of his hypertension?**
    A. Acromegaly
    B. Conn's syndrome
    C. Cushing's disease
    D. Diabetes
    E. Phaeochromocytoma

46. **A 75-year-old woman is referred to the endocrine clinic with a rapidly enlarging hard neck mass. She also has a worsening cough, pain around her neck, and shortness of breath, particularly when she lies flat. On examination there is a hard neck mass, extending out of the left side of the neck, with evidence of local lymph node enlargement. Investigations: TSH 1.3, calcium 2.41, ESR 85. Fine needle aspiration biopsy—multiple spindle cells seen. Which of the following is the most likely diagnosis?**

    A. Anaplastic thyroid carcinoma
    B. Follicular thyroid carcinoma
    C. Papillary thyroid carcinoma
    D. Medullary thyroid carcinoma
    E. Parathyroid carcinoma

47. **A 40-year-old woman presents with lethargy and tiredness six months after delivery of her fifth child. Her symptoms have been blamed on her busy family commitments and her urea, electrolytes, and liver function tests are normal. Her haemoglobin is 11.7 g/dl, free T4 6 and TSH less than 0.01 mIU/l. What is the likely cause for her symptoms?**

    A. Addison's disease
    B. De Quervain's thyroiditis
    C. Graves' disease
    D. Hashimoto's thyroiditis
    E. Sheehan's syndrome

48. **A 76-year-old woman is admitted to the hospital with a respiratory tract infection. She has had a cough for the past few days and was found by her daughter confused and rambling, sitting in her lounge. There is a past history of myocardial infarction and diet-controlled diabetes mellitus. On examination she is pyrexial 38.2 and has signs of a right lower lobe pneumonia. Investigations: Hb 11.0, WCC 13.4, PLT 214, Na 116, K 4.1, Cr 100, Alb 38, ALT 54. How would you manage the hyponatraemia?**

    A. 1.8% saline infusion
    B. 0.45% saline infusion
    C. 3% saline infusion
    D. Demeclocycline
    E. Fluid restriction

49. **A 50-year-old woman with episodic chronic diarrhoea and generalized abdominal pain was noted to have an enlarged thyroid gland. The blood pressure was 187/110 mmHg. Ultrasound study of the thyroid gland showed enlargement of both lobes of the thyroid gland with multiple lymph gland enlargement in the neck. Bowel studies were normal. The most likely diagnosis is?**

    A. Thyrotoxic multinodular goitre
    B. Multiple endocrine neoplasia
    C. Follicular cell carcinoma
    D. Riedel's thyroiditis
    E. Lymphoma

50. **You were referred a 23-year-old woman of low intelligence from whom little history was obtainable. She has been found to have a serum calcium (corrected) of 1.6 mmol/l and serum phosphate 2.2 mmol/l with normal renal function and there have been no previous hospital admissions. Her brother died of 'asthma'. What is the cause of her low serum calcium?**

    A. Hypoparathyroidism
    B. Hypocalcaemic hypercalciuria
    C. Osteomalacia
    D. Pseudohypoparathyroidism
    E. Pseudopseudohypoparathyroidism

51. **A 65-year-old woman who is under the urologists for investigation of renal stones presents with polydipsia, polyuria, and increasing fatigue. Her blood tests reveal that the albumin is 48 g/l, calcium 3.38 mmol/l, phosphate 0.49 mmol/l, urea 16 mmol/l, and creatinine 168 micromol/l. On measurement her parathyroid hormone level is 167 pmol/l. What is the most likely diagnosis?**

    A. Primary hyperparathyroidism
    B. Multiple myeloma
    C. Hypercalcaemia of malignancy
    D. Tertiary hyperparathyroidism
    E. Familial hypocalciuric hypercalcaemia

52. **Which of the following is true of Conn's syndrome?**

    A. It is associated with metabolic acidosis
    B. It iss excluded by the presence of normal serum potassium
    C. It is frequently caused by underlying malignancy
    D. It is associated with high-serum renin to aldosterone ratio
    E. It may be successfully treated with spironolactone

53. **A 33-year-old woman comes to the clinic for review a few weeks after the birth of her first baby by caesarean section. She suffered a post-partum haemorrhage and required a 3-unit blood transfusion. She is feeling tired, is gaining weight, and is increasingly nauseous. On examination her BP is 132/82. Investigations: haemoglobin 11.1 g/dl (11.5–16.5), white cells 8.0 x 10⁹/l (4–11), platelets 183 x 10⁹/l (150–400), sodium 128 mmol/l (135–146), potassium 4.9 mmol/l (3.5–5), creatinine 112 micromol/l (79–118), TSH 0.5 (0.5–5.0). What is the most likely diagnosis?**

    A. Post-partum thyroiditis
    B. Grave's disease
    C. Hashimoto's thyroiditis
    D. Pituitary failure
    E. Functional disorder

54. **A patient is found to have a phaeochromocytoma. She reports that her mother had the same thing. Which of these conditions is NOT typically associated with familial phaeochromocytoma?**

    A. Familial adenomatous polyposis (FAP)
    B. Von Hippel-Lindau (VHL) disease
    C. Neurofibromatosis type 1 (NF-1)
    D. Multiple endocrine neoplasia type 2 (MEN-2).
    E. None of the above

55. **A 53-year-old woman was initially referred because of marked weakness and hypokalaemia. She reported a history of hypertension. Further investigation showed significantly high plasma aldosterone levels. The next test you need to consider is?**

    A. A computed tomography (CT) of the abdomen
    B. Low-dose dexamethasone-suppression test
    C. 24-hour urinary catecholamines
    D. Plasma aldosterone to plasma renin ratio
    E. Adrenal venous sampling

56. **A 61-year-old man with a history of type 2 diabetes comes to the clinic complaining of hypoglycaemia in the late afternoon. His recent HbA1c is elevated at 8.4%. He takes BD mixed insulin 30/70, 22 units in the morning and 18 units in the evening. His BP is 152/72, and he has microalbuminuria. Which of the following is the correct course of action with respect to his insulin regime?**

    A. Decrease his morning mixtard to 18 units
    B. Split his morning mixtard into a breakfast and a lunchtime dose
    C. Transfer him to a basal bolus insulin regime
    D. Change him to mixtard 50:50
    E. Change him to mixtard 40:60

57. **A 17-year-old boy comes to the clinic for review with his parents. He started insulin therapy for new-onset type 1 diabetes some two weeks earlier. They have read about residual insulin production being associated with better potential outcomes and want to know about the best way to preserve their son's beta cell function. His c-peptide by mixed meal test has been measured at 1.4 nmol/l. Which of the following represents the most appropriate intervention with respect to preserving his beta cell function?**

    A. Simvastatin
    B. Anti-inflammatory agents
    C. Intensive glycaemic control
    D. ACE inhibitor use
    E. Corticosteroids

58. **A 62-year-old woman with a long history of type 2 diabetes now managed with BD mixed insulin comes to the clinic with worsening night-time pain and parasthesiae related to peripheral neuropathy. Other medication includes ramipril, atorvastatin, indapamide, and aspirin. She has tried rubbing axsain cream into her legs, but it seems to give her little benefit. Investigations: haemoglobin 10.8 g/dl (11.5–16.5), white cells 7.3 x 10^9/l (4–11), platelets 194 x 10^9/l (150–400), sodium 137 mmol/l (135–146), potassium 4.4 mmol/l (3.5–5), creatinine 138 micromol/l (79–118), HbA1c 7.4% (<5.5) (58 mmol/mol). Which of the following is the most appropriate treatment?**

    A. Carbamazepine
    B. Sodium valproate
    C. Gabapentin
    D. Duloxetine
    E. Vigabatrin

59. **A 23-year-old man with a 19-year history of type 1 diabetes comes to the clinic for review. He takes a basal bolus insulin regime, and after many years of poor blood glucose control, it has improved over the past two years. His most recent HbA1c is 7.3% and his BP is 110/72. He has background diabetic retinopathy. Which of the following managment steps is likely to have the biggest impact on his retinopathy progression?**

    A. Move to insulin pump therapy
    B. Start atenolol
    C. Start enalapril
    D. Start amlodipine
    E. Start aspirin

60. **A 23-year-old man is brought into hospital by ambulance having been found by the passers-by collapsed outside a shopping centre. Examination is unremarkable and there are no signs of trauma. During resuscitation, a colleague notes that the patient is wearing a metal bracelet with the words 'Type 1 Diabetes' engraved on it. Further tests are conducted: a capillary blood glucose reading is 'high' and an arterial blood gas demonstrates a significant metabolic acidosis. Further results become available as management continues: Na 129 mmol/l, K 4.0 mmol/l, Ur 10.0 mmol/l, C. 120 micromol/l, Cl 90 mmol/l, HC0$_3$ 18 mmol/l, glucose 32 mmol/l. Which of the following corresponds best with this patient's anion gap?**

    A. 13
    B. 17
    C. 18
    D. 25
    E. 308

61. **A 74-year-old woman is admitted from home having been found barely conscious on the floor by her home help. It looks like she has had a fall; she has a history of type 2 diabetes for which she takes metformin. On examination she is pyrexial 38.5, has a BP of 105/ 70, and a pulse of 100. She has signs of a right-sided pneumonia and appears not to be moving her left side. Investigations: haemoglobin 11.6 g/dl (11.5–16.5), white cell count 12.1 x 10^9/l (4–11), platelets 192 x 10^9/l (150–400), serum sodium 151 mmol/l (135–146), serum potassium 4.1 mmol/l (3.5–5), creatinine 172 micromol/l (79–118), glucose 38.9 mmol/l (<5.5). Which of the following represents an average recommended IV fluid replacement during the first four hours?**

    A. 0.5 litre
    B. 1 litres
    C. 3 litres
    D. 5 litres
    E. 6 litres

62. **You are reviewing a 51-year-old man with a history of type 2 diabetes who has failed to tolerate metformin monotherapy due to diarrhoea so has been started on a sulphonylurea. The reduction in HbA1C seen has been extremely impressive at 1.2% over the past four months. Which of the following is a gene thought to be involved in response to sulphonylureas?**

    A. MCR4
    B. BCAT
    C. KCNJ11
    D. OCT1
    E. TCF7L2

63. **A 36-year-old woman has been undergoing treatment for primary infertility and presents unwell with tachycardia and blood pressure 88/50 mmHg, and abdominal swelling. Blood tests show urea 15.6 mmol/l, serum creatinine 165 micromol/l, and serum albumin 20 g/l. Pregnancy test is negative. What is the cause of her abdominal swelling?**

    A. Congestive cardiac failure
    B. Hydatidiform mole
    C. Ovarian hyperstimulation syndrome
    D. Portal hypertension
    E. Nephrotic syndrome

64. **A 56-year-old man with type 2 diabetes comes to the clinic for review. He is currently taking metformin monotherapy, 1 g BD. He has recently been admitted with an anterior myocardial infarction, for which he received an LAD stent, but has a degree of cardiac failure since. Other medication now includes ramipril, furosemide, atorvastatin, aspirin, and clopidogrel. On examination his BP is 125/72, his pulse is 82, and there are bibasal crackles on auscultation of the chest. His BMI is 33. An HbA1c is measured at 8.3%, a recent creatinine is 122 micromol/l. Which of the following is the most appropriate additional medication to improve his blood glucose control?**

    A. Gliclazide
    B. Pioglitazone
    C. Long-acting insulin analogue
    D. Basal bolus insulin regime
    E. Liraglutide

65. **A 45-year-old man with long-standing type 1 diabetes comes
to the clinic for review complaining of worsening blood glucose
control. He also reports painful induration and an urticarial
rash appearing at the site of his long-acting insulin injections.
On examination you confirm multiple areas of urticaria and
induration. His HbA1c has risen from 7.4% to 9% over the last
6 months. Which of the following is the most likely diagnosis?**

    A. Lipohypertrophy
    B. Lipoatrophy
    C. Insulin allergy
    D. Hives
    E. Allergy to insulin excipients

66. **A 19-year-old anorexic woman consents to admission for
parenteral nutrition. Her BMI has fallen to 16.3 and she is
dangerously ill. She begins parenteral nutrition prepared by
the on-call dietician over the weekend. Unfortunately, a few
hours later she becomes severely unwell with muscle weakness,
hypotension, (BP 95/60), a pulse of 95, and bilateral crackles
on auscultation of her chest. Which electrolyte has not been
adequately replaced in her nutritional program?**

    A. Calcium
    B. Potassium
    C. Magnesium
    D. Phosphate
    E. Sodium

67. **A 24-year-old man with 47 XXY chromosome abnormality
attends the infertility clinic. Which of the following would be the
most likely finding on clinical examination?**

    A. An excess of facial hair
    B. Breast development
    C. Mental retardation
    D. Tall stature
    E. Ambiguous genitalia

68. **A 50-year-old diabetic man is admitted with confusion and a blood
glucose level of 2.5 mmol/l. Which of these medications does not
usually cause hypoglycaemia when used in monotherapy?**

    A. Nateglinide
    B. Gliclazide
    C. Insulin glargine
    D. Metformin
    E. Glibenclamide

69. A 25-year-old male is admitted to A&E confused and breathless. According to his housemates he has been increasingly thirsty over the past few days and waking up to pass urine many times a night. His arterial blood gas is as follows: pH 7.27, PaO$_2$ 14.8 KPa, PaCO$_2$ 2.8 KPa, HCO$_3$- 7 mEq/L. What investigation is likely to be most useful in confirming the diagnosis?

    A. CXR
    B. Blood glucose
    C. FBC
    D. Liver function test
    E. Peak flow rate

70. A 72-year-old man with a history of chronic renal failure comes to the clinic for review. He also has type 2 diabetes and despite diet and exercise measures is failing adequately to control his glucose. On examination his BP is 155/80, pulse is 80 and regular. His BMI is 31. Investigations: Hb 11.0 g/dl, WCC 7.7 x10(9)/L, PLT 192 x10(9)/L, Na+ 138 mmol/L, K+ 5.0 mmol/L, creatinine 162 μmol/L, estimated GFR 42mL/min, HbA1c 7.9%. Which of the following is the most appropriate treatment for controlling his blood glucose?

    A. Metformin
    B. Linagliptin
    C. Pioglitazone
    D. Basal insulin
    E. Glibenclamide

71. An 18-year-old woman with a history of anorexia nervosa is commenced on nasogastric feeding after admission on a Saturday morning via the psychiatry teams. You are fast bleeped to see her some three days later after she collapses and is witnessed by the nurses to suffer a tonic clonic seizure. Her BP is 105/78, pulse is 85 and regular. You note her BMI on admission to be 16.5. Which of the following is the most likely cause of her collapse?

    A. Hypocalcaemia
    B. Hypercalcaemia
    C. Hypocortisolism
    D. Hypophosphataemia
    E. Hypernatraemia

72. A 29-year-old man comes to the endocrine clinic for review having suffered a road traffic accident in which he sustained a head injury some six weeks earlier. Since then he tells you he's been passing large volumes of urine and has had difficulty keeping up with his fluid intake. On examination his BP is 120/60, pulse is 80 and regular. He has a postural drop of 15 mmHg on standing. There is mild hypernatraemia on routine U and E, urine osmolality only reaches 290 mOsm/kg after fluid deprivation, but does rise to >800 after desmopressin. Which of the following is the most appropriate treatment for him?

    A. Desmopressin
    B. Lysine vasopressin
    C. Lithium
    D. Bendroflumethiazide
    E. Demeclocycline

73. A 19-year-old woman with an eating disorder is admitted to the medical ward for re-feeding under the mental health act. Her BP is 100/60, pulse is 75 and regular; her BMI is 16.5. Which of the following is most likely to be seen on investigation?

    A. Elevated cortisol
    B. Elevated potassium
    C. Elevated sodium
    D. Elevated calcium
    E. Elevated creatinine

74. You review a 53-year-old man with type 2 diabetes who is unable to gain glycaemic control on metformin monotherapy alone. A recent HbA1c is measured at 8.4%. His BP is 155/85, pulse is 85 and regular. His BMI is 35. You elect to begin dapagliflozin. Which of the following correctly reflects its mode of action?

    A. Blocks intestinal glucose absorption
    B. Blocks renal tubular glucose reabsorption
    C. Increases GLP-1 release
    D. Increases GIP release

75. A 12-year-old boy presents to the clinic with a new diagnosis of type 1 diabetes. His 4-year-old brother and mother also have type 1 diabetes. Which of the following HLA types is he most likely to have?

    A. B6
    B. DR2
    C. DR3
    D. B27
    E. B52

76. **A 59-year-old woman presents to the clinic for review of her type 2 diabetes. She is currently taking 1g BD of metformin, but her HbA1c has steadily risen to 8.2% over the past few months. You elect to begin dapagliflozin. Which of the following is true of dapagliflozin therapy?**

    A. A small rise in blood pressure is seen with therapy
    B. It leads to excretion of approximately 70g glucose/day in patients with type 2 diabetes
    C. A small fall in haematocrit is seen with therapy
    D. Genital infections are reported in 10% of users
    E. PTH decreases are seen in conjunction with therapy

77. **An 88-year-old woman presents to the emergency department with gradually worsening stridor over a period of months. On clinical examination she has a normal respiratory rate and oxygen saturations, and is haemodynamically stable, but you note a large goitre. A CT scan is performed which confirms external compression of the trachea by the extra-thoracic goitre. Lung function tests are performed prior to bronchoscopic stenting of the trachea. What pattern would you expect to find on the lung function results?**

    A. Concave flow-volume loop with normal forced vital capacity
    B. Flattening of the expiratory flow-volume loop, with normal inspiratory flow-volume loop
    C. Normal expiratory flow-volume loop, with flattening of the inspiratory flow-volume loop
    D. Normal flow-volume loop shape with reduced forced vital capacity
    E. Normal flow-volume loop with normal force vital capacity

78. **A 31-year-old woman with recently diagnosed Graves' disease comes to the emergency department complaining of diplopia. On examination, there is obvious exopthalmos with conjunctival oedema. On testing, there is some lack of colour vision and limited upward gaze. Which of the following is the most appropriate intervention?**

    A. Stop carbimazole
    B. Stop thyroxine
    C. Start low-dose oral prednisolone
    D. Start high dose IV methylprednisolone
    E. Start azathioprine

79. **A 28-year-old man who complains of polyuria and polydipsia, comes to the endocrinology clinic some six weeks after a motorcycle accident in which he was knocked unconscious. He tells you he is thirsty all the time and drinking up to 8 litres of ice-cold water and other drinks each day. Calcium and glucose levels are normal and you arrange for him to be admitted for a water deprivation test. Urine osmolality is 280 at the end of the test; it rises to 850mOsm/kg after DDAVP is administered. Which of the following is the most likely diagnosis?**

    A. Cranial diabetes insipidus
    B. Nephrogenic diabetes insipidus
    C. Psychogenic polydipsia
    D. Diuretic abuse
    E. Partial nephrogenic diabetes insipidus

80. **A 34-year-old woman comes to the clinic for review. She has recently been diagnosed with diabetes insipidus after presenting to the clinic with polyuria and polydipsia whilst on lithium therapy. Her medication for bipolar disorder has now been changed to sodium valproate but she is still having to drink up to 7 litres/day to keep up with her fluid requirements. Which of the following is the optimal way to manage her?**

    A. Continue with increased fluid intake only
    B. Add bendroflumethiazide
    C. Add desmopressin
    D. Refer for cognitive behavioural therapy to reduce her water consumption
    E. Add demeclocycline to her regimen

81. **A 22-year-old woman comes to the clinic because she has had no menstrual periods for the past five months. On further questioning, she confirms that she has no sex drive, and experiences milk leakage from her breasts. You perform a set of investigations. These include multiple negative pregnancy tests. Her prolactin is measured at 5120mU/l. An MRI scan reveals a pituitary macroadenoma extending into the cavernous sinus. Which of the following is the most appropriate initial therapy for her?**

    A. Octreotide
    B. Cabergoline
    C. Somatostatin
    D. Bromocriptine
    E. Pergolide

82. A 28-year-old woman presents to the emergency department for the third time over the past nine months with abdominal pain and distress. She has recently begun visiting her GP because of symptoms of anxiety, and is signed off work on long-term sick leave. On examination her BP is 167/100, pulse is 100 and regular. She has abdominal pain on palpation, although the abdomen is soft, and she vomits during the examination. Of note in her investigations are a low sodium at 130 mmol/l, and a normal plain abdomen film. On reviewing her past notes, you note a low sodium on the two previous admissions. Which of the following investigations is most likely to yield the diagnosis?

    A. Faecal porphyrins
    B. Urinary porphyrins
    C. Serum lead level
    D. CT head
    E. Urinary osmolality

83. A 60-year-old taxi driver comes to the diabetes clinic for review. He has had type 2 diabetes for the past six years and is maintained on metformin 1g BD. Other past history of note is transitional cell carcinoma of the bladder for which he is under regular surveillance. His most recent HbA1c is recorded as 62 mmol/mol (7.9%) and his creatinine is 125 micromol/l. On examination his BMI is 35, BP is 155/90. Which of the following is the most appropriate next step with respect to glycaemic control?

    A. Add basal insulin
    B. Add sitagliptin
    C. Add gliclazide
    D. Add pioglitazone
    E. Add acarbose

84. A 33-year-old woman is referred to the infertility clinic by her GP. She gained 2 stone in weight over the past 9 months and has had no periods for the past 6 months. She is being monitored for borderline hypertension. She takes no regular medication. Her BP is 159/90, pulse is 70. She has a BMI of 32, Hb 12.8, WCC 8.3, PLT 190, Na 137, K 4.0, Cr 108, TSH 0.7, Prolactin 930 ng/ml, 9am cortisol 940 nmol/L, Fasting glucose 6.2, FSH and LH suppressed. Which of the following is the most likely diagnosis?

    A. Cushing's syndrome
    B. Pseudo-Cushing's
    C. Microprolactinoma
    D. Macroprolactinoma
    E. Polycystic ovarian syndrome

85. **A 22-year-old charity worker comes to the emergency department for review. She complains of polyuria and polydipsia and tells you that she needs to drink up to 12 litres of water per day to remain hydrated. Past medical history of note includes depression and anxiety which was treated with citalopram, although she no longer takes any medication. On examination her BP is 122/72, pulse is 72. There are no abnormal findings. Urine and plasma osmolality are both low. U&E are in the normal range. Corrected calcium is 2.35mmol/l (2.2-2.61), fasting glucose is 5.8 mmol/l (<7.0). Which of the following is the correct course of action?**

    A. Referral for cognitive therapy
    B. Trial of desmopressin
    C. Water deprivation test
    D. Normal saline infusion test
    E. Pituitary MRI

86. **A 28-year-old man with a history of congenital nephrogenic diabetes insipidus comes to the genetics clinic with his new partner. He is aware that his condition is caused by a mutation in the AVPR2 gene. The partner is 24 weeks pregnant with a male child and they want to know the chance of the child inheriting the condition. His partner's family are not affected by the condition. What is the chance of the child having nephrogenic diabetes insipidus?**

    A. 0%
    B. 25%
    C. 33%
    D. 50%
    E. 100%

87. **A 17-year-old man who has a history of diabetes mellitus and is partially sighted presents to the clinic for review. Despite insulin therapy and tight control of his glucose he is suffering from polyuria and polydipsia. He also wears bilateral hearing aids because of sensorineural deafness. What pattern of inheritance fits best with his underlying condition?**

    A. Autosomal dominant
    B. Autosomal recessive
    C. X-linked recessive
    D. X-linked dominant
    E. Mitochondrial

88. **A 26-year-old woman who has a diagnosis of acute intermittent porphyria (AIP) comes to the clinic with her partner. They discuss wanting to start a family and ask about the possibility of their child inheriting the disorder. Which of the following correctly reflects the inheritance of AIP?**

    A. Autosomal recessive
    B. Autosomal dominant
    C. X-linked recessive
    D. X-linked dominant
    E. Mitochondrial

89. **A 19 year old woman presents to the emergency department with an episode of anxiety, hypertension and hyponatraemia. This is the third such episode in the past year, and all investigations so far have proved negative with respect to determining the underlying cause. A arranges a porphyria screen which suggests acute intermittent porphyria. Which of the following is the enzyme defect which underlies acute intermittent porphyria (AIP)?**

    A. Uroporphyrinogen decarboxylase
    B. Ferrochelatase
    C. Porphobilinogen decarboxylase
    D. Protoporphyrinogen oxidase
    E. Aminolaevulinic acid dehydratase

1. A. Dexamethasone 20 mg should be started before week 10

In a patient with classical congenital adrenal hyperplasia, there is a risk to a female foetus of virilization. Recommended management to prevent this is dexamethasone 20 mg/day which can be discontinued once the sex of the foetus is determined (not needed in male offspring). With pre-treatment 50–75% of female foetuses do not require reconstructive surgery.

Turner H, Wass J, *Oxford Handbook of Endocrinology and Diabetes*, Second Edition, Oxford University Press, 2009, Part 4: Reproductive endocrinology, Congenital adrenal hyperplasia (CAH) in adults, Management

2. B. It has an analgesic effect

Calcitonin is a polypeptide of 32 amino acids. The parafollicular or C cells in the thyroid gland in which it is synthesized have receptors that bind calcium ions (Ca^{2+}) circulating in the blood. These cells monitor the level of circulating Ca^{2+}. A rise in its level stimulates the cells to release calcitonin. Bone cells respond by removing Ca^{2+} from the blood and storing it in the bone. Kidney cells respond by increasing the excretion of Ca^{2+}. Both types of cells have surface receptors for calcitonin. Because it promotes the transfer of Ca^{2+} to bones, calcitonin has been examined as a possible treatment for osteoporosis. In addition to its anti-resorptive effect calcitonin possesses an analgesic effect. Being a polypeptide, calcitonin cannot be given by mouth (it would be digested). However, inhaling calcitonin appears to be an effective way to get therapeutic levels of the hormone into the blood.

Boron WF, Boulpaep EL, *Medical Physiology: A Cellular and Molecular Approach*, Elsevier/Saunders, 2004, Section on endocrine system.

3. A. Prednisolone 60 mg

This patient has symptoms of acute optic neuropathy and as such requires urgent treatment to preserve her sight. Treatment of choice initially is high-dose corticosteroids +/– cyclophosphamide. Surgical decompression may be required if she fails to respond to high-dose medical intervention. Both radiotherapy and surgical techniques can be considered for severe proptosis/strabismus.

Turner H, Wass J, *Oxford Handbook of Endocrinology and Diabetes*, Second Edition, Oxford University Press, 2009, Part 1: Thyroid, Graves' ophthalmopathy, dermopathy, and acropachy, Graves' ophthalmopathy.

4. B. Serum testosterone

Being male and relatively young makes secondary osteoporosis the most likely cause for his hip fracture when pathological fractures are excluded. Basic evaluation should include a full blood count, kidney and liver function tests, vitamin D and calcium levels, measurement of sex hormones, protein electrophoresis, and thyroid hormone levels. Serum B12 deficiency, calcitonin, lipid, and vitamin E disorders are not a risk factor for the development of osteoporosis.

Poole KE, Compston JE, Osteoporosis and its management, *British Medical Journal* 2006;333(7581):1251–1256.

5. B. Primary hyperparathyroidism

Although the PTH levels are within the normal range it remains inappropriately high in the face of hypercalcaemia. In the context of hypercalcaemia normal, high-normal, or 'inappropriately detectable' PTH levels would indicate primary hyperparathyroidism as being the most likely diagnosis. A similar picture can be encountered though rarely in hypercalcaemia related to malignancy. All other listed causes of hypercalcaemia in the question are associated with suppressed and very low values for serum PTH levels.

Moosgaard B, Christensen SE, Vestergaard P et al., Vitamin D metabolites and skeletal consequences in primary hyperparathyroidism, *Clinical Endocrinology* 2008;68:707–715.

6. A. Increase her carbimazole

The intervention of choice is to increase the carbimazole, as 20 mg/day is still an appropriate dose in pregnancy. Doses of up to 150 mg BD of propylthiouracil are also used. As such, until her medication is maximized there is no reason to consider partial thyroidectomy or delivering the baby. Radioiodine is not appropriate in pregnancy.

Turner H, Wass J, *Oxford Handbook of Endocrinology and Diabetes*, Second Edition, Oxford University Press, 2009, Part 1: Thyroid, Thyrotoxicosis, Thyrotoxicosis in pregnancy.

7. E. Insulinoma

MEN-1 is suggested by the very elevated gastrin level and the hypercalcaemia which raises the possibility of hyperparathyroidism. As such a pancreatic endocrine tumour would be considered as an additional diagnosis, of which insulinomas are the most common. Phaeochromocytomas are associated with MEN-2. Anterior pituitary tumours are seen less commonly than insulinomas. They occur in 15–40% of patients with MEN-1, and prolactinomas are the commonest type seen.

Bloom S et al., *Oxford Handbook of Gastroenterology and Hepatology*, Second Edition, Oxford University Press, 2011, Chapter 3, An A to Z of gastroenterology and hepatology, Multiple endocrine neoplasia (MEN).

8. C. Ovarian failure due to low BMI

This patient's BMI is only around 18; as such it is most likely that her reduction in weight associated with exercise is the primary cause for her cessation of periods. Other possible causes include autoimmune ovarian failure but that seems less possible here. Ovarian failure due to pituitary dysfunction is associated with low levels of gonadotrophins, not the case in this patient, and there is no hypo or hyperthyroidism (TSH in normal range).

Turner H, Wass J, *Oxford Handbook of Endocrinology and Diabetes*, Second Edition, Oxford University Press, 2009, Chapter 58, Premature ovarian failure (POF), Pathogenesis.

9. C. Low molecular weight heparin should be administered

Patients with diabetic ketoacidosis (DKA) are at high risk of thromboembolus, due to dehydration and increased blood viscosity, and should receive venous thromboembolus prophylaxis. In patients DKA total body stores of potassium are depleted due to an efflux from the intracellular space and subsequent excretion due to osmotic diuresis. Potassium moves out of the cell in acidosis (competitive exchange at the cell membrane) and is unable to return to the intracellular space because it is usually transported into the cell by the action of insulin. The only reason to delay insulin therapy would be a low initial serum potassium; this is because insulin drives potassium into the cells which would consequently lower serum potassium further. In this case you would give fluids and potassium first. Intravenous sodium bicarbonate is not routinely used in DKA as it causes a paradoxical intracellular acidosis and there is little evidence that it improves outcome. Blood gases would reveal an elevated anion gap. This is because there is an elevation in the unmeasured anions and consumption of bicarbonate as a buffer to the acidosis.

Hamdy O et al., Diabetic ketoacidosis, *Medscape*, updated August 2015. http://emedicine.medscape.com/article/118361-overview

10. B. Conn's syndrome

Primary hyperaldosteronism is the overproduction of the mineralocorticoid aldosterone. Around two-thirds of cases are due to Conn's syndrome, which is a single adenoma that produces aldosterone. About one-third of cases is due to bilateral adrenal hyperplasia. There are a few other rare causes such as adrenal carcinoma and gene defects. Aldosterone is usually controlled by the renin-angiotensin system. In hyperaldosteronism, production of aldosterone becomes independent of this system. Addison's disease refers to adrenal failure and low aldosterone levels. Cushing's syndrome occurs in corticosteroid excess.

Longmore M et al., *Oxford Handbook of Clinical Medicine*, Eighth Edition, Oxford University Press, 2010, Chapter 5, Endocrinology, Hyperaldosteronism.

11. A. Autosomal dominant LDL receptor mutation which reduces cholesterol clearance

It is an autosomal dominant disorder which is mainly (>95%) caused by a mutation in the LDL receptor. LDL therefore cannot clear cholesterol adequately. Patients develop early vascular disease and should be treated aggressively to reduce their cholesterol levels. Apolipoprotein B mutations may be seen in a condition known as 'Familial defective apolipoprotein B-100 (FDB)'. It is an autosomal dominant condition and causes delayed clearance of cholesterol. Familial hypertriglyceridaemia is often autosomal dominant with elevated VLDL. Complications of this condition include eruptive xanthomata and pancreatitis. Lipoprotein lipase deficiency is a rare defect that causes hypertriglyceridaemia.

Turner H, Wass J, *Oxford Handbook of Endocrinology and Diabetes*, Second Edition, Oxford University Press, 2009, Part 12: Lipids and hyperlipidaemia, Primary hyperlipidaemias.

12. A. Graves' disease

Weight loss, anxiety, and tremor are suggestive of thyroid disease, which occurs with increasing frequency in patients who have type 1 diabetes. The absence of significant bowel symptoms counts against a diagnosis of inflammatory bowel disease or coeliac. Diagnosis is based upon thyroid autoantibodies and thyroid function testing initially.

Longmore M et al., *Oxford Handbook of Clinical Medicine*, Eighth Edition, Oxford University Press, 2010, Chapter 5, Endocrinology, Thyrotoxicosis.

13. C. Smoking

A number of factors predispose to reduced bone mineral density. These include reduced BMI, thyrotoxicosis, smoking, early menopause, and late menarche. Treatment in the first instance is with a generic weekly bisphosphonate. If these are not tolerated, more intermittent preparations can be offered, or alternatives such as PTH analogues or denosumab (a human monoclonal antibody that inhibits maturation of osteoclasts, thus reducing bone degradation).

Osteoporosis: assessing the risk of fragility fracture, NICE guidelines [CG146]. Published date: August 2012. https://www.nice.org.uk/guidance/cg146

14. C. Shortened fourth and fifth metacarpals

This man is most likely to have pseudohypoparathyroidism, as evidenced by the raised PTH accompanied by biochemical features of hypoparathyroidism. Management is with calcium and vitamin D supplementation. The condition is often associated with reduced IQ, which may account for him struggling at school, and other hormone resistance (e.g. to thyroid hormone) may also occur. Of note here is that there is mild anaemia. It is quite possible that this may be related to poor dentition (associated with pseudohypoparathyroidism), or due to poor diet, potentially associated with developmental delay.

Longmore M et al., *Oxford Handbook of Clinical Medicine*, Ninth Edition, Oxford University Press, 2014, Chapter 5, Endoclinology.

15. B. Serotonin

The case described is classical of carcinoid syndrome. The syndrome is caused by excessive levels of serotonin secreted from a neuroendocrine tumour arising from enterochromaffin cells in the gut or less frequently the lung. Carcinoid syndrome occurs in metastatic disease as the liver metabolizes the hormones secreted by gut-limited disease. The excessive release of serotonin causes symptoms of cutaneous flushing, diarrhoea, bronchoconstriction, and right-sided cardiac valve disease. Precipitation of symptoms by alcohol is common. Vasoactive intestinal polypeptide is over-produced by VIPomas which cause chronic, profound watery diarrhoea. Gastrin is produced by G cells of the stomach; its over-production leads to excessive acid production and Zollinher–Ellison syndrome. Somatostatin-producing tumours are extremely rare; the classical pentad of symptoms is diabetes, steatorrhoea, gallstones, weight loss, and achlorhydria. Patients may also experience symptoms related to mechanical obstruction—biliary or duodenal. Somatostatinomas are associated with neurofibromatosis. Cholecystokinin-producing tumours are extremely rare.

Lips CJ et al., The spectrum of carcinoid tumours and carcinoid syndromes, *Annals of Clinical Biochemistry* 2003;40:612–627.

16. C. 50%

Studies of sporadic medullary thyroid carcinoma where there is no history of MEN-2 or others in the family with the condition, suggest that *RET* mutations approach 50%. As such, they may be at risk from the other features associated with MEN-2 such as phaeochromocytoma and parathyroid hyperplasia. Unfortunately 50% have local lymph node involvement at diagnosis, 15% distant metastases. The *RET* gene codes for a tyrosine kinase receptor that is expressed in cell lineages derived from the neural crest. The RET receptor plays a crucial role in processes including regulating cell proliferation, migration and differentiation. Activating mutations in *RET* lead to the development of several inherited and sporadic diseases.

Groot JW et al., RET as a diagnostic and therapeutic target in sporadic and hereditary endocrine tumors, *Endocrine Reviews* 2006;27:535–560, Epub 2006 Jul 18.

17. C. Six months post radioiodine

Guidelines generally suggest a gap of six months post radioiodine before pregnancy. Exposure before 12 weeks gestation to radioiodine is thought to be most harmful, with clinicians usually giving anti-thyroid drugs in an attempt to protect the fetal thyroid gland. Even with these there is not insignificant risk of chromosomal breakages and malformation. Post week 12, exposure is associated with increased risk of fetal hypothyroidism.

Gleicher N et al., *Principles and Practice of Medical Therapy in Pregnancy*, Third Edition, Appleton and Lange, 1998, pp. 436–441.

18. A. MRI abdomen

The aldosterone:renin ratio fits with a diagnosis of primary hyperaldosteronism, which may be related to bilateral adrenal hyperplasia, or to an aldosterone-secreting adenoma. As such an abdominal MRI is the initial investigation of choice, rather than moving to additional anti-hypertensive medication. CT adrenals may also be useful as an alternative to MRI. Where there is doubt as to the source of aldosterone, adrenal vein sampling may be of help.

Wass J, Turner H, *Oxford Handbook of Endocrinology and Diabetes*, Second Edition, Oxford University Press, 2009.

19. A. Stop his doxycycline

This presentation is consistent with nephrogenic diabetes insipidus, one cause of which is recognized to be use of some tetracycline-based antibiotics. The degree of nephrogenic DI is thought to be related to the degree of protein binding of the compound. In the case of tetracyclines this is most with demeclocycline, then doxycycline, and least with tetracycline and oxytetracycline. Hence nephrogenic DI is a recognized effect of demeclocycline, rarely seen with doxycycline, and unheard of with tetracycline and oxytetracycline. In the first instance he should be told to stop the doxycycline, whereupon an improvement in the ability of the kidney to reabsorb water may occur over subsequent days. Where there is no pharmacological cause underlying nephrogenic DI, thiazide diuretics may be of some value in treating the condition. There is nothing here to suggest cranial DI.

Longmore M et al., *Oxford Handbook of Clinical Medicine*, Eighth Edition, Oxford University Press, 2010.

20. B. Low renin, high aldosterone

The low serum potassium in an otherwise fit patient with hypertension raises the possibility of Conn's syndrome, a primary aldosteronoma. The biochemical findings are a low serum renin and a high serum aldosterone.

Warrell DA et al., *Oxford Textbook of Medicine*, Fifth Edition, Oxford University Press, 2010, Section 16.17.3, Secondary hypertension.

21. A. Carcinoid tumour

The history of diarrhoea and flushing is characteristic of a carcinoid syndrome. Twenty-five percent of such tumours arise in the appendix, but it may also be found in the terminal ileum and rectum. In those in whom the appenidx is the origin, then 10% present with symptoms and signs suggestive of acute appendicitis. Thus all appendicectomy specimens should be examined for a carcinoid tumour. Symptoms usually only occur when metastases are present. Clinically, carcinoid tumours may present with flushing, diarrhoea, nausea, vomiting, and abdominal pain. A small percentage may develop congestive cardiac failure secondary to tricuspid incompetence and pulmonary stenosis. Whilst the menopause may cause flushing, diarrhoea is not a symptom. Thyrotoxicosis may present with diarrhoea but sweating rather than flushing accompanies the symptoms.

Longmore M et al., *Oxford Handbook of Clinical Medicine*, Eighth Edition, Oxford University Press, 2010, Chapter 6, Gastroenterology, Carcinoid tumours.

22. D. Growth hormone estimation following an insulin stress test

The definitive investigation of growth hormone deficiency is to attempt to stimulate release of this hormone. Stress is one mechanism for this and hypoglycaemia is one way of achieving this. Growth hormone estimations using clonidine and exercise are used when the potential for a hypoglycaemic fit preclude the use of insulin stress test in susceptible individuals and in children.

Turner H, Wass J, *Oxford Handbook of Endocrinology & Diabetes*, Second Edition, Oxford University Press, 2009, Part 7: Paediatric endocrinology, Growth and stature, Growth hormone deficiency.

23. D. Nelson's syndrome

Nelson's syndrome is characterized by increased pigmentation due to excessive ACTH being secreted by the pituitary. Hence patients with Addison's disease may become pigmented. In this patient, to treat Cushing's, bilateral adrenalectomy has removed the excess cortisol (driven by a pituitary tumour), although not treated the primary cause. Such surgery was not uncommon formerly when synthetic gonadotrophins were not available and patients wished to retain their fertility by not removing gonadotrophin secretion. Nowadays, bilateral adrenalectomy for pituitary-dependent Cushing's is reserved for those with no demonstrable pituitary tumour and Nelson's syndrome may occur when pituitary surgery has failed or recurrence has occurred.

Longmore M et al., *Oxford Handbook of Clinical Medicine*, Eighth Edition, Oxford University Press, 2010, Chapter 5, Endocrinology, Adrenal cortex and Cushing's syndrome.

24. C. Phaeochromocytoma

The previously normal first pregnancy, in the light of a normal weight, makes pre-eclampsia in the first pregnancy unlikely and for the condition to occur in a second pregnancy and the presence of hypertension in the second trimester makes pregnancy-associated hypertension unlikely. Coarctation would have been noted in the first pregnancy with hypertension. Whilst thyrotoxicosis may cause systolic hypertension, the degree of systolic blood pressure in that condition is rare. The associated symptoms of headaches and sweating and palpitations in a hypertensive individual makes phaeochromocytoma highly likely. All pregnant women with hypertension in the first or second trimester should be screened for this condition.

Longmore M et al., *Oxford Handbook of Clinical Medicine*, Eighth Edition, Oxford University Press, 2010, Chapter 5, Endocrinology, Phaeochromocytoma.

25. E. Globally increased uptake

The most likely diagnosis is Grave's disease (the commonest cause of thyrotoxicosis which is strongly associated with other autoimmune disorders), and as such a homogeneous increase in thyroid uptake would be expected. Treatment of choice for Grave's is radioiodine, after a period of stabilization of thyroid function, typically with a block replace regime, although it's important to exclude pregnancy first, of course. Surgery is the second-choice option, but may be considered depending on some personal circumstances, such as imminent plans to start a family.

Longmore M et al., *Oxford Handbook of Clinical Medicine*, Eighth Edition, Oxford University Press, 2010

26. B. Vitamin B1

Inadequate intake of vitamin B1 (thiamine) may lead to Wernicke–Korsakoff syndrome. In the UK the commonest cause of thiamine deficiency is alcohol dependency associated with an inadequate dietary thiamine intake, but has also been reported due to starvation/dieting, cancer, bariatric surgery, total parenteral nutrition, and hyperemesis gravidarum.

Warrell DA et al., *Oxford Textbook of Medicine*, Fifth Edition, Oxford University Press, 2010, Section 24.19, Acquired metabolic disorders and the nervous system.

27. A. Cerebral sarcoidosis

The history is significant for erythema nodosum, one cause of which is sarcoidosis. Sarcoidosis may affect every organ system in the body. One of the features of cerebral sarcoidosis is a lymphocytic meningitis which predominantly affects the hypothalamus and may manifest by polyuria and polydipsia secondary to diabetes insipidus. The normal calcium precludes an alternative complication of sarcoidosis, notably hypercalcaemia, which may also cause polyuria and polydipsia.

Warrell DA et al., *Oxford Textbook of Medicine,* Fifth Edition, Oxford University Press, 2010, Section 24.20, Neurological complications of systemic disease.

28. E. Thyroid storm

A thyroid storm is characterized by the features of this patient, acutely exaggerated signs of thyrotoxicosis, when surgery is undertaken in a patient not medically rendered euthyroid prior to surgery. Treatment is aimed at decreasing thyroid production and release of T4 and T3, blocking the effects of remaining but excessive circulating free T4 and T3, and treating the systemic decompensation which occurs. Treatment to prevent further release of T3 and T4 includes Lugol's iodine and propylthiouracil, while management of the storm itself includes oxygen therapy, control of heart rate with beta-blockers, sedation with chlorpromazine, antipyretic (patients are usually pyrexial), dexamethasone, and anti-coagulation (in view of atrial fibrillation).

Longmore M et al., *Oxford Handbook of Clinical Medicine,* Eighth Edition, Oxford University Press, 2010, Chapter 20, Emergencies, Thyroid emergencies.

29. D. Atenolol

Atenolol is not typically associated with abnormalities in thyroid function tests. However, it is used to treat the symptoms of thyrotoxicosis. Symptoms of thyrotoxicosis may be masked if a patient is already taking a beta-blocker. Acetylsalicylic acid is metabolized to salicylate. This is an inhibitor of thyroid hormone binding to serum transport proteins and reduces serum total thyroxine (T4) and triiodothyronine (T3) in vivo. Amiodarone has a variety of possible effects on the thyroid. Usually, T4 to T3 conversion is inhibited. T4 is usually raised, T3 low and reverse T3 raised. TSH may also be raised. These effects can be more prominent initially, then normalize. With carbamezapine, again, the levels of T4 and T3 are often reduced, but with normal TSH. With phenytoin the serum levels of T4 and, less often, T3 tend to be reduced. TSH is usually normal. It is not clear why this is, but possible theories include increased T4 to T3 conversion, and the fact that phenytoin may act as a weak T3 agonist. Patients are usually euthyroid clinically and do not require treatment.

Gopalan M et al., Thyroid dysfunction induced by amiodarone therapy, *Emedicine.* http://emedicine.medscape.com/article/129033-overview

30. B. Iodine deficiency

The clues here are that this patient has come from central Africa, has a goitre, and that the TSH is just above the upper limit of normal. As these are coupled with symptoms of lethargy, the likely diagnosis is one of iodine deficiency. Particularly in mountainous areas, where there is low intake of sea fish and high intake of beans and pulses, the risk of iodine deficiency is increased. Dietary supplementation with iodized salt to be used in cooking can reverse the problem. In this patient's case, supplementation of iodine in the diet is likely rapidly to improve symptoms.

Wass J, Turner H, *Oxford Handbook of Endocrinology and Diabetes,* Second Edition, Oxford University Press, 2009.

31. A. Papillary carcinoma

Papillary carcinoma is the commonest cause of thyroid carcinoma. It constitutes more than 80% of thyroid cancers and is commoner in women (3:1 ratio). It is slow growing and usually non-encapsulated, may be multi-focal in 30% of cases, and spreads to regional lymph nodes. Over 95% of cases are confined to the neck. Surgery is the primary therapy of choice with adjuvant radioiodine therapy in high-risk patients with differentiated tumours.

Wass J, Turner H, *Oxford Handbook of Endocrinology and Diabetes*, Second Edition, Oxford University Press, 2009.

32. E. Denosumab

As this patient has not tolerated generic bisphosphonate therapy, she is also likely to suffer significant symptoms of reflux in response to the monthly preparations. As such, the alternatives of strontium or denosumab are the most appropriate. Strontium ranelate was associated with a small increased risk of venous thrombosis in randomized clinical trials, so is not recommended in patients with a previous history of venous thromboembolism, so denosumab is the logical choice. Denosumab is given by six-monthly subcutaneous injection and is an inhibitor of RANK ligand, leading to downregulation of osteoclast activity.

emc+, Prolia. http://www.medicines.org.uk/EMC/medicine/23127/SPC/Prolia/

33. B. Insulin glargine

NICE guidelines for the management of type 1 diabetes endorse the use of insulin analogues such as glargine or detemir ahead of NPH insulin in patients who have troublesome nocturnal or early morning hypoglycaemia but are not able to reach HbA1c target. Glulisine, aspart, and lispro are all short-acting insulin analogues. Because glargine and detemir are so-called peakless insulins, with a long duration of action, they are particularly suitable for this population. NICE concluded, however, that any improvement in health outcomes did not justify the incremental cost for the general type 1 diabetes population.

Diagnosis and management of type 1 diabetes in children, young people and adults, NICE guidelines [CG15]. Published date: July 2004. http://www.nice.org.uk/CG15

34. A. Glibenclamide

Acarbose and pioglitazone do not increase insulin output, and so would not account for the hypoglycaemia seen here. Of the sulphonylureas given, glipizide is short acting, gliclazide undergoes hepatic metabolism, and glibenclamide has a long half-life and is renally excreted. Hence, it is the most likely cause of the presentation seen here. Hypoglycaemia may of course recur; as such the patient should be monitored over the next few hours for a recurrence of symptoms.

Jönsson A et al., Pharmacokinetics of glibenclamide and its metabolites in diabetic patients with impaired renal function, *European Journal of Clinical Pharmacology* 1998;53:429–435. http://www.springerlink.com/content/bhu8d9bxn1rpdgq5/fulltext.pdf

35. D. Eosinophilia

Adrenocortical insufficiency is a rare condition with an estimated incidence of 40–110 cases per million adults. It may be classified as primary or secondary depending on whether the causative pathology is at the level of the adrenal gland (primary) or at the level of the hypothalamus or pituitary (secondary). The most common cause of primary adrenal insufficiency (Addison's disease) is autoimmune destruction of the gland (70–90% of cases). Other causes include infections (e.g. TB, histoplasmosis), bilateral adrenal haemorrhage, AIDS, and metastatic disease. Common symptoms of Addison's disease include generalized weakness, lethargy, dizziness, weight loss, and vomiting. Signs include postural hypotension and reduced pubic and axillary hair growth. Pigmentation is typically generalized but may also be concentrated in areas of sun exposure and chronic friction. The diagnosis is often confirmed with a short synacthen test (SST). Simultaneous measurement of 9 am cortisol and ACTH can also be helpful as a low cortisol level found paired with an elevated ACTH is considered a sensitive method of detection. Although not widely advocated, a random cortisol, particularly in the acute setting, can also be diagnostically useful if found to be inappropriately low or undetectable. In Addison's disease, further investigations may also reveal hyponatraemia (90%), hyperkalaemia (65%), elevated urea levels, and eosinophilia. Plasma renin levels tend to be elevated. On imaging, adrenal calcification is much more suggestive of an infective or metastatic pathology than autoimmune disease. VLCFAs are elevated in the genetic condition adrenoleukodystrophy—a rare cause of adrenal insufficiency.

Addison's Disease Self Help Group. http://www.addisons.org.uk/

36. B. It is more common in women

Graves' disease is an organ-specific autoimmune condition which may be found in association with (other autoimmune) conditions such as pernicious anaemia, vitiligo, and alopecia. Biochemically, TSH receptor antibodies, directed against the TSH receptor on the thyroid cell membrane, are elevated and, clinically, the condition is characterized by hyperthyroidism, opthalmopathy, pretibial myxoedema, and, rarely, thyroid acropachy. Opthalmopathy develops in 20–50% of patients with Graves' disease and is more common in women. There are many established links with cigarette smoking and it is recognized that the risk of developing eye disease increases with the number of cigarettes smoked per day whilst smoking cessation appears to reduce this risk. The characteristic signs of Graves' opthalmopathy are proptosis and periorbital oedema. Proptosis is often asymmetrical. Common symptoms include pain, photophobia, and diplopia. The severity of eye changes can be classified using the 'NO SPECS' system. In clinical practice, it is important to be vigilant to the features of optic neuropathy such as impaired colour perception and reduced visual acuity although loss of vision is a rare occurrence.

Cawood T et al., Recent developments in thyroid eye disease, *British Medical Journal* 2004;329:385. doi: 10.1136/bmj.329.7462.385. http://www.bmj.com/content/329/7462/385.full

37. D. Primary hyperparathyroidism

Hypercalcaemia is a common biochemical abnormality which may be caused by a broad range of conditions but is secondary to primary hyperparathyroidism or malignancy in the vast majority of cases. Measurement of parathyroid hormone (PTH) helps to target investigation as an elevated or normal level in the context of hypercalcaemia (as seen here) is considered 'inappropriate' and suggestive of autonomous or dysregulated parathyroid activity. Hypercalcaemia associated with malignancy tends to result in a suppressed PTH and is a common occurrence, seen in 20–39% of cancer patients during the course of their illness. Often it is due to the production of parathyroid hormone-related protein (PTHrP) from an advanced squamous malignancy. Alternative mechanisms include osteolysis with bony metastases (20%) as well as secretion of 1,25-(OH) vitamin D and PTH (<1%). In this case, the smoking history may suggest a diagnosis of malignancy but the PTH levels do not. Hypercalcaemia has been described in 5–10% of patients with sarcoidosis. Various factors have been implicated including endogenous overproduction of 1,25-(OH) vitamin D by the alveolar macrophage as well as PTHrP production within the sarcoid granulomas. PTH levels are typically normal or reduced. Serum ACE levels tend to be elevated to very high levels in the majority of patients (with untreated sarcoidosis) although false positive rates mean that this test cannot be reliably used in the diagnostic process. Therefore, in the absence of any characteristic clinical features of sarcoidosis, the mildly elevated ACE level seen in this case should not sway us from the two most frequent causes of hypercalcaemia—primary hyperparathyroidism and malignancy. BHH is a benign cause of hypercalcaemia, much less common that primary hyperparathyroidism. Patients are often diagnosed incidentally and tend to be relatively asymptomatic. Biochemically, hypercalcaemia is typically mild, urinary calcium excretion is low, and PTH levels are inappropriately normal or high. The condition is inherited in an autosomal dominant fashion and it is therefore important to take a family history in all patients with hypercalcaemia, as early diagnosis of this disorder can prevent unnecessary investigation and treatment. In this case, an elevated urinary calcium excretion points away from the diagnosis. Finally, many drugs have been implicated in the aetiology of hypercalcaemia including thiazide diuretics, lithium, exogenous vitamin D, and calcium carbonate (milk-alkali syndrome). However, ACE inhibitors are not commonly thought to cause hypercalcaemia. This leaves the most likely diagnosis as primary hyperparathyroidism. This condition is frequently seen in postmenopausal females who may present asymptomatically or with a characteristic constellation of symptoms including confusion, general malaise, and abdominal pain. Often, and as seen in this case, there is an elevated urinary calcium excretion. PTH levels may be elevated or, importantly, may also be inappropriately normal (non-suppressed).

Hemphill RR, Hypercalcaemia in emergency medicine, *Medscape,* 2010. http://emedicine.medscape.com/article/766373-overview

38. D. Intravenous hydrocortisone

The combination of hypotension, hypoglycaemia, hypoatraemia, and hyperkalaemia is very suggestive of an Addisonian crisis. Of the options given the administration of intravenous hydrocortisone is most appropriate; without it many of the biochemical disturbances will prove extraordinarily difficult to correct. Hypertonic saline is not appropriate initially as resuscitation with 0.9% saline should be tried first and is usually sufficient. Both the potassium and glucose are at levels which whilst concerning do not necessarily require emergency but rather urgent intervention. Vomiting is common in such situations and the chest signs may indicate either a community-acquired pneumonia or aspiration. The majority of Addisonian crises are precipitated. Care should be taken to identify any possible source of sepsis in particular and start appropriate antibiotic therapy.

Longmore M et al., *Oxford Handbook of Clinical Medicine,* Eighth Edition, Oxford University Press, 2010, Chapter 20, Emergencies, Addisonian crisis.

39. C. Add enalapril titrated to maximal tolerated dose

Adding ACE inhibition is effective in slowing progression of renal disease in normotensive patients with established microalbuminuria. A number of trials have looked at the effect of ACE inhibition versus placebo and ACE inhibition versus other agents with similar blood pressure lowering ability. One example trial, the link for which is provided, trialed perindopril versus amlodipine versus placebo, but a number of others exist. In patients treated with perindopril the albumin excretion rate decreased around 45% over three years, versus a 17% rise in the nifedipine group, and a 27% rise in the placebo group.

Jerums G et al., Long-term comparison between perindopril and nifedipine in normotensive patients with type 1 diabetes and microalbuminuria, *American Journal of Kidney Diseases* 2001;37:890–899. http://www.ajkd.org/article/S0272-6386(05)80003-4/abstract

40. A. Serum glucose

Common causes of polyuria and polydipsia include diabetes mellitus and hypercalcaemia. Diabetes insipidus is rare (prevalence 1 in 25,000). Initial investigations for polyuria and polydipsia should include urea and electrolytes, corrected calcium, and glucose. If these are normal, further investigations should be done to look for rare causes.

Longmore M et al., *Oxford Handbook of Clinical Medicine*, Eighth Edition, Oxford University Press, 2010, Chapter 5, Endocrinology, Diabetes mellitus.

41. C. Monitor with serial imaging

The macroadenoma is a coincidental finding. The small rise in prolactin probably reflects stalk compression and does not indicate a prolactinoma. In macroprolactinomas, the prolactin concentration is greater than 2000 mU/l. The most appropriate treatment would be observation with serial scanning to assess for any change in size that would merit surgery because this patient has no visual field defects and the tumour is distant from the chiasm. Serial MRI scans are preferable to CT if available and there are no contraindications, to avoid radiation.

Longmore M et al., *Oxford Handbook of Clinical Medicine*, Eighth Edition, Oxford University Press, 2010, Chapter 5, Endocrinology, Hyperprolactinaemia.

42. B. Graves' disease

Many of her signs are consistent with hyperthyroidism of any cause. However, pretibial myxoedema is generally associated with Graves' disease, and occasionally occurs in Hashimoto's. It is thought that it may be caused by TSH receptors in the connective tissue being activated by the antibodies that cause Graves' disease. They stimulate fibroblasts to produce excess glycosaminoglycan, leading to the clinical lesions.

Fatourechi V, Pretibial myxedema: pathophysiology and treatment options, *American Journal of Clinical Dermatology* 2005;6(5):295–309. http://www.ncbi.nlm.nih.gov/pubmed/16252929

43. C. Increase dose by 10 mg/day in the third trimester

The correct advice is to increase the dose by 10 mg/day in the third trimester. Hydrocortisone can then be reduced again in the post-partum period. With respect to labour it is usual to give 100 mg IM every six hours. As per usual, if intercurrent illness occurs, then steroid cover should be increased. If steroids are not adequately replaced during the third trimester then intrauterine growth retardation may occur.

Turner H, Wass J, *Oxford Handbook of Endocrinology & Diabetes*, Second Edition, Oxford University Press, 2009, Part 5: Endocrine disorders of pregnancy, Adrenal disorders during pregnancy, Addison's disease.

44. C. Measurement of serum calcium is a useful screening test for suspected cases

Multiple endocrine neoplasia (MEN) type 1 is a syndrome characterized by a predisposition to tumour development in a variety of endocrine glands: parathyroid (occurring in ~95% of cases); pancreatic occurring in ~75% of cases); pituitary (anterior) (occurring in ~50% of cases). All forms of MEN are inherited via an autosomal dominant pattern; the gene for MEN-1 has been mapped to chromosome 11q13. The most commonly occurring neoplastic development is a parathyroid adenoma. This may lead to development of clinical hyperparathyroidism and, as such, raised calcium. Hypercalcaemia is therefore frequently the first manifestation of MEN-1. Pancreatic manifestations of MEN-1 are most commonly insulinomas and gastrinomas. Pituitary tumours may secrete prolactin (leading to symptoms of hyperprolactinaemia), growth hormone (leading to acromegaly), or ACTH (leading to Cushing's disease). Alternatively pituitary tumours may be non-functioning and produce symptoms via compression effects (pituitary hypo-function or visual impairment). Patients with MEN-2b, not MEN-1, often demonstrate a Marfanoid habitus.

Marini F et al., Orphanet, *Journal of Rare Diseases* 2006;1:38.

45. A. Acromegaly

The combination of secondary diabetes and hypertension is seen in patients with Cushing's syndrome and acromegaly. In the former, one might have expected the serum potassium to be low, and obesity. The numbness in the patient's fingers is secondary to carpal tunnel syndrome, a not uncommon complication of acromegaly, and the cause of the accident was due to a failure to see the car as a result of bitemporal hemianopia secondary to his pituitary tumour.

Turner H, Wass J, *Oxford Handbook of Endocrinology and Diabetes*, Second Edition, Oxford University Press, 2009, Part 2: Pituitary, Acromegaly, Definition.

46. A. Anaplastic thyroid carcinoma

The age at onset for this patient, coupled with the rapidly enlarging neck mass and spindle cells seen on FNAB is most consistent with anaplastic carcinoma. Unfortunately, treatment is palliative only, with patients usually responding poorly to chemo or radiotherapy. Surgery is occasionally used in an attempt to obtain a tissue diagnosis if there is any doubt from the FNAB.

Cassidy J et al., *Oxford Handbook of Oncology*, Third Edition, Oxford University Press, 2010, Chapter19, Endocrine cancers, Thyroid cancer

47. E. Sheehan's syndrome

Chronic fatigue is too often blamed on lifestyle without appropriate investigation. In this patient it is noted that she has both low T4 and low TSH levels suggesting a secondary hypothyroidism, due to pituitary disease. One of the causes of hypopituitarism occurring in a woman post-partum is Sheehan's syndrome, which is associated with post-partum haemorrhage and pituitary infarction. Post-partum bleeds are more commonly seen in multipara and the question which might have been asked of her in the history would have been whether she had been able to breastfeed her child as, following Sheehan's syndrome, there is an inability to lactate due to failure of prolactin secretion, and secondary amenorrhoea occurs.

Warrell DA et al., *Oxford Textbook of Medicine*, Fifth Edition, Oxford University Press, 2010, Section 14.11, Endocrine disease in pregnancy.

48. E. Fluid restriction

Too rapid correction of sodium runs the risk of central pontine myelinolysis. As such, fluid restriction is the most appropriate initial treatment here. More rapid correction of sodium may be considered if there is significant impairment of consciousness or seizures. Sodium should not be increased by more than 8–10 mmol/l during any 24-hour period.

Wass J, Turner H, *Oxford Handbook of Endocrinology and Diabetes*, Second Edition, Oxford University Press, 2009.

49. B. Multiple endocrine neoplasia

Thyroid enlargement and cervical lymphadenopathy would suggest a primary thyroid cancer. The history of chronic diarrhoea would raise suspicion of the possibility of medullary carcinoma. When hypertension is identified multiple endocrine neoplasia MEN-2 and pheochromocytoma is often considered. Riedel's thyroiditis (RT) is characterized by the replacement of normal thyroid parenchyma with dense fibrotic tissue and by the extension of this fibrosis to adjacent structures of the neck. Lymph gland enlargement is not a typical feature. In lymphoma the most common clinical presentation is that of a rapidly enlarging thyroid mass, frequently in association with neck adenopathy. Hypertension and chronic diarrhoea are not features. Thyrotoxicosis could present with loose bowel motion, tremor, and anxiety. The blood pressure is often normal with wide pulse pressure. Cervical lymphadenopathy is not a feature of an overactive thyroid gland. Although follicular thyroid cancer occurs more commonly in women over 50 years of age, chronic diarrhoea and hypertension are not characteristic features.

Sippel RS, Chen H, Medullary thyroid cancer, *Endocrine Surgery* 2009;1:149–162.

50. D. Pseudohypoparathyroidism

Pseudohypoparathyroidism is an autosomal dominant condition characterized by low serum calcium, short stature, typical round facies, dental hypoplasia, and short fourth to fifth metacarpals, and it is due to PTH resistance rather than PTH deficiency. The cause of the patient's brother's death was stridor (secondary to laryngeal spasm as a consequence of hypocalcaemia), not asthma, as he suffered from the same condition. In pseudopseudohypoparathyroidism, the serum calcium is normal. Hypoparathyroidism is not associated with low intelligence, and is usually caused by autoimmune disease. Familial hypocalciuric hypercalcaemia is an asymptomatic condition, not to be confused with hypocalcaemic hypercalciuria, which does not exist. Patients with PTH-1a often have characteristic physical features known as Albright's hereditary osteodystrophy (AHO). These features are also present in pseudopseudohypoparathyroidism but these patients do not show renal PTH resistance. PTH-1b patients mainly present with renal PTH resistance and lack the features of AHO.

Wass J, Turner H, *Oxford Handbook of Endocrinology & Diabetes*, Second Edition, Oxford University Press, 2009, Part 6: Calcium and bone metabolism, Hypocalcaemia, Clinical features.

51. A. Primary hyperparathyroidism

This patient has an elevated calcium and parathyroid hormone level. This makes the diagnoses of multiple myeloma and hypercalcaemia of malignancy incorrect as in both these instances negative feedback would mean that parathyroid hormone levels would be suppressed. Familial hyocalciuric hypocalcaemia (FHH) is a rare condition which usually results from a loss of function mutation in a calcium-sensing receptor expressed in the parathyroid and kidney. FHH does cause elevated serum calcium and PTH levels; however, symptoms are uncommon and, due to low urinary calcium excretion, renal stones are very unlikely. Tertiary hyperparathyroidism occurs in the setting of long-standing renal failure and chronically low calcium levels; phosphate levels are usually elevated. A diagnosis of primary hyperparathyroidism is most likely and fits with an elevated PTH despite the markedly elevated calcium; a low phosphate is also consistent. Renal failure in this setting may be attributable to one or a combination of dehydration, stones, and/or urinary tract infection.

Longmore M et al., *Oxford Handbook of Clinical Medicine*, Eighth Edition, Oxford University Press, 2010, Chapter 5, Endocrinology, Parathyroid hormone and hyperparathyroidism.

52. E. May be successfully treated with spironolactone

Conn's syndrome is characterized by high serum levels of aldosterone in the absence of stimulation of the renin-aldosterone system. Aldosterone levels are elevated usually as a result of an adrenal adenoma that secretes aldosterone (~75% of cases). An underlying adrenal carcinoma is rare. Around a quarter of cases of Conn's syndrome are caused by bilateral adrenal hyperplasia. Biochemically, aldosterone leads to upregulation of Na+/K+ pumps in the distal tubule and collecting duct of the kidney. The consequence of this is increased sodium resorption into the blood (and with it water), with exchange of potassium into the urine (there is also hydrogen ion loss). Electrolyte analysis of patients with Conn's syndrome is therefore associated with hypokalaemia and metabolic alkalosis. Serum potassium can, however, be normal. Sodium may be normal or elevated. Conn's syndrome may frequently be entirely asymptomatic. Symptoms can be present as a consequence of the hypokalaemia: namely, muscle weakness/cramps, polyuria, polydipsia, and parasthesia. It is estimated that Conn's syndrome is the underlying cause in around 1% of cases of hypertension. Measurement of the serum levels of renin and aldosterone should confirm high aldosterone levels in the presence of low renin. These measurements are frequently skewed by intercurrent anti-hypertensive medications taken by the patient. (See the attached references for further reading regarding the investigation and diagnosis of Conn's syndrome.) Potassium sparing diuretics that antagonize the action of aldosterone (spironolactone, amiloride) are often a successful treatment for patients with underlying bilateral adrenal hyperplasia. Surgical intervention may be indicated if imaging confirms adrenal adenoma.

Funder JW et al., Case detection, diagnosis, and treatment of patients with primary aldosteronism: an Endocrine Society clinical practice guideline, *Journal of Clinical Endocrinology & Metabolism* 2008;93(9):3266–3281. http://www.endo-society.org/guidelines/final/upload/Final-Standalone-PA-Guideline.pdf

53. D. Pituitary failure

The clues here point towards pituitary failure. The significant post-partum haemorrhage may have resulted in failure of blood supply to the gland and a subsequent lack of ACTH and TSH production over the next few weeks; this is known as Sheehan's syndrome. This has resulted in failure of lactation within the post-partum period, hyponatraemia, hyperkalaemia, and low TSH despite weight gain and lethargy. Management involves corticosteroid replacement first, ahead of thyroxine replacement, as starting with thyroxine may precipitate an adrenal crisis.

Wass J, Turner H, *Oxford Handbook of Endocrinology and Diabetes*, Second Edition, Oxford University Press, 2009.

54. A. Familial adenomatous polyposis (FAP)

Phaeochromocytomas are tumours of the adrenal medulla or sympathetic chain. They occur sporadically, or as part of a syndrome. VHL disease is an autosomal dominant condition, associated with haemangioblastomas, retinal angiomas, renal cell carcinoma, and renal, pancreatic and epididymal cysts, as well as phaeochromocytoma. NF-1 is also autosomal dominant, and associated with cutaneous manifestations such as multiple neurofibromata. Phaeochromocytomas occur in 1%, and other complications include optic nerve sheath tumours, malignant peripheral nerve sheath tumours, and a small increase in malignant soft tissue tumours. MEN-2 is again autosomal dominant. MEN-2a results in parathyroid tumours, medullary thyroid carcinoma as well as phaeochromocytoma. MEN2b results in medullary thyroid carcinoma as well as phaeochromocytoma and other abnormalities (e.g. Marfanoid habitus). FAP is not associated with phaeochromocytoma (although there are reports of a small increase in incidental adrenal masses). This condition is associated with multiple bowel polyps, which usually become malignant when the individual is in their twenties.

Bradley-Smith et al., *Oxford Handbook of Genetics*, Oxford University Press, 2010, Chapter 7, Cancer, Phaeochromocytoma.

55. D. Plasma aldosterone to plasma renin ratio

Conn's syndrome, also known as primary hyperaldosteronism, is the result of increased aldosterone secretion leading to hypernatraemia, hypokalaemia, and HTN. Increased aldosterone production may also be the result of an adenoma or adrenal hyperplasia. Routine laboratory studies can show hypernatraemia, hypokalaemia, and metabolic alkalosis resulting from the action of aldosterone on the distal tubule of the kidney (i.e. enhancing sodium reabsorption and potassium and hydrogen ion excretion). In order to improve the sensitivity of a screening test for primary hyperaldosteronism, a ratio of plasma aldosterone (PA) activity to PRA can be calculated. High aldosterone and low renin with a significantly increased ratio is consistent with primary hyperaldosteronism. Once the diagnosis of primary hyperaldosteronism is confirmed, the next step is to differentiate the subtypes and to identify surgically curable disease. Abdominal CT scanning is considered the procedure of choice. Because of the difficulties in distinguishing hyperplastic lesions from adenomatous lesions, adrenal venous sampling has become the preferred diagnostic approach in patients with equivocal findings after CT scanning. Low-dose dexamethasone-suppression test and 24-hour urinary catecholamines are often performed in the context of hypertension and hypokalaemia to exclude the possibility of Cushing's syndrome or phaeochromocytoma. In both disorders, the aldosterone levels are often within normal limits.

Tzanela M, Effremidis G, Vassiliadi D et al., The aldosterone to renin ratio in the evaluation of patients with incidentally detected adrenal masses, *Endocrine* 2007;32(2):136–142.

56. C. Transfer him to a basal bolus insulin regime

The most appropriate option is to change him to basal bolus insulin, with mealtime injections of short-acting insulin and a long-acting insulin injection in the evening. Increasing his mixtard to gain HbA1c target would further increase his risk of hypoglycaemia, and decreasing his morning mixtard would result in an increase in his HbA1c. Moving to a basal bolus regime will allow him flexibility, particularly with respect to his lunchtime insulin, allowing him to reach target without significant hypos. You should note, however, that in type 2 diabetes, according to NICE guidance, patients should try standard long-acting insulin before insulin analogues.

Nice guidelines [CG66], Type 2 diabetes. http://guidance.nice.org.uk/CG66

57. C. Intensive glycaemic control

Evidence from the DCCT (diabetes control and complications trial), which tested an intensive multi-injection low HbA1c target versus a higher one (2% difference) suggests that in the group given intensive blood glucose-lowering therapy, beta cell function was preserved for signficantly longer versus the standard glycaemic control group. As a whole, the study showed that the intensive control group experienced significantly reduced microvascular complications. The DCCT was conducted in patients with established type 1 diabetes, but this result is supported by other data from smaller Scandinavian intensive diabetes control studies. The mixed meal test is a standardized method of assessing beta cell function, where patients are usually given an milkshake-style drink containing pre-specified amounts of carbohydrate, protein and fat, glucose and insulin, and are then measured every 15 minutes to generate a glucose/insulin profile.

Steffes MW et al., β-cell function and the development of diabetes-related complications in the Diabetes Control and Complications Trial, *Diabetes Care* 2003;26:832–836. http://care. diabetesjournals.org/content/26/3/832.full

58. D. Duloxetine

NICE clinical guideline no. 96 deals with the management of peripheral neuropathy. Duloxetine is the first-line treatment of choice, with pregabalin a reasonable alternative in patients who fail to tolerate duloxetine. Other agents that are used in the management of neuropathic pain include amitryptilline and carbamazepine. Routine bloods are an important part of the workup to exclude B12 deficiency and subsequent anaemia, and renal impairment as alternative causes of peripheral neuropathy which may drive differences in clinical management.

Nice guidelines [CG96], Neuropathic pain in adults: pharmacological management in non-specialist settings. http://guidance.nice.org.uk/CG96

59. C. Start enalapril

There is a long-standing debate about the benefits of inhibition of the angiotensin pathway in normotensive patients with type 1 diabetes. The debate has been partially resolved by a multi-centre prospective study in 285 subjects with type 1 diabetes who were normotensive with normal urinary albumin excretion. Patients were randomized to receive losartan or enalapril, and neither showed any impact on renal progression. In contrast, both losartan and enalapril demonstrated a 65–70% reduction in retinopathy progression.

Mauer M et al., Renal and retinal effects of enalapril and losartan in type 1 diabetes, *New England Journal of Medicine* 2009;361:40–51. http://www.nejm.org/doi/full/10.1056/NEJMoa0808400?hits=10& andorexactfulltext=and&FIRSTINDEX=10&FIRSTINDEX=10&SEARCHID=1&searchid=1&COLLEC TION_NUM=32&resourcetype=HWCIT&resourcetype=HWCIT&andorexacttitleabs=and

60. A. 13

The anion gap is calculated with the formula: [Na + K]—[Cl + HCO] and a normal gap is 6–16 mmol/l. The correct answer is A. Levels are raised in most cases of metabolic acidosis with a few exceptions such as distal renal tubular acidosis. Other causes of a (raised anion gap) metabolic acidosis include: lactic acidosis, salicylate, and methanol poisoning. Diabetic ketoacidosis (DKA) is a serious and potentially life-threatening complication seen most often in patients with type 1 diabetes. It occurs as a result of absolute or relative insulin deficiency which then leads to a rise in counter-regulatory hormones. Increased hepatic gluconeogenesis, glycogenolysis, and lipolysis subsequently follow and lead to the metabolism of free fatty acids as fuel (and ketone formation). Signs and symptoms of DKA include: vomiting, abdominal pain, confusion, fatigue, polyuria. Cerebral oedema is a rare but potentially lethal complication. When identified, patients should be managed as 'medical emergencies' with close adherence to guidelines and intensive monitoring. The diagnosis of DKA is confirmed with the triad of: ketonaemia, hyperglycaemia, and acidaemia.

Joint British Diabetes Societies, *The Management of Diabetic Ketoacidosis in Adults*, March 2010. http://www.diabetes.org.uk/About_us/Our_Views/Care_recommendations/ The-Management-of-Diabetic-Ketoacidosis-in-Adults/

61. C. 3 litres

Fluid replacement in hyperosmolar non-ketotic coma is more cautious than in DKA. Average recommended fluid replacement is 1 litre during the first hour, followed by 2 litres in the subsequent 3–4 hours. More rapid fluid replacement runs the risk of precipitating cardiac failure as these patients often have underlying LV dysfunction. Normal saline is hypotonic relative to the patient's own serum and remains the fluid replacement of choice. When blood glucose reaches 15 mmol/l, IV insulin is usually ceased, and fluid replacement changed to 5% dextrose.

Ramrakha P et al., *Oxford Handbook of Acute Medicine*, Third Edition, Oxford University Press, 2010.

62. C. KCNJ11

KCNJ11 is a gene coding for a potassium channel which is responsible for beta cell insulin release in response to sulphonylurea stimulation. It is well known that mutations in the *KCNJ11* gene can lead to a reduction or enhancement of the therapeutic effect of sulphonylureas. *OCT1* is a gene which codes for the transporter which allows metformin to enter hepatocytes or enterocytes. Mutations in *OCT1* lead to a reduction or enhancement in the effect of metformin. *TCF7L2* is involved in the incretin effect. *MCR4* and *BCAT* are genes which govern the development of obesity.

Reitman ML et al., Pharmacogenetics of metformin response: a step in the path toward personalized medicine, *Journal of Clinical Investigation* 2007;117(5):1226–1229. http://www.ncbi.nlm.nih.gov/pmc/ articles/PMC1857273/

63. C. Ovarian hyperstimulation syndrome

Ovarian hyperstimulation syndrome is a complication of excessive ovarian stimulation by exogenous gonadotrophin administration (hCG) to obtain eggs for in vitro fertilization. This results in marked enlargement of the ovaries with a protein-rich transudate from them resulting in ascites and hypoalbuminaemia. Renal failure and shock secondary to hypovolaemia may also occur. Treatment involves infusion of 20% albumin to correct the circulating blood volume and diuretics.

Budev MM, Arroliga AC, Falcone T, Ovarian hyperstimulation syndrome, *Critical Care Medicine* 2005;33(Suppl.):S301–S306

64. E. Liraglutide

In this situation, liraglutide, a daily GLP-1 analogue, is the most appropriate option. The presence of heart failure rules out pioglitazone, and the potential for weight gain means that gliclazide is also not appropriate. With respect to insulin, either basal bolus or the addition of basal insulin is going to promote further weight gain, which may exacerbate fluid retention and problems controlling blood pressure. In addition, mortality was increased in association with hypoglycaemia in the VADT and ACCORD studies. As such liraglutide, which promotes modest weight loss and improves glycaemic control without particular problems with hypoglycaemia, is the best option. The class may also be cardioprotective by reducing cardiac myocyte apoptosis.

emc+, Victoza 6 mg/ml solution for injection in pre-filled pen.
http://www.medicines.org.uk/emc/medicine/21986/SPC/

65. C. Insulin allergy

Insulin allergy is thankfully rare, but may still occur with human insulins when they are combined with agents that cause them to precipitate, such as zinc used in some long-acting insulin preparations. Historically, insulin allergy was much more common during the time that porcine and bovine insulins were the only products available. The indurated skin and local urticaria is typical of this. In this case his long-acting insulin should be switched, potentially to a formulation which does not rely on precipitating out in the subcutaneous tissue, such as detemir (which becomes long-acting because of binding to human albumin). Where allergy persists, desensitization regimes can be pursued. These may involve giving insulin via another route (e.g. orally), which promotes a non-IgE-mediated respones to insulin, or giving topical corticosteroids with the injection.

Spickett G, *Oxford Handbook of Clinical Immunology and Allergy*, Second Edition, Oxford University Press, 2006, Chapter 3, Allergic disease, Drug allergy 1: penicillin, other antibiotics, and insulin.

66. D. Phosphate

Refeeding in anorexia, as in other conditions associated with severe malnutrition such as alcoholism, is associated with significant reactive hyperinsulinaemia. This drives very rapid movement of phosphate from the extra-cellular to the intra-cellular space. Hypophosphataemia then leads to skeletal muscle weakness and low output heart failure. In this situation, the make-up of feeds should be carefully balanced by an experienced dietician, to ensure that phosphate replacement is adequate.

Refeeding syndrome: what it is, and how to prevent and treat it, *British Medical Journal* 2008;336:1495. doi: http://dx.doi.org/10.1136/bmj.a301; http://www.bmj.com/content/336/7659/1495.short

67. D. Tall stature

This man has Klinefelter's syndrome. Patients have scanty body hair and little facial hair growth. About 40% develop gynaecomastia. Klinefelter's syndrome does not cause mental retardation. Most patients present later in life with either delayed puberty or reporting difficulties forming relationships with women.

Longmore M et al., *Oxford Handbook of Clinical Medicine*, Eighth Edition, Oxford University Press, 2010, Chapter 5, Endocrinology, Hirsutism, virilism, gynaecomastia & impotence/ED.

68. D. Metformin

Metformin is a biguanide, which increases sensitivity to insulin. It does not, however, cause hypoglycaemia. Nateglinide is a sulphonylurea receptor binder which increases beta cell insulin release, and can therefore lead to hypoglycaemia. Glargine is a long-acting insulin and is usually administered once daily. It can therefore cause hypoglycaemia for some hours after the dose is given. This can be particularly important in treating a patient who has taken an overdose of insulin glargine, as treatment of the hypoglycaemia needs to be ongoing for at least 24 hours. Glibenclamide is a sulphonyluria which stimulates beta cells to release insulin, and can therefore lead to hypoglycaemia.

Longmore M et al., *Oxford Handbook of Clinical Medicine*, Eighth Edition, Oxford University Press, 2010, Chapter 6, Endocrinology, Treating diabetes mellitus.

69. B. Blood glucose

This man has a metabolic acidosis and an extremely rapid respiratory rate. A common cause of this presentation in a young patient is diabetic ketoacidosis. This may be the first presentation of diabetes, or the patient may not be able to give a history if he is confused or unconscious, so clinical vigilance is required. The diagnosis is confirmed by finding a high-serum glucose in combination with a metabolic acidosis and urinary ketones (which may also be detected by their characteristic smell on the patient's breath). The collateral history from his flatmates is supportive of ketoacidosis as the diagnosis.

Longmore M et al., *Oxford Handbook of Clinical Medicine*, Eighth Edition, Oxford University Press, 2010, Chapter 20, Emergencies, Diabetic ketoacidosis.

70. B. Linagliptin

Metformin is not recommended in patients with a GFR of <60 mL/min due to risk of accumulation and possible lactic acidosis. Similarly, glibenclamide is renally excreted and is at risk of accumulation and subsequent hypoglycaemia. Pioglitazone leads to fluid retention and is ill advised for this reason in patients with renal impairment. Given his HbA1c is only just above target, linagliptin is the most appropriate option because it is excreted via the enterohepatic circulation and therefore does not need dose adjustment in renal impairment.

emc+, Trajenta 5 mg film-coated tablets. http://www.medicines.org.uk/emc/medicine/25000/SPC

71. D. Hypophosphataemia

The history given here, in a patient with significant malnutrition, is consistent with re-feeding syndrome. It is thought that reactive hyperinsulinaemia in response to carbohydrate loading leads to a massive intracellular shift of magnesium, phosphate and potassium, leading to a fall in extracellular concentration of these ions. It can be avoided by tailoring calorie replacement with the risk of re-feeding syndrome in mind, by increasing the protein content of the feed, coupled with daily electrolyte monitoring and necessary replacement.

Nutrition support for adults: oral nutrition support, enteral tube feeding and parenteral nutrition, NICE guidelines [CG32], Published date: February 2006

72. A. Desmopressin

Diabetes insipidus is an uncommon finding after head injury, but is the most likely diagnosis here, given the symptoms and findings on water deprivation test. Desmopressin is the treatment of choice because it acts predominantly on V2 receptors in the kidney, and does not have a substantial pressor effect. This is in contrast to lysine vasopressin which is shorter acting and less specific. Lithium is a cause of nephrogenic diabetes insipidus, bendroflumethiazide is a treatment for nephrogenic diabetes insipidus, and demeclocycline is a treatment for SIADH.

Capatina C, Paluzzi A, Mitchell R, Karavitaki N, Diabetes Insipidus after traumatic brain injury, *Journal of Clinical Medicine* 2015 Jul 13;4(7):1448–1462.

73. A. Elevated cortisol

Patients with low weight due to anorexia usually have raised cortisol, in keeping with a stress response to the period of low calorific intake. In keeping with use of purgatives/induced vomiting or use of diuretics, potassium is usually reduced or normal. Calcium may well be low due to dietary deficiency of vitamin D or calcium. Elevated sodium or creatinine are not usual findings. When feeding is commenced it is crucial to take specialist dietician advice to ensure the ratio of protein to carbohydrate is appropriate, and phosphate replacement is adequate to avoid re-feeding syndrome. Magnesium levels also go down and need careful monitoring during re-feeding.

Schorr M, Lawson EA, Dichtel LE, Klibanski A, Miller KK, Cortisol measures across the weight spectrum, *Journal of Clinical Endocrinology & Metabolism* 2015 Sep;100(9):3313–3321.

74. B. Blocks renal tubular glucose reabsorption

Dapagliflozin is an SGLT-2 inhibitor which blocks reabsorption of glucose from the glomerular filtrate, leading to excretion of approximately 30% of the filtered glucose load. In patients with type 2 diabetes this corresponds to approximately 70g of excreted glucose per day. It is associated with increased risk of candidiasis and urinary tract infection, particularly in women. SGLT-1 inhibitors block intestinal absorption of glucose. The incretin effect leads to increased levels of GLP-1 and GIP in response to an oral glucose challenge. Subcutaneous GLP-1 analogues exist for the treatment of type 2 diabetes, as do DPPIV inhibitors, which block GLP-1 breakdown.

emc+, Dapagliflozin: pharmacodynamic properties. http://www.medicines.org.uk/emc/medicine/27188#PHARMACODYNAMIC_PROPS

75. C. DR3

It is highly likely, given the strong family history of type 1 diabetes, that this patient carries one or both of these antigens. HLA-B27 is associated with seronegative arthritis and inflammatory bowel disease. HLA-B6 is associated with unexplained infertility, HLA-B52 with Takayasu's arteritis and ulcerative colitis. DR2 is associated with reduced incidence of diabetes.

Longmore M et al., *Oxford Handbook of Clinical Medicine*, Eighth Edition, Oxford University Press, 2010.

76. B. It leads to excretion of approximately 70g glucose/day in patients with type 2 diabetes

Dapagliflozin is an SGLT-2 inhibitor which blocks glucose reabsorption in the proximal tubule. In trials of dapagliflozin in patients with type 2 diabetes, approximately 70 g of glucose was excreted in the urine per day (corresponding to 280 kcal/day) at a dapagliflozin dose of 10 mg/day in subjects with type 2 diabetes mellitus for 12 weeks. An osmotic diuresis occurs in conjunction with therapy which leads to approximately a 2% rise in haematocrit and a small fall in blood pressure. Rates of genital infection approximate to around 5% in patients on therapy. Modest weight loss is also seen. With respect to PTH, dapagliflozin therapy is associated with a small rise.

emc+, Dapagliflozin: pharmacodynamic properties. http://www.medicines.org.uk/emc/medicine/27188#PHARMACODYNAMIC_PROPS

77. C. Normal expiratory flow-volume loop, with flattening of the inspiratory flow-volume loop

Extra-thoracic extrinsic compression of the large airways will cause a flattening of the inspiratory component of the flow-volume loop; the expiratory component is normal as the obstruction is pushed outwards on expiration but on inspiration the obstruction is sucked into the trachea causing partial obstruction. Concave flow-volume loops with normal forced vital capacity (FVC) is typical of obstructive (small airways) lung disease. Flattening of the expiratory flow-volume loop with normal inspiration would be seen in intra-thoracic large airway obstruction. Normal flow-volume loop shape with reduced FVC would be typical of restrictive lung disease.

Spirométrie. http://www.spirometrie.info/fvc.html

78. D. Start high-dose IV methylprednisolone

The loss of colour vision and problems with upward gaze are signs of significant thyroid eye disease. As such urgent intervention is required. High-dose methylprednisolone is superior to oral prednisolone and is therefore the intervention of choice. Steroid sparing therapy may be required for disease which is resistant to steroid therapy, and in this situation azathioprine is a reasonable choice. Surgical decompression is used for severe sight-threatening disease, or for cosmetic reasons once the activity of eye disease has reduced (via an inferior orbital approach, using space in the ethmoidal, sphenoidal, and maxillary sinuses). Patients are typically managed with thyroxine and carbimazole in a block and replace regimen, as maintaining stable thyroxine levels may reduce the risk of deterioration of thyroid eye disease.

Longmore M et al., *Oxford Handbook of Clinical Medicine*, Eighth Edition, Oxford University Press, 2010, Chapter 5, Endocrinology.

79. A. Cranial diabetes insipidus

DDAVP is a synthetic vasopressin (also known as the anti-diuretic hormone ADH) that acts on renal collecting ducts to increase water absorption. The fact that this patient is passing dilute urine at the end of the water deprivation test, and is able to concentrate his urine following DDAVP, is highly suggestive of a diagnosis of cranial diabetes insipidus. The significant head injury at the time of his motor-cycle accident is the most likely cause. Whilst desmopressin is certainly indicated at this stage, endogenous production of ADH may recover, so his serum sodium should be re-tested every few months. Passing dilute urine at the end of the test which fails to concentrate after DDAVP is suggestive of nephrogenic diabetes insipidus. Elevated urine osmolality at the end of the test without DDAVP fits best with psychogenic polydipsia. We ave no indication that this patient abuses diuretics.

Wass J, Turner H, *Oxford Handbook of Endocrinology and Diabetes*, Second Edition, Oxford University Press, 2009, Chapter 33, Nephrogenic diabetes insipidus.

80. B. Add bendroflumethiazide

This patient has residual diabetes insipidus despite having stopped the lithium therapy. Leaving her requiring to drink substantial amounts of fluid per day is suboptimal, therefore a logical next step is to add bendroflumethiazide to her regime which reduces free water loss in this situation.

This is a paradoxical effect seen in nephrogenic DI versus what you would expect in the normal situation. If she fails to respond to the diuretic, an NSAID can also be added which promotes salt and water retention. In cases which are resistant to initial therapy, nephrogenic DI may respond to high-dose DDAVP although where there is significant intrinsic renal damage this is usually ineffective. Demeclocycline induces renal resistance to ADH and is therefore used as a treatment for SIADH resistant to fluid restriction. Demclocycline is used for the treatment of resistant SIADH.

Wass J, Turner H, *Oxford Handbook of Endocrinology and Diabetes*, Second Edition, Oxford University Press, 2009, Chapter 33, Diabetes insipidus.

81. B. Cabergoline

The different treatment options for a pituitary adenoma include surgery, radiotherapy, and medical therapy. However, a pituitary adenoma extending into the cavernous sinus presents increased operative risk. Prolactinomas are highly responsive to drug therapy, and therefore, in this patient pharmacological intervention should be attempted first. Of the options given, prolactinomas are poorly responsive to somatostatin analogues, but respond well to dopamine agonists. The greatest evidence base is for cabergoline and bromocriptine, and of the two, better efficacy data exists for cabergoline, and it has a superior adverse event profile.

Wass J, Turner H, *Oxford Handbook of Endocrinology and Diabetes*, Second Edition, Oxford University Press, 2014, Chapter 17, Prolactinomas.

82. B. Urinary porphyrins

Whilst porphyria is a rare condition, it can be considered in patients presenting with a psychiatric illness, abdominal pain, hypertension, and hyponatraemia. Out of the various porphyrias, it is acute intermittent porphyria which has the highest incidence, and is the most likely diagnosis here. The diagnosis can be confirmed by raised levels of urinary porphobilinogen. Haem arginate and carbohydrate supplementation are the treatments of choice in this situation. A number of medications potentially increase the risk of acute attacks (a list can be found on the European Porphyria initiative website), but they include oestrogens which women commonly use as part of the oral contraceptive pill.

European porphyria initiative website. http://www.porphyria-europe.com/

83. B. Add sitagliptin

This patient's job as a taxi driver means that exposure to hypoglycaemia should be minimized if possible. As such, neither basal insulin or addition of a sulphonylurea are ideal choices to gain glycaemic control. Acarbose can cause significant GI upset and is also best avoided in patients who spend many hours driving for a living. This leaves sitagliptin and pioglitazone as possible options. Pioglitazone is contraindicated in patients with a history of bladder cancer. These leaves sitagliptin as the most appropriate glucose lowering option, it is not associated with significant hypoglycaemia, and is associated with modest weight loss as well as an improvement in HbA1c.

Type 2 diabetes: The management of type 2 diabetes, NICE guidelines [CG87]. Published date: May 2009, Last updated: December 2014

84. A. Cushing's syndrome

The key first fact to take away here is that the morning cortisol is significantly elevated. As such Cushing's disease is a main consideration with respect to the underlying diagnosis. Pituitary dependent Cushing's occurs due to elevated ACTH, which in turn leads to elevated cortisol. This in turn drives massive weight gain, hypertension, and a picture of insulin resistance, which eventually in most cases leads to the development of diabetes mellitus. The initial investigation of choice is 24-hour urinary free cortisol as it can be carried out as an outpatient. This is followed by a low-dose dexamethasone suppression test, coupled with imaging of the pituitary and/or adrenals according to clinical suspicion. The prolactin seen here, whilst elevated, is not likely to be due primarily to a prolactin-producing tumour, instead being due to release of prolactin as a result of local pressure effects. Given the endocrine abnormalities seen, PCOS is unlikely to be the underlying diagnosis. Pituitary MRI is a logical next step with respect to investigation.

Wass J et al., *Oxford Handbook of Endocrinology and Diabetes*, Second Edition, Oxford University Press, 2011, Chapter 5.7, Cushing's syndrome.

85. A. Referral for cognitive therapy

The low urine and plasma osmolality raise the possibility that this patient's symptoms are due to psychogenic polydipsia, which is much more common than diabetes insipidus that has a combined incidence (cranial and nephrogenic) of 1 in 25,000. The normal calcium and glucose effectively rule out hypercalcaemia and hyperglycaemia as possible causes of her symptoms. Where there is diagnostic confusion, a water deprivation test could be considered. If the diagnosis is still in doubt after a water deprivation test, vasopressin and osmolality in response to 5% saline infusion is an option. Management of choice in this case would be referral for cognitive behavioural therapy, to encourage her to progressively reduce her fluid intake. This in turn is likely to be associated with an improvement in her symptoms.

Turner H, Wass J, *Oxford Handbook of Endocrinology and Diabetes*, Second Edition, Oxford University Press, 2009, Chapter 33, Diabetic insipidus (DI).

86. A. 0%

Answering this question relies on knowing that it is an X-linked recessive disorder. As such any male children fathered by the affected patient cannot by definition have the condition and the percentage chance of them inheriting it is therefore 0. All-female offspring of this male will carry the gene but not suffer from the condition. If the condition were X-linked dominant then all female offspring would suffer from the condition. Congenital nephrogenic diabetes insipidus may also carry an autosomal dominant or autosomal recessive pattern of inheritance due to a mutation in the *AQP2* gene; both dominant and recessive mutations exist.

Turner H, Wass J, *Oxford Handbook of Endocrinology and Diabetes*, Second Edition, Oxford University Press, 2009, Chapter 33, Diabetes insipidus.

87. B. Autosomal recessive

This patient has the DIDMOAD or Wolfram syndrome. It is characterized by diabetes insipidus, diabetes mellitus, optic atrophy, and sensorineural deafness. Diabetes mellitus, usually requiring insulin therapy, is the first manifestation, usually followed by optic atrophy and evidence of hearing loss. The condition is rare, has a prevalence of only 1 in 500,000, and is caused by a mutation in the *WFS1* gene, which is inherited in autosomal recessive fashion. The mutation leads to production of abnormal wolframin protein, which is thought to regulate calcium homeostasis within cells. Abnormal calcium homeostasis is in turn thought to lead to progressive apoptosis of beta cells, cells within the optic and vestibulocochlear nerve, and in neurones responsible for producing ADH.

Turner H, Wass J, *Oxford Handbook of Endocrinology and Diabetes*, Second Edition, Oxford University Press, 2009, Chapter 33, Diabetes insipidus.

88. B. Autosomal dominant

All of the porphyrias are associated with an autosomal dominant inheritance pattern apart from aminolaevulinic acid dehydratase porphyria (ADP) and congenital erythropoietic porphyria (CEP), which follow an autosomal recessive inheritance pattern and X-linked dominant protoporphyria (XLDPP). Given this woman has a copy of the affected gene on only one of her chromosome 11s, the possibility of a child of her's inheriting the disorder is 50%. She also has a 50% chance of having a normal child. Diagnosis of AIP is based on demonstration of elevated urinary porphobilinogen during an acute attack, as levels may be normal in the intervening period.

Warrell DA et al., *Oxford Textbook of Medicine*, Oxford University Press, 2010, Section 12.5, The Porphyrias.

89. C. Porphobilinogen decarboxylase

AIP is an autosomal dominant disorder which is related to a deficiency of porphobilinogen deaminase. The defect is on the short arm of chromosome 11. AIP is associated with acute attacks of hypertension, abdominal pain, anxiety, and hyponatraemia. A number of drugs may precipitate attacks including the combined oral contraceptive pill. Treatment is with haem arginate and carbohydrate replacement. Uroporphyrinogen decarboxylase deficiency is associated with the development of porphyria cutanea tarda. Ferrochelatase deficiency is associated with the development of erythropoietic protoporphyria. Protoporphyrinogen oxidase deficiency is associated with the development of variegate porphyria. Aminolaevulinic acid dehydratase deficiency is associated with the development of Aminolaevulinic acid dehydratase porphyria (ADP).

Warrell DA et al., *Oxford Textbook of Medicine*, Oxford University Press, 2010, Section 12.5, The Porphyrias.

1. **Regarding Crohn's disease, which one of the following is true?**
   A. There is no increased risk of colonic cancer in those with colonic Crohn's disease
   B. Post-operative recurrence leads to re-operation in around 10% of patients at five years
   C. Smoking status is the most well-characterized environmental factor associated with disease susceptibility and outcome
   D. Is a monogenic disorder related to carriage of the *NOD2* gene
   E. Anti-TNF alpha therapy is indicated for those with a perianal abscess

2. **Which of the following supports a diagnosis of hereditary haemochromatosis in a male patient (select the single most appropriate response)?**
   A. Serum ferritin levels of 251 mcg/l accompanied by fasting transferrin saturation of 19%
   B. Serum ferritin levels of 351 mcg/l accompanied by fasting transferrin saturation of 58%
   C. Serum ferritin levels of 642 mcg/l accompanied by fasting transferrin saturation of 31%
   D. Serum ferritin levels of 764 mcg/l accompanied by fasting transferrin saturation of 24%
   E. Serum ferritin levels of 366 mcg/l accompanied by fasting transferrin saturation of 14%

3. **Which of the following statements regarding hereditary haemochromatosis is true (select the single most appropriate response)?**
   A. Liver biopsy is required for diagnosis in all cases
   B. Cardiac failure due to dilated cardiomyopathy is a common complication
   C. Chondrocalcinosis may be visible on X-ray films
   D. Universal screening for haemochromatosis is currently recommended in the UK
   E. Liver histology does not improve despite effective venesection

4. **In a 54-year-old man with Crohn's disease confined to the terminal ileum, deficiency in which of the following is expected?**

   A. Folic acid
   B. Vitamin B12
   C. Iron
   D. Calcium
   E. Magnesium

5. **Which one of the following is about gastrin hormone?**

   A. It is secreted from the parietal cells in the stomach
   B. Levels are undetectable in chronic atrophic gastritis
   C. Proton pump inhibitors suppress gastrin secretion
   D. High levels of gastrin can lead to peptic ulcers
   E. Gastrinomas are usually located in the stomach

6. **Regarding the management of inflammatory bowel disease during pregnancy, which of the following statements is correct (select the single most appropriate response)?**

   A. Treatment of active disease with corticosteroids is contraindicated
   B. Treatment of active disease with aminosalicylates is contraindicated
   C. Maintenance therapy with azathioprine/mercaptopurine should be discontinued during pregnancy
   D. Maintenance therapy with aminosalicylates should be discontinued during pregnancy
   E. Maintenance therapy with azathioprine should be continued during pregnancy if recurrent relapse is likely

7. **A 30-year-old woman with severe ulcerative colitis is being consented for an elective laparotomy and hemicolectomy operation. Her Hb is 10 and she has received intravenous iron for a few years. She is a Jehovah's witness and says she does not want any blood transfusion because of her religious belief. Her boyfriend is not happy with this. With regards to the risks of intra-operative bleeding, which one of the following is the most appropriate in her case?**

   A. Give the maximum dose of iron infusion possible prior to her operation
   B. Explain the risks of bleeding and document her wishes in the notes
   C. Having explained the risks, plan for autologous transfusion
   D. If she bleeds in theatre, liaise with the boyfriend and get his consent
   E. Ask the boyfriend to speak to the patient prior to the operation

8. **A 32-year-old man who has been diagnosed with acromegaly is referred to the gastroenterology clinic for review as he has been told he may be at increased risk of colon cancer and needs a colonoscopy. Which of the following correctly reflects the increased risk of colon cancer in patients with acromegaly?**

   A. No increased risk
   B. Two-fold increase
   C. Five-fold increase
   D. 10-fold increase
   E. 20-fold increase

9. **A 20-year-old man has a six-month history of intermittent episodes of lower colicky abdominal pain. He reports weight loss of 1 stone in the same period. His appetite is as per usual. He complains of intermittent constipation and abdominal bloatedness. He reports no diarrhoea. He is Caucasian and travelled to Barbados for a holiday one year ago. The systemic enquiry of note was that he reports short episodes of painful ankles associated with circular erythematous skin lesions on the shin. On examination, he looked thin and mildly clubbed. His pulse was 80 and regular. His blood pressure was 108/60 mmHg. A BCG scar was noted on his right upper arm. Cardiorespiratory examination was normal. There was some tenderness over the hypogastrium and the right iliac fossa. Blood tests are as follows: Hb 10 (13.5–17.5 g/dl), WBC 11 x 10^9/l (4–11), Plt 498 x 10^9/l (150–400), ESR 55 (0–10 mm in the first hour), Na 138 (137–144), K 4.0 (3.5–4.9), U 5.0 (2.5–7.5), Cr 80 (60–110), bilirubin 13 micromol/l (2–17), ALP 40 U/l (30–130), ALT 28 U/l (5–30), albumin 36 g/l (35–55). Stool sample was negative. Chest X-ray was normal. Which is the most likely diagnosis?**

   A. Tropical sprue
   B. Whipple's disease
   C. Ulcerative colitis
   D. Crohn's disease
   E. Intestinal tuberculosis

10. **A 24-year-old man presented to his GP because of weight loss and abdominal pain. Subsequent evaluation by a consultant gastroenterologist led to colonoscopy which revealed endoscopic and histopathological features consistent with Crohn's disease. Which one of the following is most consistent with a diagnosis of Crohn's disease?**

    A. Severe crypt architectural distortion
    B. Epithelioid granulomata
    C. Rectal inflammation/involvement
    D. Cobblestone mucosal appearance
    E. Crypt abscesses

11. **A 32-year-old woman presented to her GP complaining of bloody diarrhoea. Subsequent evaluation by a consultant gastroenterologist led to investigations including colonoscopy, which reported 'erythema and mild continuous ulceration confined to the rectum'. Associated biopsies confirmed histopathological features in keeping with ulcerative colitis. Of the following, which is the most appropriate treatment? Select the single most appropriate answer.**

    A. Oral mesalazine
    B. Rectal mesalazine suppository
    C. Oral prednisolone
    D. Oral metronidazole
    E. Dietician referral

12. **Which of the following HFE mutations occurs most frequently in confirmed hereditary haemochromatosis?**

    A. *C282Y/H63D* compound heterozygote
    B. *C282Y/C282Y* homozygote
    C. *H63D/H63D* homozygote
    D. *H63D* heterozygote
    E. *C282Y* heterozygote

13. **Which of the following statements regarding hereditary haemochromatosis is true (select the single most appropriate response)?**

    A. Universal screening for haemochromatosis is currently recommended in the UK
    B. Universal screening for haemochromatosis is currently recommended in the United States
    C. Symmetrical polyarthropathy is a recognized feature
    D. Venesection is curative
    E. The condition is autosomal dominant

14. **Which of the following statements regarding Wilson's disease is true (select the single most appropriate response)?**

    A. Neuropsychiatric features usually precede liver disease in children
    B. The condition is autosomal dominant
    C. Corneal Kayser–Fleischer rings (detected by slit lamp) are diagnostic
    D. The condition is characterized by excessive deposition of iron in the liver, brain, and other tissues
    E. Lifelong therapy with a chelating agent such as penicillamine is required

15. **A 41-year-old man with a history of alcohol excess is admitted via the emergency department. He is unkempt, tremulous, and physical examination reveals him to be underweight with scattered spider naevi. No organomegaly is detected. His laboratory investigations are as follows: ALT 123, alkaline phosphatase 164 IU/l, bilirubin 96 micromol/l, Hb 12.0, WCC 16.0, urea 5.6 mmol/l, PT ratio 2.1. What is the most appropriate diagnosis from the list below (select the single most appropriate answer)?**

    A. Decompensated alcoholic liver disease
    B. Alcoholic encephalopathy
    C. Delerium tremens
    D. Alcoholic hepatitis
    E. Portal vein thrombosis

16. **Regarding ulcerative colitis (UC), which of the following statements is accurate? Select the single most appropriate response.**

    A. Ulcerative colitis is typically characterized by diffuse mucosal inflammation limited to the colon
    B. An uncommon symptom of UC is bloody diarrhoea
    C. Abdominal pain and weight loss are more consistent with ulcerative colitis than Crohn's disease
    D. Fistulation is a feature of UC
    E. UC, in contrast to Crohn's colitis, is not associated with an increased risk of colonic carcinoma

17. **A 39-year-old male with a history of alcohol abuse is admitted with abdominal distension, jaundice, and malaise. The admitting team initiate treatment with pabrinex, lactulose, and a withdrawal regime of chlordiazepoxide. His renal function and serum electrolytes are within the normal range. Which of the following represent appropriate first-line management of this patient's ascites? Select the single most appropriate response.**

A. Initiate diuretic therapy with furosemide 40 mg/day
B. Initiate diuretic therapy with spironolactone 100 g/day
C. Intravenous colloid 500 ml/4 h
D. Oral fluid restriction
E. Initiate diuretic therapy with spironolactone 200 mg/day

18. **A 62-year-old woman presents to the gastroenterology clinic complaining of chronic watery diarrhoea which has persisted for the past 18 months. She has a history of osteoarthritis for which she takes regular ibuprofen. On examination her BMI is 23. General physical examination is unremarkable. Flexible sigmoidoscopy is macroscopically normal. Investigations: Hb 12.4, WCC 5.9, PLT 203, Na 138, K 3.9, Cr 109. Stool microscopy is negative for blood but positive for white cells. Which of the following is the most likely diagnosis?**

A. Ulcerative colitis
B. Crohn's disease
C. Coeliac disease
D. Irritable bowel syndrome
E. Microscopic colitis

19. **Regarding the dietary management of proven coeliac disease, select the single most appropriate response from the following five:**

A. Gluten should be strictly avoided for life
B. Small amounts of gluten may be permitted once symptoms are controlled
C. Oats must be strictly avoided
D. Rye does not contain gluten, and therefore may be consumed freely
E. Barley contains small amounts of gluten, and may be ingested in small quantities

20. **A 37-year-old man is referred to the gastroenterology clinic because he is noted to have abnormal LFTs whilst volunteering for a phase 1 drug study. Further serology testing revealed that he is hepatitis C positive. Which of the following is with respect to hepatitis C?**

    A. Genotype 1 requires 24 weeks of anti-viral therapy
    B. Genotype 5 has a response rate of 38–50% to anti-viral therapy
    C. Genotype 2 has a response rate of 90% to anti-viral therapy
    D. Genotype 3 requires 48 weeks of anti-viral therapy
    E. A 50-fold reduction in viral load at 12 weeks is required to continue therapy

21. **Regarding Barrett's oesophagus:**

    A. The condition is present in 0.2% of the population in the Western World
    B. The absolute lifetime risk of progression to oesophageal adenocarcinoma is around 3–5%
    C. White ethnicity and female sex are associated with progression to adenocarcinoma
    D. Surveillance has been shown, in a randomized controlled trial, to improve mortality
    E. Laparoscopic fundoplication has been proven to be superior to long-term proton pump inhibitor therapy for symptom control in the longer term

22. **A 51-year-old publican comes to the clinic complaining of epigastric pain, nausea, weight loss, and chronic diarrhoea, which he says is difficult to flush away. You wonder whether he has pancreatic insufficiency and arrange a faecal elastase test. Which of the following is true of the faecal elastase test?**

    A. Pancreatic supplements interfere with the analysis
    B. Levels less than 200 mcg/g of stool are diagnostic of insufficiency
    C. Levels greater than 50 mcg/g of stool are diagnostic of insufficiency
    D. ELISA is used to detect elastase in a single stool sample
    E. 24 hours' worth of stool sample is required for the test

23. **A 49-year-old man with a history of inflammatory bowel disease comes to the clinic complaining of increasing jaundice, nausea, and anorexia over the past few weeks. On examination he is thin, with a BMI of 20. There is discomfort on palpation of the epigastrium. Investigations: Hb 10.9 g/dl (13.5–17.7), WCC 9.9 x10⁹/l (4–11), PLT 201 x 10⁹/l, Na 138 (137–145) mmol/l, K 4.5 (3.5–5) mmol/l, ALT 82 (7–50) U/l, bilirubin 95 (<25) micromol/l, alkaline phosphatase 425 (38–126) U/l, ultrasound abdomen suggests an intrahepatic mass lesion. Which of the following is likely to be the most effective intervention?**

    A. Biliary stenting
    B. Resection of the mass
    C. Chemotherapy
    D. Radiotherapy
    E. Immunotherapy

24. **Regarding variceal haemorrhage, which one of the following statements is:**

    A. Vasopressin analogues are of no proven mortality benefit
    B. A patient who has lost 1000 ml of blood may be normotensive
    C. In patients with chronic liver disease who present with variceal haemorrhage, empirical antibiotic use does not alter mortality rates
    D. Endoscopic sclerotherapy is superior to band ligation in preventing re-bleeding
    E. In the presence of coagulopathy, transjugular intrahepatic portosystemic shunt insertion (TIPSS) is contraindicated

25. **A 75-year-old man presents with haematemesis. You wish to estimate his prognosis, and use the Rockall score. Which of these features of his condition will NOT add any additional points to the score?**

    A. Diagnosis: Mallory–Weiss tear
    B. Pulse rate: 110 per minute
    C. Age: 75 years
    D. Past medical history: Ischaemic heart disease
    E. None of the above, i.e. they all add to the score

26. **A 17-year-old man presents to the clinic with evidence of chronic GI blood loss. He is noted on clinical examination to have peri-oral pigmentation which resembles freckling. Upper GI endoscopy is unremarkable, but a barium follow-through is suspicious for multiple polyps in the small bowel. Investigations: Hb 10.9, WCC 8.0, PLT 193, Na 137, K 4.3, Cr 101. Where is the defect that is responsible for this disorder most likely to lie?**

    A. Chromosome 5
    B. Chromosome 6
    C. Chromosome 7
    D. Chromosome 11
    E. Chromosome 19

27. **A 45-year-old live-in carer is referred to the A&E department by her GP with one week of generalized itching. Her GP had noted that she appeared jaundiced. On further questioning, she admits to losing weight over the last few months but says she has been trying to lose weight recently. She also suffers from back pain that started a few weeks ago, which she had put down to her work. She does not have any other medical history but is a smoker with 20-pack-years history. Her clinical examination is unremarkable apart from jaundice and a few scratch marks. What is the most likely diagnosis?**

    A. Cancer of tail of pancreas
    B. Hepatocellular carcinoma
    C. Cholangiocarcinoma
    D. Acute pancreatitis
    E. Gallstones

28. **A 60-year-old woman presents with abdominal distention and jaundice. She also complains of itching and some weight loss. Her only past medical history is ulcerative colitis which has not been well controlled for a few years. Her blood tests show bilirubin 50 (3–17 mmol/l), ALP 230 (30–150 iu/l), ALT 50 (5–35 iu/l), Hb 9.8 (11.5–16 g/dl), MCV 71 (76–96 fl), PLT 560 (150–400). On clinical examination she has hepatomegaly and ascites. What is the most appropriate first-line investigation?**

    A. MRCP
    B. ERCP
    C. CT abdomen
    D. Colonoscopy
    E. Abdominal ultrasound

29. **A 45-year-old man undergoes laparoscopic resection of his terminal ileum for Crohn's disease refractory to medical treatment. Twenty-five centimetres of inflamed bowel are resected, and a primary anastamosis formed. His initial post-operative course is uneventful and he is swiftly discharged. However, when seen in clinic six weeks later, he complains of ongoing troublesome diarrhoea, opening his bowels up to six times during the day, and once or twice at night. There is no blood in the stool, and he does not experience any abdominal pain. He is otherwise in good health, does not smoke, and admits to drinking around 20 units of alcohol per week. He notices that his symptoms tend to be worse after eating. What is the most likely diagnosis?**

    A. Neoterminal ileal Crohn's disease
    B. Chronic pancreatitis
    C. Intestinal lymphangiectasia
    D. Bile salt malabsorption
    E. Irritable bowel syndrome

30. **In chronic hepatitis C, which of the following factors is NOT associated with increased risk of progression to cirrhosis?**

    A. Male sex
    B. Infection at young age
    C. Excess alcohol consumption
    D. Obesity
    E. HIV co-infection

31. **A 40-year-old man presents to the A&E department after a heavy night of drinking. It is difficult to get much history from him as he is under the influence of alcohol. His vomit bowl contains fresh blood. On clinical examination his BP is 99/58, HR 100, slightly clammy but otherwise unremarkable. His friend who comes with him does not know much about the patient's past medical history, but says he has been wretching and vomiting significantly prior to presenting to the emergency department. What is the most appropriate step?**

    A. He is most likely suffering from a Mallory–Weiss tear and just needs fluid replacement
    B. He requires upper GI endoscopy after resuscitation and high-dose proton pump inhibitors
    C. He needs urgent upper GI endoscopy as soon as possible
    D. He needs anti-emetics and fluid resuscitation
    E. He needs a sengstaken tube inserted urgently

32. **A 50-year-old woman has scleroderma, and is managed with a number of medications including amlodipine for Raynaud's phenomenon and omeprazole for reflux presumed to be related to oesophageal dysmotility. Although her symptoms have been well controlled for many months, for the past 4–6 weeks she has begun to suffer from increasing abdominal bloating with mild tenderness and worsening nausea. On examination, there is obvious peripheral calcinosis and mild abdominal distension. Haematology and biochemistry investigations are normal, but the barium swallow confirms severe oesophageal dysmotility. A hydrogen breath test is positive. Which of the following is the most appropriate treatment?**

    A. Metronidazole
    B. Ciprofloxacin
    C. Prednisolone
    D. Gluten-free diet
    E. Mesalazine

33. **A 46-year-old man who has vague epigastric pain which radiates to his back, worsening over the past few months, presents to the clinic with new symptoms of jaundice. He also has itching and is passing dark urine. On examination he looks thin, his BP is 134/72, his pulse is 74 and regular. He has epigastric tenderness on palpation of his abdomen. Investigations: haemoglobin 10.4 g/dl (13.5–17.7), white cell count 8.3 x 10⁹/l (4–11), platelets 191 x 10⁹/l (150–400), serum sodium 136 mmol/l(135–146), serum potassium 4.2 mmol/l(3.5–5), creatinine 112 micromol/l (79–118), alkaline phosphatase 292 U/l (39–117), bilirubin 210 micromol/l (<17), alalanine aminotransferase 83 U/l (5–40), ultrasound abdomen—mass in the head of pancreas. Which of the following is the most appropriate initial chemotherapy (the tumour is inoperable)?**

    A. 5-fluorouracil
    B. Gemcitabine
    C. Erlotinib
    D. Rituximab
    E. Etopiside

34. **A 60-year-old diabetic patient complains of frequent vomiting and weight loss. His symptoms started about three months ago. He denies any dysphagia or acid-reflux-type symptoms but does get bloating and early satiety. On clinical examination, there is no lymphadenopathy but you note that his vision is poor and that he has peripheral neuropathy. Which of the following is most likely to provide you with the diagnosis?**

   A. Barium swallow
   B. Barium meal
   C. OGD
   D. Abdominal ultrasound
   E. HbA1c

35. **Regarding risk factors for gastric cancer, which one of the following statements is not true?**

   A. *H. pylori* infection represents the strongest known environmental risk factor for gastric cancer
   B. Smoking increases risk of gastric cancer around 1.5-fold
   C. Truncating mutations of the E.-cadherin gene (*CDH1*) are detected in 50% of diffuse-type gastric cancers
   D. Previous gastric surgery is implicated as a risk factor for gastric cancer
   E. Type O blood group is associated with a small increase in risk of gastric cancer

36. **A 19-year-old man who is normally fit and well has had bloody diarrhoea for the past four days. He has been doing work experience at a daycare centre for children as part of his university nursery nursing course. Apparently some children within the centre have also been ill with diarrhoea. On examination his BP is 110/70, with a postural drop of 20 mmHg. He looks dehydrated and there is diffuse pain on abdominal palpation. Blood tests reveal mild hypokalaemia with a potassium of 3.0 mmol/l, and an elevated creatinine. Which is the following is the most likely diagnosis?**

   A. Salmonella
   B. Shigella
   C. Campylobacter
   D. *E. coli*
   E. Giardiasis

37. **A 63-year-old man presented with a short history of two weeks of abdominal pain, swelling, nausea, and vomiting. On examination, he was plethoric and had ascites and mild tender hepatomegaly. Initial investigations revealed a haemoglobin of 19.2 mg/l, but other results are not yet available. What condition would you suspect?**

    A. Amyloidosis
    B. Budd–Chiari syndrome
    C. Haemochromatosis
    D. Hydatid cyst
    E. Portal vein thrombosis

38. **A 46-year-old female with known coeliac disease has a series of blood tests performed as part of a routine outpatient appointment. Which one of the following laboratory findings is not consistent with her clinical history? (Normal ranges are given in square brackets.)**

    A. Hb 10.3 g/dl [13.0–17.0]
    B. PT 13.6 s [9–12]
    C. IgA 0.3 g/l [0.8–4.0]
    D. Ca^{2+} 2.98 mmol/l [2.2–2.65]
    E. PTH 102 ng/l [<65 ng/l]

39. **A 53-year-old man presents with haematemesis and on examination is found to have ankle swelling, ascites, and splenomegaly. He does not drink or smoke, and there is no family history of liver disease. His mother died of bronchial carcinoma and his father of respiratory failure secondary to emphysema—he was a smoker. What further blood tests would help to elucidate the cause of his liver pathology?**

    A. Alpha-fetoprotein
    B. Alpha-1-antitrypsin levels
    C. Autoantibodies
    D. Caeruloplasmin levels
    E. Ferritin

40. A 51-year-old man presented with arthritis, foul-smelling diarrhoea, abdominal pain, and weight loss of 15 kg over two years. A previous barium meal and follow-through and a colonoscopy showed no significant abnormality. Urinary 5HIAA was normal. On examination he was cachectic. There was no abdominal swelling but he had a pyrexia of 37.8°C. Haemoglobin was 10.5 g/dl, serum ferritin 20 ng/ml, and albumin 20 g/l. Routine urinalysis was negative. What is the likely cause for his illness?

A. Chronic pancreatitis

B. Coeliac disease

C. Lymphoma

D. Maltoma

E. Whipple's disease

41. Please read the following statements regarding serologic testing in coeliac disease and indicate which single answer is true.

A. The first step in pursuing a diagnosis of coeliac disease is a distal duodenal biopsy

B. IgA tissue transglutaminase (TTG) and IgA endomysial antibody (EMA) tests do not have equivalent diagnostic accuracy

C. The sensitivity of IgA tissue transglutaminase (TTG) and IgA endomysial antibody (EMA) tests is impaired in the presence of selective IgA deficiency

D. Antigliadin antibody (AGA) tests are still routinely recommended because of their high sensitivity and specificity

E. When serologic testing provides indeterminate results, HLA haplotyping for the DQ2 and/or DQ8 marker can be utilized due to their high positive predictive value in coeliac disease

42. A 47-year-old woman complaining of pruritus is found to have the following blood results: bilirubin 45 mmol/l, alkaline phosphatase 256 IU/l, GGT321 IU/l, anti-mitochondrial antibody positive. What is the most appropriate treatment for her?

A. Colchicine

B. Ursodeoxycholic acid

C. Chlorambucil

D. Ciclosporin

E. Prednisolone

43. Anti-*Saccharomyces cerevisiae* antibodies are most commonly found in:

A. Ulcerative colitis

B. Crohn's disease

C. Sarcoidosis

D. *C. difficile* colitis

E. Ischaemic colitis

44. **The risk of hepatocellular carcinoma is highest in liver cirrhosis due to:**
    A. Primary biliary cirrhosis
    B. Alcohol
    C. Hepatitis B
    D. Hepatitis C
    E. Autoimmune hepatitis

45. **A 41-year-old woman comes to the clinic for review of her coeliac disease. She tells you that she is compliant with her gluten-free diet and currently has no problems with diarrhoea. On examination her BMI is 23 and she looks well. When considering follow-up measures for her, which of the following is required?**
    A. DEXA scan should be performed at the menopause
    B. Yearly pneumococcus vaccination
    C. Calcium and vitamin D. supplementation
    D. Prophylactic penicillin
    E. Ferritin supplementation

46. **A 47-year-old woman presents with painless jaundice. She is a non-drinker and there is no family history of liver problems. At health screening one year previously, she was told that her liver enzymes were abnormal but since she felt well, she did not see her general practitioner, and she is taking no medication. Investigations revealed: haemoglobin 11.8 g/dl; urea and electrolytes normal; albumin 36 g/l; globulin 42 g/l; serum bilirubin 45 micromol/l; alkaline phosphatase 289 U/l; ALT 43 U/l; GGT 321 U/l. Liver ultrasound was normal. A diagnosis of primary biliary cirrhosis is suspected. What investigation is the best to confirm this?**
    A. Anti-nuclear factor
    B. Anti-mitochondrial antibodies
    C. Anti-Ro antibodies
    D. Anti-smooth muscle antibodies
    E. Anti-double-stranded DNA antibodies

47. **A 42-year-old man undergoes a Whipple's procedure for very early pancreatic carcinoma. He has recovered well from this major operation, but wants to know how the oncologists can monitor him for a recurrence of his disease. Which of the following is the best tumour marker to look for recurrence of pancreatic carcinoma?**
    A. Alpha-fetoprotein
    B. CA-125
    C. Carcino-embryonic antigen
    D. CA-19-9
    E. Beta-HCG

48. **A 24-year-old woman is referred for further investigation of weight loss and increasing pallor and fatigue. Physical examination followed by abdominal ultrasound reveals no abnormalities. The results of blood investigations are as follows: Hb 9.8 g/dl, MCV 80 fl, serum ferritin 4 micrograms/l (normal value 15–300 micrograms/l), and the serum folate 0.5 micrograms/l (normal value 2.0–12.0 micrograms/l) with normal B12. What is the most likely diagnosis?**

    A. Crohn's disease
    B. Coeliac disease
    C. Adenocarcinoma of the colon
    D. Haemolytic anaemia
    E. NSAIDS therapy

49. **A 51-year-old man with a history of ulcerative colitis comes to the clinic for review. Over the past few months he has had progressive symptoms of lethargy, nausea, and itching. His bowel disease has been relatively quiescent. Examination reveals scratch marks and right upper quadrant tenderness, and liver function testing is consistent with an obstructive picture. MRCP is suggestive of primary sclerosing cholangitis (PSC). When considering therapies for PSC, which of the following is?**

    A. Ursodeoxycholic acid is proven to impact on clinical progression
    B. Rituximab reduces increase in alkaline phosphatase over time
    C. No therapies are proven to impact on clinical progression
    D. High-dose corticosteroids are the initial therapy of choice
    E. Liver transplant is of no value

50. **A 62-year-old man presents to the oncology clinic with metastatic pancreatic carcinoma. He has decided to pay privately for erlotinib in combination with gemcitabine as he still feels relatively well and wants to give himself the possibility of a few months more survival. Which of the following correctly describes the mode action of erlotinib?**

    A. Tyrosine kinase inhibitor
    B. Serine protease inhibitor
    C. PDGFR inhibitor
    D. Serine kinase inhibitor
    E. Protease inhibitor

51. A 45-year-old man is being treated by his GP for dyspepsia. Despite a one-month course of a proton-pump inhibitor, he remains symptomatic and his GP suspects he may have *Helicobacter pylori* infection. Which one of the following statements is true?

A. The GP should send a blood sample for serological testing for IgG antibodies to *H. pylori*

B. Faecal urease testing, when performed in a community setting, carries a high positive predictive value

C. Carbon-13 urea breath testing is not suitable for primary care, because of exposure to ionizing radiation

D. *H. pylori* testing should not be offered in this situation, because of the low pre-test probability.

E. Carbon-13 urea breath testing represents a suitable test to confirm *H. pylori* eradication after antimicrobial therapy

52. Bile acid deficiency, such as that seen following terminal ileal resections, can be complicated by deficiencies of the fat-soluble vitamins. Which of the following is not a fat-soluble vitamin?

A. Vitamin A

B. Vitamin C

C. Vitamin D

D. Vitamin E

E. Vitamin K

53. Which of the following disorders is associated with a deficiency of one of the fat-soluble vitamins?

A. Anaemia

B. Cardiomyopathy

C. Encephalopathy

D. Night blindness

E. Peripheral neuropathy

54. Regarding carcinoid syndrome:

A. It is typically caused by a fast growing neuroendocrine tumour with liver metastases

B. The primary tumour is typically bronchial in origin

C. The most common clinical features are periodic facial flushing, diarrhoea, and wheezing

D. Twenty-four hour urinary 5-hydroxyindoleacetic acid (5-HIAA) assay is unaffected by diet

E. The five-year overall survival rate is around 5%

55. Regarding colorectal neoplasia:

A. Adenocarcinoma of the colon and rectum is the third commonest cause of cancer in the UK

B. Colonoscopy has been proven to improve mortality as the primary screening tool for a colorectal neoplasia

C. The liver condition, primary sclerosing cholangitis, is associated with an increased risk of colon cancer unless the patient has undergone a liver transplant

D. Hereditary non-polyposis colon cancer (HNPCC) is inherited as an autosomal recessive condition

E. Familial adenomatous polyposis (FAP) is due to a mutation in the mismatch repair genes

56. Regarding proton pump inhibitor (PPI) therapies:

A. They are all pro drugs requiring activation by the parietal cells in the stomach

B. They inhibit the parietal cells' ability to produce sulphuric acid

C. The drugs work topically and immediately when they come into contact with the parietal cells in the gastric lumen

D. Of all the drugs in the class, omeprazole seems to cause the fewest drug interactions

E. There appears to be no increase in the risk of *Clostridium difficile*-associated diarrhoea in users

57. Regarding upper GI cancer:

A. Increased body mass index is a recognized risk factor for oesophageal squamous carcinoma

B. At the present time, endoscopic ultrasound for oesophageal cancer is done to specifically judge the nodal stage for the TNM classification

C. Patients with widespread metastatic disease should not be undergoing radical surgical resection

D. Ulcerated gastric tumours can typically be cured with endoscopic mucosal resection

E. Cases are most effectively managed by a single consultant

58. Regarding non-alcoholic fatty liver disease (NAFLD):

A. It is the commonest cause of what is often termed cryptogenic cirrhosis

B. It is not a recognized cause of cirrhosis

C. It is usually associated with type 1 diabetes mellitus

D. It does not recur post orthotopic liver transplantation

E. It is decreasing in incidence in the Western world

59. A 67-year-old lady with poorly controlled COPD starts to complain of difficulties swallowing. She describes intense pain and retrosternal discomfort when consuming both liquids and solids. Her appetite is normal and weight is below normal but steady. She has been admitted to hospital several times in the last eight months with exacerbations of her respiratory disease. She no longer smokes and does not drink any alcohol. Her current medications include salbutamol, salmeterol, fluticasone, tiotropium, and Adcal-D3. She has recently had a course of nystatin. A chest X-ray demonstrates hyperexpansion of both lung fields and osteopenia. Which is the most likely cause of her symptoms?

    A. Oesophagitis
    B. Achalasia
    C. Pharyngeal pouch
    D. Oesophageal candidiasis
    E. Oesophageal cancer

60. A 46-year-old man with known chronic liver disease secondary to hepatitis B. presents with increasing abdominal distension, pain, and confusion. He has previously had a variceal bleed. A diagnostic ascitic tap confirms spontaneous bacterial peritonitis and he is started on ciprofloxacin. His abnormal blood tests reveal that the Hb is 11.2 g/l, WCC is 13.7 x 10⁹/l, bilirubin is 54 micromol/l, INR 1.5, sodium is 131 mmol/l, urea 9.2 mmol/l, and creatinine 138 micromol/l. Despite drainage of his ascitic fluid he continues to complain of abdominal pain. Which of the following is the most appropriate analgesic agent?

    A. Ibuprofen
    B. Paracetamol
    C. Codeine phosphate
    D. Morphine sulphate
    E. Diclofenac

61. A 61-year-old man gives a history of weight loss and lethargy. He is a smoker with a 40-pack-year history and drinks at least 18 pints of lager per week and some spirits. On examination he is cachetic and has jaundiced sclera. His liver function tests reveal the bilirubin is 78 mg/l, ALP 247 IU/l, ALT 72 IU/l, and AST 55 IU/l. His albumin is 28 g/l and INR 1.3. What is the most likely diagnosis?

    A. Alcoholic cirrhosis
    B. Pancreatic carcinoma
    C. Cholangiocarcinoma
    D. Gallstone disease
    E. Acute alcoholic hepatitis

62. **A 42-year-old man who has recently begun treatment for idiopathic epilepsy has come to the clinic complaining of severe epigastric pain and vomiting. On examination he has features consistent with acute pancreatitis, and this is confirmed with an amylase of 1800. Which of the following anti-epileptics is most likely to be associated with the development of pancreatitis?**

    A. Gabapentin
    B. Vigabatrin
    C. Topiramate
    D. Lamotrigine
    E. Sodium valproate

63. **A 45-year-old man returns from an assignment in Vietnam working for a mining company. He has diarrhoea which is difficult to flush away, passing up to eight motions per day. He also has abdominal bloating and pain, and says he has been losing kilograms in weight over the past few months. On examination his BMI is 20, his abdomen is distended but soft, he has bilateral pitting oedema. Investigations: potassium 3.4 mmol/l, albumin 24 g/l, 72-h faecal fat 9.2 g (normal <7.0), small bowel biopsy—villous atrophy with PAS positive macrophages. Which of the following is the most appropriate treatment?**

    A. Cotrimoxazole for 12 months
    B. Amoxycillin for six months
    C. Ciprofloxacin for three months
    D. Metronidazole for six months
    E. Co-trimoxazole for three months

64. **Which of the following statements regarding primary biliary cirrhosis (PBC) is true (select the single most appropriate response)?**

    A. Oesophageal varices are an uncommon complication
    B. Treatment with ursodeoxycholic acid is curative in some patients
    C. Treatment with immunosuppressive agents such as azathioprine has a proven survival advantage
    D. End stage liver disease does not occur
    E. Liver transplantation is curative in appropriately selected patients

65. **A 47-year-old man, with a 20-year history of alcohol excess, presents with sudden onset of jaundice. Clinically, he has stigmata of chronic liver disease, is febrile, and has a palpable, enlarged, tender liver. The patient has grade 2 encephalopathy. Blood tests are as follows: WCC 14 x 10⁹/l (neutrophils 13 x 10⁹/l), CRP 100 mg/l, bilirubin 120 micromol/l, AST 1200 IU/l, ALT 400 IU/l, PT 20 seconds, creatinine 170 micromol/l. Ultrasound of the liver reveals ascites, no evidence of biliary obstruction, normal hepatic/portal vessel blood flow, and no evidence of hepatic abscess. Ascitic tap results exclude spontaneous bacterial peritonitis. Urinalysis, serial blood cultures, and a chest radiograph are unremarkable. Which drug is proven to reduce short-term mortality in such a patient?**

   A. Lactulose
   B. Infliximab
   C. Pabrinex
   D. Rifaximin
   E. Prednisolone

66. **A 60-year-old Iranian patient presents with symptoms of difficulty swallowing which started 3–4 months ago. The symptoms are progressive and are worse with solids than liquids. He is a smoker, drinks alcohol as well as tea, which he says he likes piping hot. He has lost some weight in the last few months but he says he has been trying to lose weight for a few years. What is the most likely diagnosis?**

   A. Oesophageal squamous cell carcinoma
   B. Oesophageal adenocarcinoma
   C. Achalasia
   D. External oesophageal compression from lung cancer
   E. Severe oesophagitis

67. **A 50-year-old man with a history of alcohol abuse is referred by his GP for management of his ascites. He admits to still drinking 5–6 cans of strong lager per day. As part of his investigations, he undergoes an upper GI endoscopy that showed varices. He has never had any bleeding. How would you manage this patient?**

   A. Propranolol
   B. Variceal banding
   C. Repeat endoscopy in six months
   D. Repeat endoscopy in one year
   E. Terlipressin

68. **A 60-year-old man presents with intermittent dysphagia and unintentional weight loss. He also complains of intermittent chest pain. On further questioning, he tells you he has been having difficulty in belching, and also has been getting trouble with food regurgitation, especially at nights. He undergoes an upper GI endoscopy which is normal. His blood tests are all normal—these include full blood count, liver function tests, and renal function. What is the most likely diagnosis?**

    A. Oesophageal carcinoma
    B. Gastroesophageal reflux disease
    C. Achalasia
    D. Barrett's oesophagus
    E. Cardiac disease

69. **A 40-year-old woman presents to you complaining of hot flushes, watery diarrhoea, and crampy abdominal pain. On clinical examination you notice that she has a pansystolic murmur and a raised JVP. The initial blood tests done by her GP included full blood count, renal function, and thyroid function, and were all normal. What is the most likely diagnosis?**

    A. Tropical sprue
    B. Coeliac disease
    C. Crohn's disease
    D. Carcinoid syndrome
    E. Pancreatic insufficiency

70. **A 56-year-old Irish woman presents to the gastroenterology clinic for investigation of intermittent diarrhoea, abdominal pain, and cramps. She has tried to have a gluten-free diet as much as possible given that she has a strong family history of coeliac disease, including her sister, mother, and aunt. Her symptoms have improved greatly on this diet but she would now like formal confirmation that she has coeliac disease. How would you manage this lady?**

    A. Referral to dietitian for further education of which foods contain gluten
    B. OGD and jejunal biopsies as soon as possible
    C. Send off anti-TTG antibody levels in the clinic
    D. Advise her to start eating normal bread for 4–6 weeks prior to investigations
    E. Empirically give a two-week course of antibiotics for small bowel bacterial overgrowth

71. **A 50-year-old man presents to your clinic with a 3–4-month history of diarrhoea, with pale, foul-smelling stools that float easily on water. He denies any past medical history or recent foreign travel. On further questioning he says he has been drinking 2–3 bottles of wine in the evening for many years. Clinical examination is normal. Full blood count and renal function are normal. Which of the following is most likely to provide you with the diagnosis?**

    A. Stool culture
    B. Stool microscopy
    C. Faecal elastase
    D. Trial of cholestyramine
    E. Serum amylase

72. **A 45-year-old man presents to the A&E department with a lower respiratory tract infection. You note on his blood tests that his bilirubin is 40. Apart from a raised WCC and CRP the rest of his bloods are normal. He denies any past medical history or abdominal pain. His systemic enquiry is normal. Which one of the following will give you the diagnosis?**

    A. Abdominal USS
    B. ERCP
    C. Hepatitic viral serology
    D. Autoimmune antibodies
    E. None of the above

73. **Which of the following is NOT a cause of abdominal ascites? Select the single most appropriate response.**

    A. Isolated portal vein thrombosis
    B. Cardiac failure
    C. Chronic liver disease due to alcohol
    D. Budd–Chiari syndrome
    E. Meig's syndrome

74. **Considering the hepatorenal syndrome (HRS), which of the following statements is accurate?**

    A. HRS is usually due to volume depletion
    B. HRS is due to parenchymal renal disease
    C. HRS usually occurs in patients with early cirrhosis
    D. HRS can often be corrected by intravenous fluid administration
    E. The pathophysiology of HRS is related to splanchnic vasodilatation

75. **A 73-year-old lady is admitted with rigors. On examination her pulse is 124 sinus rhythm and blood pressure 100/60 mmHg. Her chest radiograph is clear. She has some diffuse abdominal tenderness and absent bowel sounds. A plain abdominal radiograph shows gas in the biliary tree. What is the likely cause of her illness?**

   A. Acute pancreatitis
   B. Ascending cholangitis
   C. Cholecysto-duodenal fistula
   D. Cholecystitis
   E. Systemic candidiasis

76. **A 50-year-old man presents to the clinic for investigation of ascites. He also complains of lethargy and, on direct questioning, he tells you he has joint aches and pains. His past medical history includes diabetes. He drinks about 10 units of alcohol per week and has smoked 20 cigarettes per day since the age of 15. His ferritin is raised at 1200. Which ONE of the following tests will be diagnostic for this patient's condition?**

   A. HFE gene testing
   B. Transferrin/saturation
   C. Liver biopsy
   D. MRI scan
   E. Liver ultrasound

77. **A 45-year-old man is referred by his GP with deranged liver function tests. He has a history of diabetes controlled with insulin and reports a number of episodes of admission to hospital with abdominal pain. On inspection there is evidence of malnutrition, Dupytren's contracture of the right hand, and gynaecomastia. The liver is palpable 3 cm below the costal margin. He has an unsteady wide-based gait. His blood tests show that his bilirubin is 21 micromol/l, AST 96 IU/l, ALT 44 IU/l, and ALP 35 IU/l. His ferritin is 400 micrograms/l with a C.-reactive protein of 25 and serum caeruloplasmin is 20 mg/dl. What is the most likely diagnosis?**

   A. Alcoholic liver disease
   B. Wilson's disease
   C. Haemochromatosis
   D. Autoimmune polyglandular syndrome
   E. Metastatic hepatocellular carcinoma

78. **A 39-year-old woman presents with generalized itching and fatigue. She also reports having dry eyes and a dry mouth. Examination reveals widespread scratch marks. On testing her Hb is 11.2 g/dl, WCC is 6.7 x 10⁹/l, Plts are 387 x 10⁹/l. Her renal function is normal and her liver function tests show her bilirubin is 24 micromol/l, ALT is 37 IU/l, AST is 40 IU/l and ALP 208 IU/l. Which autoantibody is most likely to be positive?**

    A. Anti-scl-70
    B. Anti-centromere
    C. Anti-mitochondrial
    D. Anti-liver kidney microsomal
    E. Anti-smooth muscle

79. **A 32-year-old woman with a previous history of intravenous drug abuse presents with abnormal liver function tests. She denies any high risk exposures for over six years. Her viral hepatitis screen reveals the following results: hepatitis B surface antigen (HBsAg) = negative; hepatitis B surface antibody (anti-HBs) = positive; hepatitis B anti-core IgM (anti-HBc IgM) = negative; hepatitis B anti-core (anti-HBc IgG) = positive; hepatitis C antibody = positive; hepatitis C RNA = detected. What is the most appropriate interpretation of these serological results?**

    A. Chronic hepatitis B infection, chronic hepatitis C infection
    B. Acute hepatitis B infection, chronic hepatitis C infection
    C. Previous hepatitis B vaccination, acute hepatitis C infection
    D. Previous hepatitis B infection, chronic hepatitis C infection
    E. Chronic hepatitis B infection, acute hepatitis C infection

80. **A 54-year-old man with a history of ulcerative colitis for the past 15 years comes to the clinic complaining of increasing tiredness, lethargy, night sweats, and itchiness over the past few months. He has no symptoms of diarrhoea, his bowel motions have been stable over recent times. He takes regular mesalazine. On examination his BP is 135/72, his pulse is 83 and regular. His BMI is 22. There are some scratch marks on his skin and he has vague right upper quadrant tenderness. Investigations: haemoglobin 12.6 g/dl (13.5–17.7), white cell count 8.1 x 10⁹/l (4–11), platelets 197 x 10⁹/l (150–400), serum sodium 136 mmol/l (135–146), serum potassium 4.4 mmol/l (3.5–5), creatinine 93 micromol/l (79–118), alkaline phosphatase 343 U/l (39–117), alanine aminotransferase 110 U/l (5–40), ANCA positive. Which of the following is the most likely diagnosis?**

    A. Autoimmune hepatitis
    B. Primary sclerosing cholangitis
    C. Primary biliary cirrhosis
    D. Cholangiocarcinoma
    E. Hepatocellular carcinoma

81. **A 41-year-old woman presents with fatigue, joint pains, and mild itching which have increased over the past 18 months. There is also a history of gradual weight loss. On examination her BP is 138/88, her pulse is 74 and regular, and her BMI is 27. She has a two-finger-breadth liver edge. Investigations: haemoglobin 10.5 g/dl (11.5–16.5), white cell count 9.1 x 10⁹/l (4–11), platelets 142 x 10⁹/l (150–400), serum sodium 136 mmol/l (135–146), serum potassium 4.1 mmol/l (3.5–5), creatinine 90 micromol/l (79–118), alanine aminotransferase 377 U/l (5–40), alkaline phosphatase 145 U/l (39–117), anti-smooth muscle antibody positive. Which of the following is the most likely diagnosis?**

    A. Autoimmune hepatitis type 1
    B. Autoimmune hepatitis type 2
    C. Primary sclerosing cholangitis
    D. Primary biliary cirrhosis
    E. Non-alcoholic steatohepatitis

82. **All of the following statements regarding autoimmune hepatitis are true, except:**

    A. Progression to cirrhosis is more common in type 2 than in type 1 autoimmune hepatitis
    B. Females are more commonly affected than males
    C. A homogeneous pattern of anti-nuclear antibody staining is seen in type 1 autoimmune hepatitis
    D. Anti-liver-kidney microsomal antibodies are found in type 2 autoimmune hepatitis
    E. Type 1 autoimmune hepatitis typically affects elderly or immunosuppressed individuals

83. **A 35-year-old former user of intravenous drugs requests testing for bloodborne viruses. HIV and hepatitis C viral serology is negative, but the laboratory reports a positive hepatitis B test, with following additional information: hepatitis B surface antigen (HBsAg): detected; hepatitis B E antigen (HBeAg): not detected; anti-E antigen (anti-HBe): detected; liver function tests are all within normal range. Which of the following is the most appropriate next step?**

    A. Reassure; these tests are compatible with viral clearance
    B. Arrange measurement of hepatitis B viral DNA load
    C. Offer hepatitis B. immune globulin (HBIg)
    D. Arrange liver biopsy to guide treatment planning
    E. Offer treatment with antiviral agents

84. **Which one of the following statements about hereditary haemochromatosis is correct?**

    A. Inheritance of mutant HFE is autosomal dominant
    B. The HFE C282Y mutation accounts for over 80% of cases among persons of northern European descent
    C. Inheritance of mutant HFE is X-linked recessive
    D. The HFE gene product promotes renal iron excretion
    E. Transferrin saturation greater than 60% in women is highly specific

85. **Which of the following statements regarding primary biliary cirrhosis (PBC) is true (select the single most appropriate response)?**

    A. Clinical onset is usually within the first four decades of life
    B. It is more common in men
    C. Anti-mitochondrial antibody (AMA) in not diagnostically useful
    D. Pruritis is a common symptom
    E. Associated fatigue is easily treated

86. **A man presents to his GP complaining of intermittent bouts of loose stool over the past year. He has no previous history of any gastroenterological problems. Which of the following features would be least compatible with a diagnosis of irritable bowel syndrome?**

    A. Passage of more than five loose stools/day
    B. Passage of mucus
    C. Temporary relief of abdominal pain upon defecation
    D. Abdominal distension
    E. Patient age over 60

87. **A 27-year-old student gives a history of nine days of bloody diarrhoea which has gradually been worsening. He reports that he is currently opening his bowels six times per day with blood in each motion. Three weeks ago he returned from a four-week holiday in India. Whilst abroad he ate food from a number of street vendors. He denies any dietary indiscretion since his return. On examination his temperature is 37.9°C and there is generalized abdominal tenderness, most marked in the left lower quadrant. Of the following, which is the most likely infectious agent?**

    A. *Campylobacter jejuni*
    B. *Bacillus cereus*
    C. *Giardia duodenalis*
    D. *Entamoeba histolytica*
    E. *Salmonella enteritidis*

88. **Regarding *Clostridium difficile* (*C. difficile*), which of the following statements is not correct?**

   A. The bacterium may be detected in the bowel flora of 15% of the adult population
   B. Widespread use of broad spectrum antibiotics is associated with increased risk of *C. difficile*-associated diarrhoea
   C. Clinical diagnosis is based upon enzyme-linked immunoabsorbent assay (ELISA) for *C. difficile* toxin A or B
   D. Disease recurrence after successful treatment of *C. difficile*-associated diarrhoea can occur in 10–25% of patients
   E. Intravenous metronidazole may be used to treat *C. difficile*-associated diarrhoea when the oral route in not suitable

89. **A 28-year-old woman is seen on the post-take ward round. She has been admitted following several days of vomiting without haematemesis. She has mild abdominal discomfort. This is her third episode of this type in the past 12 months. After each episode (usually lasting approximately three days) she has returned to normal health. Her past medical history is unremarkable. This condition may be associated with all of the following except?**

   A. Metabolic acidosis
   B. Family history of migraine
   C. Chronic cannabis use
   D. Onset during menstrual period
   E. Food allergy

90. **A 26-year-old woman has a five-year history of constipation. Colonic transit studies reveal slow transit, and lower GI endoscopy was unremarkable. Multiple laxative remedies have failed to improve her symptoms, and she is opening her bowels once per week. Which of the following would be most appropriate at this stage?**

   A. Pelvic floor exercises
   B. Prucalopride
   C. Dietetian referral
   D. SSRI anti-depressant
   E. Surgical referral

91. **A 28-year-old woman is seen on the post-take ward round. She has been admitted following several days of vomiting without haematemesis. She has mild abdominal discomfort. This is her third episode of this type in the past 12 months. After each episode (usually lasting approximately three days) she has returned to normal health. Her past medical history is unremarkable except for social use of cannabis. What is the likely diagnosis?**

    A. Cannabis toxicity
    B. Duodenal ulcer
    C. Gastric ulcer
    D. Cyclical vomiting syndrome
    E. Anorexia nervosa

92. **A 46-year-old woman sees you because of diarrhoea. This has been occurring for several months. She describes passing four to six loose, watery motions throughout the day and occasionally at night, sometimes accompanied by feelings of bloating. She has not noticed rectal bleeding and her weight has been stable. She has diet-controlled diabetes, and had a cholecystectomy for gallstone disease six months ago. What is the most appropriate inverstigation?**

    A. Thyroid function test
    B. Barium enema
    C. Small bowel barium meal
    D. Faecal elastase
    E. Selenium-homocholic acid taurine (SeHCAT) test

93. **A 32-year-old man with known ulcerative colitis is admitted to hospital. He has experienced five days of bloody diarrhoea (seven stools per day). He is normally treated with mesalazine 800 mg TDS and azathioprine 150 mg OD. Which one of the following statements concerning azathioprine is most accurate?**

    A. Belongs to the category of calcineurin inhibitor drugs
    B. Has a rapid onset of therapeutic effect in inflammatory bowel disease
    C. Is metabolized to mercaptopurine in vivo
    D. Is metabolized predominantly by the enzyme folylpolyglutamyl synthase
    E. Belongs to US FDA pregnancy category X

94. **A 34-year-old woman with terminal ileal and colonic Crohn's disease is reviewed in clinic. She has been managed with azathioprine 125 mg OD for the past 12 months. Prior to this she required a course of oral prednisolone to achieve remission. At review she complains of loose stool and abdominal discomfort. Her CRP is elevated at 64 mg/dl. A subsequent computed tomography scan of the abdomen and pelvis reveals some thickening of the distal ileum, but no abdominal or pelvic collection. Colonoscopy reveals patchy ulceration with intervening areas of normal mucosa. You are now considering escalating her treatment to infliximab. Which of the following statements regarding infliximab is true?**

A. It is a fully human monoclonal antibody
B. It is a first-line treatment in inflammatory bowel disease
C. It has excellent oral bioavailability
D. It is administered as a subcutaneous injection
E. It is a monoclonal antibody against tumour necrosis factor alpha

95. **A 61-year-old man comes to the joint oncology/surgery clinic for review. He has a 5 mm oesophageal adenocarcinoma identified on a recent endoscopy performed for worsening symptoms of indigestion against a background of chronic reflux. Workup has demonstrated no evidence of local lymph node involvement or distant metastases. He has a good functional status and works full time as a builder. Which of the following is the correct management of his disease?**

A. Progress immediately to oesophagectomy
B. Plan cisplatin-based chemotherapy pre and postoesophagectomy
C. Plan cisplatin-based chemotherapy post oesophagectomy
D. Plan cisplatin-based chemotherapy and radiotherapy post oesophagectomy
E. Arrange for him to be stented when symptoms of obstruction become severe

96. **You are asked to see a 74-year-old woman who has been admitted from a nursing home to the elderly care ward with a urinary tract infection. Unfortunately she has developed profuse watery diarrhoea and C. *difficile* toxin testing is positive. Which of the following antibiotics is most likely to have been responsible?**

A. Trimethoprim
B. Ciprofloxacin
C. Amoxicillin
D. Co-amoxiclav
E. Cephalexin

97. **A 72-year-old woman is admitted to the emergency department following an upper GI haemorrhage. According to her husband she has filled the toilet with fresh blood. She has been started on diclofenac some 10 days earlier after a left knee arthroscopy. There is a past history of treated cardiac failure. Her BP is 95/60 on admission and her pulse is 95 and regular. Investigations reveal an Hb of 9.8 g/dL (was 12.0 at pre-admission clinic), and a urea of 12.2. What is her Blatchford score?**

   A. Between 0 and 3
   B. Between 3 and 6
   C. Between 6 and 9
   D. Between 9 and 12
   E. >12

98. **A 28-year-old woman who is 33 weeks pregnant presents to the emergency department with jaundiced sclerae. She admits to increasing itchiness over the past 3–4 weeks and says that her stools have become increasingly pale. Her bilirubin is measured at 65 micromol/L, AST is 200 IU/L, alkaline phosphatase is 280 IU/L. Which of the following is the treatment of choice?**

   A. Ursodeoxycholic acid
   B. Prednisolone
   C. Low molecular weight heparin
   D. Urgent delivery
   E. Azathioprine

99. **A 42-year-old man is referred to the gastroenterology clinic with a diagnosis of genotype 1 hepatitis C after presenting for blood donation. On further questioning he admits to using intravenous drugs on three occasions whilst a student. Blood workup is normal apart from an ALT of 180. Liver biopsy reveals evidence of inflammation and early fibrosis. Which of the following is the most appropriate treatment for him?**

   A. Boceprevir
   B. Peginterferon alpha-2a and ribavirin
   C. Peginterferon alpha-2a and boceprevir
   D. Peginterferon alpha-2a, ribavirin and boceprevir
   E. Peginterferon alpha-2a and amantadine

100. **A 29-year-old man with known ulcerative pan-colitis is admitted to hospital. He has experienced five days of bloody diarrhoea (seven stools per day). He is normally treated with mesalazine 800 mg TDS. On examination he is slightly pale, pulse 85/min. His initial blood tests reveal a CRP of 86, and a Hb of 10.2. Which is the most appropriate strategy?**

    A. Admit, oral ciprofloxacin 500 mg BD, OD
    B. Admit, oral prednisolone 40 mg OD
    C. Admit, IV hydrocortisone 100 mg BD
    D. Admit, IV hydrocortisone 100 mg QDS
    E. Admit, await immediate surgical review

101. **You are asked to review a 21-year-old woman with a history of anorexia nervosa who has recently begun feeding. The nurses are concerned as she has developed worsening lethargy, muscle weakness, and shortness of breath. She is hypotensive with a BP of 95/60 and a pulse of 95. Correction of serum levels of which of the following would have (in all likelihood) avoided this problem?**

    A. Sodium
    B. Potassium
    C. Calcium
    D. Phosphate
    E. Sulphate

102. **Prucalopride is a new drug treatment licensed for treatment of women with chronic constipation. What is the correct mechanism of action?**

    A. 5HT3 receptor agonist
    B. H2 receptor agonist
    C. 5HT4 receptor agonist
    D. Bile acid sequestration
    E. Osmotic laxative effect

103. **A 62-year-old man is seen in clinic because of intermittent small-volume rectal bleeding, and a feeling of urgency to pass stool. He has not experienced diarrhoea or weight loss. His past history includes hypertension, eczema, and pelvic radiotherapy for prostatic carcinoma one year ago. Physical examination including rectal exam are normal. Initial investigations reveal Hb 12.8g/dL, CRP <5. What is the most likely diagnosis?**

    A. Rectal carcinoma
    B. Inflammatory bowel disease
    C. Lymphocytic colitis
    D. Radiation proctitis
    E. Bile acid malabsorption

104. **A 17-year-old woman is referred to outpaients because of lethargy. On further questioning she admits to intermittent, moderately severe central and right-sided abdominal pain over the past 12 months. She also describes some weight loss, which she is unable to quantify further. She has not experienced night sweats, diarrhoea, or rectal bleeding. Physical examination reveals her to be slim but is otherwise unremarkable. Early investigations reveal: Hb 11.2 g/dL, MCV 82fl, Plts 284, and WCC 6.8. Renal function and electrolytes are normal. Choose the most appropriate initial test:**

    A. Pancreatic function testing
    B. Upper GI endoscopy with duodenal biopsies
    C. Barium enema
    D. Faecal calprotectin
    E. Trial of antispasmodic medication

105. **A 63-year-old woman is admitted to hospital complaining of diarrhoea and a rash. She has undergone a small bowel resection some six months earlier for ischaemic bowel and is now receiving parenteral nutrition. Other past history of note is type 1 diabetes managed with insulin. On examination she is afebrile, and hypertensive with a BP of 180/80, pulse is 85 and regular. Her abdomen is soft, and there is a widespread crusting rash affecting her upper body and limbs. Investigations reveal an Hb of 11.0g/dL (11.5–16.0), and an MCV of 79 fl (80–96). What is the most likely diagnosis?**

    A. Amyloidosis
    B. Coeliac disease
    C. Pellagra
    D. Small bowel lymphoma
    E. Zinc deficiency

1. C. Smoking status is the most well-characterized environmental factor associated with disease susceptibility and outcome

Smoking is the most well-established and replicated environmental factor implicated in Crohn's disease. Current smoking increases the chance of disease onset. Furthermore, it increases the disease severity and reduces the likelihood of successful pharmacological therapy. In addition, the chances of post-operative relapse of disease are far higher in smokers. Patients with colonic Crohn's disease do indeed have an increased risk of colorectal cancer. The risk is related to disease extent, duration of disease, activity (macro and microscopic inflammatory score), family history of colorectal cancer, presence of primary sclerosing cholangitis, presence of pseudopolyps, and presence of colonic strictures. Post-operative recurrence leads to re-operation in around 50% of patients at five years. Crohn's disease is a multigenic disorder with environmental modulating factors. Numerous genes, each conferring a small individual susceptibility, have been identified to confer increased risk of disease susceptibility. The *NOD2* gene, the first Crohn's susceptibility gene to be identified, increases the risk of ileal Crohn's disease, but the absolute risk is small and many carriers of the mutant gene do not develop disease. Perianal Crohn's disease is a complex disease phenotype often requiring a multi-disciplinary approach to management and initial steps include draining active sepsis and antibiotic therapy. Seton emplacement and diverting colostomy are often useful as adjunctive therapies. Medical options include traditional immunosuppressants and biological anti-TNF alpha therapies. The latter two medications should only be started after active sepsis has been drained.

Vavricka SR, Rogler G, Recent advances in the etiology and treatment of Crohn's disease, *Minerva Gastroenterologica e Dietologica* 2010;56(2):203–211.

2. B. Serum ferritin levels of 351 mcg/l accompanied by fasting transferrin saturation of 58%

High transferrin saturation provides the earliest evidence of haemochromatosis. A value greater than 60% in men and 50% in women is highly specific. Elevated ferritin is also suggestive, but since ferritin is an acute phase protein, it can be elevated in a variety of other conditions.

Duchini A, Haemochromatosis, *Medscape*. http://emedicine.medscape.com/article/177216-overview

3. C. Chondrocalcinosis may be visible on X-ray films

Although a recognized complication, cardiac failure due to dilated cardiomyopathy is rare. Population screening is not recommended for this condition. Venesection can control symptoms, prevent complications, and lead to improvement in liver histology. Chondrocalcinosis is a recognized result of haemochromatosis.

Duchini A, Haemochromatosis, *Medscape*. http://emedicine.medscape.com/article/177216-overview

4. B. Vitamin B12

The distal 100 cm of the ileum is the only region of the small bowel where vitamin B12-intrinsic factor complex is absorbed. The bulk of nutrient absorption takes place in the first 150 cm of the small bowel in the region of the duodenum and proximal jejunum. The length of the small bowel in adults ranges from 365 to 600 cm. The duodenum is the site where calcium, magnesium, iron, and folate are preferentially absorbed.

Steger GG et al., Folate absorption in Crohn's disease, *Digestion* 1994;55:234–238.

5. D. High levels of gastrin can lead to peptic ulcers

Gastrin is a hormone that regulates the production of acid in the stomach. It is produced by G cells in the stomach. Gastrin in turn stimulates parietal cells to produce stomach acid. As stomach and intestinal acidity rises, gastrin production normally decreases. G-cell hyperplasia and Zollinger–Ellison (ZE) syndrome can cause an over-production of gastrin and stomach acid. These conditions can lead to peptic ulcers that can be difficult to treat. Greater than normal levels may indicate: use of antacids or other acid-suppressive medications (PPIs), chronic atrophic gastritis, massive small bowel resection, or renal failure. Gastrinomas are neuroendocrine tumours, usually located in the pancreas.

Campana D et al., Zollinger–Ellison syndrome. Diagnosis and therapy, *Minerva Medica Jun* 2005;96(3):187–206.

6. E. Maintenance therapy with azathioprine should be continued during pregnancy if recurrent relapse is likely

Active disease poses the greatest risk to the pregnancy, therefore maintenance therapy with 5 ASA or azathioprine can be safely continued, especially if recurrent relapse is expected. Flares can be safely treated with steroids or 5 ASA if necessary.

Carter MJ et al., Guidelines for the management of inflammatory bowel disease in adults, *Gut* 2004;53(Suppl V):v1–v16. http://www.bsg.org.uk/images/stories/docs/clinical/guidelines/ibd/ibd.pdf

7. C. Having explained the risks, plan for autologous transfusion

Jehovah's witness patients are against any sort of blood products. However, most will consent to an autologous transfusion, in which their own blood is taken and stored, and their body given time to replace that blood. Then, during the operation, if they need transfusion, they will receive their own blood. Because this is a planned operation, an autologous transfusion is the best option. Obviously, in the emergency setting this option is not viable. If the patient refused an autologous transfusion, then giving the maximum dose of iron infusion is an option. Explaining the risks of bleeding and documentation is a must anyway. The boyfriend does not have any legal powers to consent for the patient. It is unethical to ask a relative to put pressure on the patient just because we do not agree with them.

Vanderlinde ES et al., Autologous transfusion, *British Medical Journal* 2002;324:772.

8. B. Two-fold increase

Acromegaly is recognized to be associated with increased risk of colonic polyps and subsequent colon cancer, but the precise increased risk has not been quantified. Most guidelines recommend initial colonoscopy by age 40, and then every five years thereafter. Large cohort studies put the increased risk at 2–3 times that of controls.

Bloom S et al., *Oxford Handbook of Gastroenterology and Hepatology*, Second Edition, Oxford University Press, 2011, Section 3, An A to Z, Acromegaly and GI tract.

9. D. Crohn's disease

Abdominal cramps, weight loss, erythema nodosum, and raised inflammatory markers are highly suggestive of inflammatory bowel disease. Right iliac fossa tenderness points to the possibility of terminal ileal disease and hence Crohn's disease is the most likely diagnosis. Diarrhoea is not always a prominent symptom of Crohn's disease. His ethnic origin and the BCG scar goes against the diagnosis of intestinal tuberculosis.

Longmore M et al., *Oxford Handbook of Clinical Medicine*, Eighth Edition, Oxford University Press, 2010, Chapter 6, Gastroenterology, Crohn's disease.

10. B. Epithelioid granulomata

Granulomata are the key distinguishing histopathological hall mark of CD. The others are all common features of UC.

Carter MJ et al., Guidelines for the management of inflammatory bowel disease in adults, *Gut* 2004;53(Suppl V):v1–v16. http://www.bsg.org.uk/images/stories/docs/clinical/guidelines/ibd/ibd.pdf

11. B. Rectal mesalazine suppository

The European Crohn's and Colitis Organisation (ECCO) guidelines (2008) make it clear that the treatment of choice in mild or moderately active proctitis is rectal mesalazine in suppository form. This formulation is better tolerated than enemas. The combination of oral and rectal preparations is effective, but suppositories alone are better than oral 5 ASA alone. The other therapies are not supported by evidence in this setting and rectal mesalazine is the preferred answer.

Stange EF et al., European evidence-based Consensus on the diagnosis and management of ulcerative colitis: definitions and diagnosis, *Journal of Crohn's & Colitis* 2008;2:1–23. http://www.ecco-ibd.eu/images/stories/docs/guidelines/2007_uc_definitions_diagnosis.pdf

12. B. *C282Y/C282Y* homozygote

C282Y homozygotes account for 82–90% of clinical diagnoses of hereditary haemochromatosis among persons of northern European descent.

Duchini A, Haemochromatosis, *Medscape*. http://emedicine.medscape.com/article/177216-overview

13. C. Symmetrical polyarthropathy is a recognized feature

Population screening is not recommended for this condition. Venesection can control symptoms and prevent complications, but is not curative. The condition is autosomal recessive.

Duchini A, Haemochromatosis, *Medscape*. http://emedicine.medscape.com/article/177216-overview

14. E. Lifelong therapy with a chelating agent such as penicillamine is required

Excessive deposition of copper occurs in the liver and brain. Although Kayser–Fleischer rings are a useful diagnostic sign, they are no longer considered diagnostic of Wilson's disease in isolation (the sign must be accompanied by neurological manifestations). Although children usually present with liver disease, young adults most commonly present due to neuropsychiatric features. The condition is autosomal recessive.

Gilroy RK, Wilson disease, *Medscape*. http://emedicine.medscape.com/article/183456-overview

15. D. Alcoholic hepatitis

The raised transaminases, bilirubin, and clinical setting are most consistent with a diagnosis of alcoholic hepatitis. In fact, the combination of raised WCC, urea, and deranged clotting render this severe enough for corticosteroid therapy to be considered. There is no radiological evidence to support portal vein thrombosis, and no hallucinations or sensory disturbance to support delirium tremens. Alcoholic hepatitis is more accurate in this setting than the diagnosis of decompensated liver disease.

AASLD guidelines, Alcoholic liver disease. http://www.aasld.org/practiceguidelines/Documents/ Bookmarked%20Practice%20Guidelines/AlcoholicLiverDisease1-2010.pdf

16. A. Ulcerative colitis is typically characterized by diffuse mucosal inflammation limited to the colon

Ulcerative colitis is typified by bloody diarrhoea, and is associated with an increased risk of colonic carcinoma. In contrast to Crohn's disease, it is not typically associated with abdominal pain and weight loss, and is not a transmural condition; therefore fistulation is not a feature.

Carter MJ et al., Guidelines for the management of inflammatory bowel disease in adults, *Gut* 2004;53(Suppl V):v1–v16. http://www.bsg.org.uk/images/stories/docs/clinical/guidelines/ibd/ibd.pdf

17. B. Initiate diuretic therapy with spironolactone 100 g/day

Spironolactone (an aldosterone antagonist) is the first-line therapy in ascites due to cirrhosis (initial dose 100 mg/day, increased according to response). Furosemide (a loop diuretic) can be added as an adjunct if spironolactone alone is ineffective. Intravenous colloid treatment is usually only needed when renal impairment occurs in the setting of ascites due to cirrhosis. Fluid restriction is no longer recommended.

Moore KP, Aithal GP, BSG 2005 guideline—management of acsites in cirrhosis. http://www.bsg.org.uk/ images/stories/docs/clinical/guidelines/liver/ascites_cirrhosis.pdf

18. E. Microscopic colitis

The macroscopic appearance of this woman's flexible sigmoidoscopy makes ulcerative colitis extremely unlikely. Equally, the normal bloods make both coeliac and Crohn's disease unlikely. The age of the patient, use of NSAIDs, and presence of stool leucocytes (found in 50%) fit with a diagnosis of microscopic colitis. Biopsy may reveal an increase in T cells, plasma cells, and macrophages. A range of treatments including metronidazole, bismuth, 5-ASA compounds, and corticosteroids have been tried for the condition. In this case it would be optimal to withdraw her non-steroidals if possible.

Bloom S et al., *Oxford Handbook of Gastroenterology and Hepatology*, Second Edition, Oxford University Press, 2011, Section 3, An A to Z, Microscopic colitis.

19. A. Gluten should be strictly avoided for life

A gluten-free diet (GFD) is defined as one that excludes wheat, rye, and barley. Even small amounts of gluten may be harmful, so these grains should be totally avoided for life in coeliac patients. There is some debate about the safety of oats for coeliac patients: the general consensus is that they are probably safe, but in practical terms their inclusion in a GFD is problematic because of potential contamination with gluten during processing. Serologic testing may take some time to normalize (up to one year), but persistently abnormal serology beyond this stage should prompt concerns over adherence to a gluten-free diet.

NIH Consensus Development Conference on Celiac Disease, National Institutes of Health, Consensus Development Conference Statement, June 28–30, 2004. http://consensus.nih.gov/2004/ 2004CeliacDisease118html.htm

20. B. Genotype 5 has a response rate of 38–50% to anti-viral therapy

Treatment of genotypes 1, 4, 5, and 6 requires 48 weeks of pegylated interferon and ribavirin and leads to sustained viral response rates of 38–50%. Treatment of genotypes 2 and 3 requires 24 weeks of pegylated interferon and ribavirin and leads to sustained viral response rates of 75–80%. A minimum of a 100-fold drop in viral load is required to continue treatment beyond 12 weeks. Repeat courses of treatment are not recommended in patients who have not responded to the first course of treatment.

Bloom S et al., *Oxford Handbook of Gastroenterology and Hepatology*, Second Edition, Oxford University Press, 2011, Section 3, An A to Z, Hepatitis C.

21. B. The absolute lifetime risk of progression to oesophageal adenocarcinoma is around 3 to 5%

The incidence of Barrett's oesophagus is rising and is now present in 2% of the Western population. However, the lifetime risk of progression to adenocarcinoma is small at around 3–5%. Factors associated with the disease progression include male sex, white ethnicity, length of the Barrett's segment, poor diet, obesity, and smoking. Endoscopic surveillance for dysplasia in Barrett's oesophagus has never been proven in a randomized control to improve mortality and, furthermore, the cost-effectiveness of such programmes is controversial. Effective treatment of reflux disease eliminates symptoms and heals oesophagitis in gastro-oesophageal reflux disease. At the present time, either long-term proton pump inhibitor therapy or a Nissen fundoplication appear to be equivalent options for symptom control in the longer term. It should be highlighted that neither of these options have been proven to reduce the risk of progression to oesophageal adenocarcinoma.

Watson A et al., Guidelines for the diagnosis and management of Barrett's columnar-lined oesophagus, British Society of Gastroenterology. http://www.bsg.org.uk/pdf_word_docs/Barretts_Oes.pdf

22. D. ELISA is used to detect elastase in a single stool sample

Levels of faecal elastase less than 50 mcg/g of stool are diagnostic of the condition; levels less than 200 mcg/g may occur in watery diarrhoea due to another underlying cause. The test is monoclonal antibody and ELISA-based and can be conducted on a single stool sample. It has a sensitivity/specificity >90% for pancreatic exocrine insufficiency. Measurement is not affected by use of pancreatic supplements.

Bloom S et al., *Oxford Handbook of Gastroenterology and Hepatology*, Second Edition, Oxford University Press, 2011, Section 2, Clinical practice and diagnostics, Blood tests and special investigations.

23. A. Biliary stenting

Given this patient's history of inflammatory bowel disease, and the presence of a mass on ultrasound, the most likely diagnosis is of cholangiocarcinoma. Only 10–15% of patients have a resectable tumour, and for the remainder, stenting is the best possible option for relieving hepatic obstruction. With respect to chemotherapy, gemcitabine has an impact in some cases. CA19-9 is elevated in 85% of cases and may therefore be useful as a tumour marker for some patients. It is likely that this tumour is the end result of a prolonged course of primary sclerosing cholangitis, which occurs with greatly increased frequency in this population.

Bloom S et al., *Oxford Handbook of Gastroenterology and Hepatology*, Second Edition, Oxford University Press, 2011, Section 3, An A to Z, Cholangiocarcinoma.

24. B. A patient who has lost 1000 ml of blood may be normotensive

Variceal haemorrhage is frequently associated with large volume blood loss, often in the context of coagulopathy. As a consequence, it carries a high mortality and therefore swift recognition and treatment is key. Haemodynamic compensation may be sufficient to maintain a normal blood pressure (particularly in younger patients) despite large volume blood loss (see further reading). Evidence of tachycardia should therefore be taken seriously. Beware also the beta-blocked patient (frequently propranolol is used for secondary prevention of variceal bleeding) as tachycardia may be masked. Such patients require aggressive resuscitation and optimization prior to proceeding to endoscopic evaluation and treatment. Vasopressin analogues such as terlipressin have been shown to improve survival and should therefore be given prior to endoscopy in patients with suspected variceal bleeding. Likewise, antibiotics should be administered prior to endoscopic intervention as studies have shown proven survival benefit. The incidence of aspiration is high in such patients, hence the requirement for empirical antibiotics. Current evidence suggests that endoscopic band ligation of varices is superior, compared to sclerotherapy, in terms of re-bleeding and mortality. In patients with variceal bleeding not controlled by endoscopy, balloon tamponade is frequently used as a temporary measure prior to proceeding to further endoscopic intervention, surgical intervention, or the insertion of a transjugular intrahepatic portosystemic shunt (TIPSS). Coagulopathy is frequently encountered in this situation and should be corrected; it is however not a contraindication to TIPSS.

Baskett PJF, ABC of major trauma: management of hypovolaemic shock, *British Medical Journal* 1990;300:1453–1457.

25. A. Diagnosis: Mallory–Weiss tear

This patient presents with upper GI bleeding. Since the initial description in 1996, the Rockall score has been used to help assess the need for urgent endoscopy and to stratify the risk of re-bleeding after this initial endoscopy (see Table 3.1). An initial score is based upon the patient's age, comorbidities, and degree of haemodynamic compromise at presentation. Higher scores correspond to increasing risk and the more urgent need for informing the gastroenterology and/ or surgical teams. After a definitive endoscopic diagnosis, additional information is used to generate the complete score, which is informative for re-bleed and mortality rates.

All the features listed (age of 75, pulse rate of 100, and ischaemic heart disease) will score this particular patient points: in this case his total initial score would be 4 or 5, depending upon the systolic BP at presentation, which we are not told. This would support the need for an urgent endoscopy after appropriate resuscitation. Indeed, in Rockall's original report, this predicted a 25–40% mortality

Table 3.1 Rockall score

Rockall Score				
	Score			
Variable:	**0**	**1**	**2**	**3**
Age (years)	<60	60–79	>/= 80	
Shock	No shock BP < 100 HR > 100	Tachycardia Syst BP > 100 HR > 100	Hypotension Syst BP < 100	
Comorbidity	Nil major		Cardiac failure, IHD	Renal failure, disseminated malignancy
Post-endoscopy:				
Diagnosis	Mallory—Weiss tear, no lesion, no stigmata	All other diagnoses	Upper GI malignancy	
Major Stigmata	None, or dark spots		Blood in upper GI tract, clot, visible vessel	

Reproduced from Bloom S et al., *Oxford Handbook of Gastroenterology and Hepatology*, Second Edition, 2011 with permission from Oxford University Press; Data from *Gut*, 38, Rockall TA et al., 1996, 'Risk assessment after acute upper gastrointestinal haemorrhage'.

rate. However, an endoscopic diagnosis of a Mallory–Weiss tear would not add any points, leaving his complete Rockall score unchanged, with an associated mortality rate of around 5–10%.

Bloom S, Webster G, *Oxford Handbook of Gastroenterology and Hepatology*, Second Edition, Oxford University Press, 2011, Section 5, Emergencies: Acute upper gastrointestinal bleeding.

26. E. Chromosome 19

The clinical picture here is consistent with Peutz–Jegher's syndrome, which is caused by a mutation on chromosome 19 because of a germline mutation of a serine-threonine kinase gene. There is a high risk of GI bleeding, and cancer occurs in 90% by the age of 65 years. Risk of colon cancer is 40%, with similar rates seen for gastric and pancreatic cancers. Breast, uterine, and testicular cancers also occur with increased frequency.

Bloom S, Webster G, *Oxford Handbook of Gastroenterology*, Oxford University Press, 2006, Chapter 3, An A to Z of gastroenterology and hepatology: Peutz–Jeghers syndrome.

27. C. Cholangiocarcinoma

The most likely diagnosis here is cholangiocarcinoma. Cancer of the tail of the pancreas should not cause jaundice as it will not cause obstruction of the biliary drainage. Cancer in the head of pancreas will cause jaundice; however, patients almost always complain of a boring pain which is the result of invasion of the coeliac plexus. Up to 50% of patients with cholangiocarcinoma do not experience pain. The diagnosis is with CT or MRI and ERCP is useful for tissue diagnosis. The five-year survival is very poor, in the region of 5%. Acute pancreatitis and gallstones are most acute, cause pain, and do not fit with the weight loss. Hepatocellular carcinoma does not usually present with jaundice.

Longmore M et al., *Oxford Handbook of Clinical Medicine*, Eighth Edition, Oxford University Press, 2010, Chapter 6, Gastroenterology, Liver tumours.

28. A. MRCP

This patient is suffering from primary sclerosing cholangitis. It is a condition in which the medium and large bile ducts (both intra and extra-hepatic) undergo inflammation and fibrosis, resulting in structuring. This leads to a characteristic multi-focal structuring and dilatation of the biliary tree, showing as the 'beading' sign in MRCP and ERCP. The resulting obstruction of biliary flow results in a cholestatic picture in the liver function tests with raised alkaline phosphatase and bilirubin. PSC has a much higher prevalence in patients with ulcerative colitis. The first choice study here should be MRCP because it can be diagnostic, and it can potentially avoid an invasive procedure for the patient. ERCP is too invasive as first line and nowadays MRCP should be performed first. CT abdomen is not of high enough resolution to clearly show the beading pattern of the bile ducts. Colonoscopy will only provide information regarding the activity of the ulcerative colitis and would not be helpful in the diagnosis of the patient's deranged LFTs and symptoms. Abdominal ultrasound is not of high enough resolution to clearly show the beading pattern of the bile ducts.

Longmore M et al., *Oxford Handbook of Clinical Medicine*, Eighth Edition, Oxford University Press, 2010, Chapter 6, Gastroenterology, Primary biliary cirrhosis, Primary sclerosing cholangitis.

29. D. Bile salt malabsorption

All of the diseases listed can be associated with chronic diarrhoea. Recurrence of Crohn's disease so soon after surgery would be unlikely, and the absence of abdominal pain makes this less likely. Chronic pancreatitis is characterized by recurrent disabling bouts of abdominal pain. Risk factors include chronic alcohol excess (at higher levels than described here), recurrent gallstone pancreatitis, and autoimmune pancreatitis. The associated diarrhoea is usually malodorous steatorrhoea. Diagnosis is based upon pancreatic imaging (typically CT pancreas) and pancreatic enzymatic assays (faecal elastase). Non-invasive testing of exocrine pancreatic function may be performed using the Fluorescein dilaurate test, based upon the ability of pancreatic enzymes to cleave a fatty acid to release a fluorescein molecule which is renally excreted and can readily be detected. Intestinal lymphangiectasia leads to protein-losing enteropathy and diarrhoea secondary to malabsoprtion due to defective bowel lymphatic drainage. Peripheral oedema is usually present, reflecting impaired lymphatic draining outside the gut. Primary forms present in childhood with diarrhoea and growth retardation, whilst secondary causes presenting in adulthood include infiltrative diseases of the bowel lymphatics, including malignancy, lymphoma, sarcoidosis, and mesenteric tuberculosis. Irritable bowel syndrome represents chronic, recurrent abdominal pain or discomfort associated with altered bowel habit in the absence of structural gastrointestinal abnormalities to account for these symptoms. The diagnostic criteria have been refined in a series of international symposia meeting in Rome ('The Rome Criteria'); Rome III, the most recent definitions from 2006, define irritable bowel syndrome as: Recurrent abdominal pain or discomfort at least three days a month in the past three months, associated with two or more of the following: improvement with defecation; onset associated with a change in frequency of stool; onset associated with a change in form (appearance) of stool. Criteria should be fulfilled for the past three months, with symptom onset at least six months before diagnosis. Other well recognized features in irritable bowel syndrome include the passage of mucus with stool, and the sensation of abdominal bloating or visible distension (more common in women than men). Symptoms may be made worse by eating. The presence of nocturnal symptoms, the recent onset, and the significant medical history make a diagnosis of irritable bowel syndrome less likely in this case. Bile salt malabsorption is an under-recognized cause of chronic diarrhoea. Under normal physiology, bile acids are largely reabsorbed in the distal ileum. Following terminal ileal resection, as in this patient, or post-cholecystectomy, increased levels of bile acid may enter the colon, leading to colonic irritation and diarrhoea. Accepted techniques for detection of bile salt malabsorption include quantification of retained bile salts, following ingestion of synthetic radiolabelled bile salts, in the 75Se-HCAT test. Poor retention of radiolabel suggests bile salt malabsorption. As in this case, symptoms are often worse after eating, and relieved by fasting. Treatment is with bile acid sequestrants, such as cholestyramine.

Thomas PD et al., British Society of Gastroenterology Guidelines for the investigation of chronic diarrhoea, *Gut* 2003;52(Suppl V):v1–v15. http://www.bsg.org.uk/images/stories/docs/clinical/guidelines/sbn/cd_body.pdf

30. B. Infection at young age

Although progression to cirrhosis in chronic hepatitis C typically takes at least two decades, rates of progression are higher in those infected at an older age, as well as in all the other groups above. After infection with hepatitis C virus, between 15–45% of individuals will clear the virus, with undetectable viral RNA levels upon repeat testing. However, the remainder of infected individuals will continue to have detectable viral RNA. In these individuals with chronic viral carriage, 5–20% will progress to develop cirrhosis, typically over 25–30 years. Progression to cirrhosis occurs more frequently in males, those infected at an older age, those who consume in excess of 50 grams of alcohol/day (approx. 6 UK units), those with obesity of hepatic steatosis, and those with HIV co-infection. Of those patients who do develop hepatitis C-related cirrhosis, approximately 30% will progress to end-stage liver disease over the following decade. There is also a 1–3% chance per year of developing hepatocellular carcinoma. Successful treatment for chronic hepatitis C viral infection reduces the risk of these complications.

AALSD practice guidelines, Diagnosis, management, and treatment of hepatitis C: an update. http://www.aasld.org/practiceguidelines/Documents/Hepatitis%20C%20UPDATE.pdf

31. B. He requires upper GI endoscopy after resuscitation and high-dose proton pump inhibitors

The most likely diagnosis in this patient is Mallory–Weiss tear after repeated vomiting. However, we do not know much about his past medical history and he could well have been a heavy alcohol drinker for years and have cirrhosis and oesophageal varices which are now bleeding. The other differential is that he has a stomach or duodenal ulcer that is bleeding. His observations suggest that he is in hypovolaemic shock with hypotension and tachycardia. The most important and urgent treatment for him is fluid resuscitation to correct his hypovolaemic shock. You cannot be certain that this is only a Mallory–Weiss tear, and even if it is, it may need active treatment. Hence he actually needs an OGD. Upper GI endoscopy after resuscitation is the most appropriate option. He should be treated with high-dose PPI. This has been shown to reduce mortality. Urgent OGD in the setting of a patient with hypovolaemic shock can be detrimental. It is more important to fluid resuscitate this patient first. His history does not suggest that his bleeding is so profuse that he needs a sengstaken tube which is usually used when patients have profuse variceal bleeding unable to wait for urgent OGD after fluid resuscitation.

Longmore M et al., *Oxford Handbook of Clinical Medicine*, Eighth Edition, Oxford University Press, 2010, Chapter 6, Gastroenterology, Upper gastrointestinal bleeding.

32. A. Metronidazole

Bacterial overgrowth syndrome occurs either where there is abnormal gut anatomy such as post abdominal surgery or where there is gut dysmotility, for instance due to systemic sclerosis. Patients complain of symptoms of abdominal bloating, nausea/indigestion, and intermittent diarrhoea. Metronidazole is the initial treatment of choice, although antibiotics may actually be rotated over a period of a few months. In this scenario, the recent change in symptoms on a background of stable symptom control imply that the new symptoms are due to bacterial overgrowth.

Bloom S et al., *Oxford Handbook of Gastroenterology and Hepatology*, Second Edition, Oxford University Press, 2011, Section 3, An A to Z of gastroenterology and hepatology, Bacterial overgrowth.

33. B. Gemcitabine

NICE guidance suggests that gemcitabine should be first-line palliative therapy where pancreatic carcinoma is associated with reasonable functional status. Combinations with capcitabine/platinum-based agents may be associated with prolongation of survival, although increased toxcity often means there is little additional advantage overall. Erlotinib may offer benefit in some patients, although it is not recommended by NICE as the additional survival benefit gained was only an average ten days overall. For the future, vaccine-based antigenic modulation may offer further survival advantage.

Nice guidelines [TA25], Guidance on the use of gemcitabine for the treatment of pancreatic cancer. http://guidance.nice.org.uk/TA25

34. B. Barium meal

This patient is suffering from gastroparesis. Generally, in diabetics, it takes ten years of poorly controlled diabetes before symptoms develop. It is due to autonomic neuropathy. Other causes of gastroparesis include Parkinson's disease, scleroderma, and medication such as opiates. A barium meal is most likely to show delayed gastric emptying from the list provided. X-rays are taken at various times, showing delayed gastric emptying. Still better, but not provided as an option here, is gastric emptying studies using radioactive isotopes. None of the other options provided here will give any suggestion of delayed gastric emptying, which is required for diagnosis of gastroparesis. An OGD may show food in the stomach despite several hours of fasting, giving suggestion of gastroparesis, but barium meal is far superior.

Colledge NR et al., *Davidson's Principles and Practice of Medicine,* Twenty-first Edition, Churchill Livingstone Elsevier, Dysphagia, p. 876.

35. E. Type O blood group is associated with a small increase in risk of gastric cancer

Type O blood group is NOT associated with a small increase in risk of gastric cancer. Epidemiological studies have shown an increased prevalence of blood type A in patients with gastric cancer. Although rates of gastric cancer have declined sharply in the Western world in recent decades, it remains the second most common cause of cancer-related death worldwide, with the highest incidence in Asia and South America. In common with most common diseases, gastric cancer risks appear to be multi-factorial, involving both inherited predisposition and environmental factors. Chronic bacterial infection with *H. pylori* is the strongest known environmental risk factor. In particular, *H. pylori* infection is associated with chronic atrophic gastritis. Prolonged gastritis is associated with a six-fold increased risk of developing gastric cancer, particularly tumours of the gastric antrum and fundus. Smoking increases the risk of gastric cancer in a dose-dependent manner, by around 1.5-fold. Approximately 10% of cases of gastric cancer show a familial pattern. Most genetic factors remain poorly understood, but certain specific mutations have been identified. Of these, the best recognized are truncating mutations of the E-cadherin gene (*CDH1*), which have been detected in 50% of the subset of gastric cancers with a diffuse-type histology. Previous surgery is implicated as a risk factor from epidemiological data. This may be related to pH changes following previous surgery, increasing the risk of metaplasia. Epidemiological studies have shown an increased prevalence of blood type A in patients with gastric cancer. Numerous other epidemiological associations have been demonstrated. A diet rich in pickled vegetables, salted fish, and smoked meats is associated with an increased risk of gastric cancer. Pernicious anaemia, presumably through predisposition to chronic atrophic gastritis, also increases risk, as does obesity and prior exposure to ionizing radiation.

Guidelines for the management of oesophageal and gastric cancer. http://www.bsg.org.uk/pdf_word_docs/ogcancer.pdf

36. B. Shigella

Shigellosis causes a dysentery-type picture with severe bloody diarrhoea with mucus. It is highly infectious, and outbreaks are relatively common in children's daycare centres. Giardiasis tends to result in an irritable bowel-type picture with diarrhoea, abdominal bloating, and increased bowel gas. *Staphylococcus aureus* food poisoning is associated with toxin ingestion and leads to vomiting a few hours after it is eaten. *Salmonella* and *campylobacter* are associated with diarrhoea and vomiting and occur most commonly after ingestion of contaminated meat or diary products.

Longmore M et al., *Oxford Handbook of Clinical Medicine,* Eighth Edition, Oxford University Press, 2010, Chapter 9, Infectious diseases, Bacillary dysentery.

37. B. Budd–Chiari syndrome

Budd–Chiari syndrome is a type of venous outflow obstruction caused by occlusion of the hepatic veins. The liver becomes engorged resulting in portal hypertension and ascites. The stretching of the liver capsule gives tender hepatomegaly. No cause may be found in 50% of patients, but it may be due to compression of the hepatic veins by tumour or thrombosis due to a hypercoagulability state secondary to polycythaemia or the oral contraceptive pill.

Bloom S et al., *Oxford Handbook of Gastroenterology and Hepatology,* Second Edition, Oxford University Press, 2011, Section 3, An A to Z, Budd–Chiari syndrome (BCS).

38. D. Ca^{2+} 2.98 mmol/l [2.2–2.65]

Coeliac disease is associated with electrolyte deficiencies and malabsorption, leading to hypokalaemia, hypocalcaemia, and hypomagnesaemia. Hypoalbuminaemia, hypoproteinaemia, and hypocholesterolaemia may also be present. Coeliac disease is an inflammatory disease characterized by a T-cell response to the gluten-derived peptide gliadin. Inflammation within the small bowel leads to loss of intestinal villi and resulting malabsorption. Most of the laboratory abnormalities seen can be understood in terms of failure to absorb vitamins, minerals, and nutrients. Anaemia is a relatively common finding, that typically reflects iron deficiency due to failure of iron absorption in the proximal small bowel. Folate malabsorption is also common. In more severe disease, ileal inflammation will lead to vitamin B12 deficiency. Prothrombin time prolongation reflects malabsorption of the fat-soluble vitamin K. Selective IgA deficiency is present in approximately 1% of the general population. Clinical manifestations range from no symptoms to recurrent infections and autoimmunity. IgA is normally secreted into the gut lumen and plays a role in host defence against enteric pathogens. IgA anti-endomysial and anti-tissue transglutaminase antibodies are sensitive and specific for coeliac disease and reflect mucosal damage. When testing for the presence of these antibodies, it is important to check total IgA levels, since individuals with coeliac disease but selective IgA deficiency will have a false negative result. Furthermore, the incidence of selective IgA deficiency in coeliac disease appears to be higher than the general population (perhaps as high as 8%). Metabolic bone disease is common in coeliac disease with osteopenia and osteoporosis reflecting malabsorption of dietary calcium, phosphate, and vitamin D. Therefore hypocalcaemia and secondary hyperparathyroidism are sometimes seen. Hypercalcaemia is not a feature of coeliac disease, and should prompt a search for an underlying diagnosis, which should always start with measurement of a paired parathyroid hormone.

NICE guideline [CG86], Coeliac disease: recognition and assessment, Issue date: May 2009. http://www.nice.org.uk/CG86

39. B. Alpha-1-antitrypsin levels

A deficiency of alpha-1-antitrypsin may be associated with liver disease and emphysema. The deficiency is inherited as autosomal dominant and the enzyme inhibits neutrophil elastase, a proteolytic enzyme capable of destroying alveolar wall connective tissue. Such deficiency may progress to cirrhosis in 10–15% of patients. About 2% of patients with emphysema have the enzyme deficiency.

Bloom S et al., *Oxford Handbook of Gastroenterology and Hepatology*, Second Edition, Oxford University Press, 2011, Section 3, An A to Z, Alpha-1-antitrypsin deficiency.

40. E. Whipple's disease

This rare condition, caused by an actinobacterium, *Tropheryma whipplei*, may affect any organ but most commonly affects the gastro-intestinal system with consequent malaise, weight loss, diarrhoea, and arthralgia. The arthritis is migratory, predominantly affecting peripheral joints. Jejunal biopsy with the characteristic histological picture is the easiest way to make a diagnosis. Treatment with antibiotics is recommended although treatment may need to be continued for a year.

Bloom S et al., *Oxford Handbook of Gastroenterology and Hepatology*, Second Edition, Oxford University Press, 2011, Section 3, An A to Z, Whipple's disease.

41. C. The sensitivity of IgA tissue transglutaminase (TTG) and IgA endomysial antibody (EMA) tests is impaired in the presence of selective IgA deficiency

The first step in investigation is almost never an invasive investigation such as a gastrointestinal endoscopy (which is required to obtain a distal duodenal biopsy). After basic steps such as history and examination, the initial diagnostic test of choice is a serologic test such as that for IgA tissue transglutaminase (TTG) and IgA endomysial antibody (EMA). Both tests have approximately the same diagnostic accuracy, and have largely superseded the less sensitive and specific antigliadin antibody (AGA) test. However, these investigations must be used with caution as their sensitivity is impaired in the presence of selective IgA deficiency. It is good practice to check IgA levels at the same time as requesting either of these serological tests to reduce the likelihood of a false negative result. Greater than 97% of coeliac disease patients are positive for the DQ2 and/or DQ8 marker, compared to approximately 40% of unaffected individuals. Therefore, an individual negative for DQ2 or DQ8 is extremely unlikely to have coeliac disease (the tests have high negative predictive value).

NIH Consensus Development Conference on Celiac Disease, National Institutes of Health, Consensus Development Conference Statement, June 28–30, 2004. http://consensus.nih.gov/2004/2004CeliacDisease118PDF.pdf

42. B. Ursodeoxycholic acid

The blood investigations are entirely compatible with a diagnosis of primary biliary cirrhosis. Treatment with ursodeoxycholic acid (13–15 mg/kg/day) is the treatment of choice. It may improve biochemistry and delay progression to cirrhosis.

Warrell DA et al., *Oxford Textbook of Medicine*, Fifth Edition, Oxford University Press, 2010, Section 15.21.3, Primary biliary cirrhosis. http://www.otm.oxfordmedicine.com/cgi/content/full/med-9780199204854-chapter-152103

43. B. Crohn's disease

Antibodies to the budding yeast Saccharomyces cerevisiae are common in patients with Crohn's disease. They are also found less frequently in those with ulcerative colitis. Anti-neutrophil cytoplasmic antibodies are more common in ulcerative colitis.

Baumgart DC, Sandborn WJ, Inflammatory bowel disease: clinical aspects and established and evolving therapies, *Lancet* 2007;369:9573, 1641.

44. D. Hepatitis C

The risk of HCC is highest in cirrhosis due to hepatitis C, followed by haemochromatosis. Other risk factors include cirrhosis with associated alcohol abuse or NASH, coinfection with multiple viruses, aflatoxin exposure, and type 2 diabetes. Screening for HCC is a key component of management of cirrhosis.

Schuppan D, Afdhal NH, Liver cirrhosis, *Lancet* 2008;371:9615, 838.

45. A. DEXA scan should be performed at the menopause

Considerations for patients with coeliac disease include hyposplenism, possible increased risk of osteoporosis, and anaemia due to low levels of ferritin (most common), folate, and less commonly B12. With respect to osteoporosis risk, DEXA scan should be considered at the point of diagnosis, at the menopause for women, at the age of 55 for men, and earlier if an osteoporotic fragility fracture occurs. Hyposplenism dictates vaccination against *Haemophilus influenzae B*, influenza, and pneumococcus, but not routine prophylactic antibiotics. If there is poor compliance with diet and significant anaemia, then dietary supplementation of B vitamins and iron may be required.

NICE guidelines: Coeliac disease: recognition, assessment and management, NICE guidelines [NG20]. Published date: September 2015.

Osteoporosis: assessing the risk of fragility fracture, NICE guidelines [CG146]. Published date: August 2012.

46. B. Anti-mitochondrial antibodies

Anti-mitochondrial antibodies are positive in primary biliary cirrhosis. Anti-double-stranded DNA antibodies are seen in lupus and anti-Ro antibodies in Sjogren's syndrome.

Warrell DA et al., *Oxford Textbook of Medicine*, Fifth Edition, Oxford University Press, 2010, Section 15.21.3, Primary biliary cirrhosis.

47. D. CA-19-9

CA 19-9 testing is designed to detect a monosialoganglioside found in patients with gastrointestinal adenocarcinoma. It is found in 20–40% of patients with colonic or gastric adenocarcinoma. With respect to pancreatic carcinoma it is present in 70–90% of cases, and is more likely to be present where the cancer is of the excretory ductal type. Clearly, if the original tumour was positive for CA 19-9, then it is possible to use the test for monitoring for tumour recurrence.

Hernandez JM et al., CA 19-9 Velocity predicts disease-free survival and overall survival after pancreatectomy of curative intent, *Journal of Gastrointestinal Surgery* 2009;13:349–353. http://www.springerlink.com/content/p3558rgq635g64p6/

48. B. Coeliac disease

The combination of iron deficiency anaemia and reduced serum folic acid levels indicate impaired absorption in the upper small intestine and malabsorption syndrome. An FBC count may reveal microcytic anaemia due to iron deficiency or macrocytic anaemia due to folate malabsorption. Sometimes the picture is dimorphic. Coeliac disease is a common cause of malabsorption caused by inflammation of the mucosal lining of the upper small intestine and results from gluten ingestion in genetically susceptible individuals. It is now estimated that coeliac disease may affect 1 in 200 individuals. Endomysial antibodies are closely associated with gluten-sensitive disease, and in an appropriate clinical setting coeliac disease can be diagnosed with 100% specificity. Vitamin B12 is absorbed in the terminal ilium and therefore is more a feature of Crohn's disease. In haemolytic anaemia the folate levels are also low and iron overload due to RBC disintegration is expected. NSAIDS use and large bowel malignancy are often associated with iron loss but serum folate levels are not particularly altered.

Green PH, Jabri B, Coeliac disease, *Lancet* 2003;362(9381):383–391.

49. C. No therapies are proven to impact on clinical progression

As yet no medical therapies have been seen to significantly impact on the progression of primary sclerosing cholangitis (PSC). Studies have included the use of a number of agents including corticosteroids and ursodeoxycholic acid. Only ursodeoxycholic acid has been shown to impact on changes in liver function tests, although this was not correlated with an improvement in clinical status. Other therapies including anti-B-cell agents such as rituximab are undergoing clinical trials. Cholangiocarcinoma develops with increased frequency in patients with PSC, one case series putting the rate at 7% over an 11-year period of follow-up. Liver transplant is successful in managing end-stage PSC, with five-year survival rates at 75–80%.

Chen W, Gluud C, Bile acids for primary sclerosing cholangitis, *Cochrane Database of Systematic Reviews* 2003;(2):CD003626. http://www.ncbi.nlm.nih.gov/pubmed/12804480?dopt=Abstract

50. A. Tyrosine kinase inhibitor

Erlotinib is a tyrosine kinase inhibitor, which inhibits intracellular phosphorylation of the EGFR type 1 receptor. The major indication for erlotinib is in the treatment of non-small cell lung cancer, although it is also associated with a very modest improvement in survival in pancreatic carcinoma. This improvement in survival has not been deemed large enough for many healthcare providers to pay for it as part of standard therapy, however. In respect of NICE, it is only currently recommended as second-line therapy for the treatment of non-small cell lung cancer.

Moore et al., Erlotinib plus gemcitabine compare with gemcitabine alone in patients with adavnced pancreatic cancer, *Journal of Clinical Oncology* 2007;25:1960–1966.

51. E. Carbon-13 urea breath testing represents a suitable test to confirm *H. pylori* eradication after antimicrobial therapy

Testing for *H. pylori* after eradication therapy has been given should be done using carbon-13 urea breath testing. *H. pylori* is a curved, Gram-negative rod found in the upper gastrointestinal tract of more than 50% of the world's population. Most infections occur in childhood, with risk factors including low socio-economic status, crowded living conditions and lack of access to clean water. Infection with *H. pylori* is associated with chronic gastritis, which is thought to explain the positive association with gastric and duodenal ulceration, gastric lymphomas, and gastric adenocarcinoma. This question tests knowledge of testing methods for *H. pylori*. Gold standard tests all involve endoscopy and collection of gastric mucosal biopsies. Culture of this material for *H. pylori* requires special techniques and is rarely necessary. Histological identification of characteristic organisms requires additional input from a histopathologist and incurs diagnostic delay, but can provide useful additional information regarding the presence of gastritis or metaplastic changes. Tests for the presence of the urease enzyme, produced by Helicobacter depend upon colorimetric detection of pH changes in the presence of urea. Various commercial urease detection kits are available, including several that provide rapid detection within 30–60 minutes; these may give false negative results in patients on acid-suppressing medications, particularly proton pump inhibitors. Serological tests are available for *H. pylori* but suffer from a low specificity which lessens their diagnostic utility in primary care. Testing for IgG will remain positive, even after eradication therapy has been successful. Two non-invasive tests are widely used and suitable for primary care. Faecal testing for *H. pylori* antigens in the stool depends upon ELISA. Sensitivity and specificity are both high; however, there are conflicting data regarding the reliability of the test after successful eradication therapy, with high rates of both false negatives and false positives reported. Carbon-13 urea breath testing involves ingestion of urea labelled with carbon-13. Bacterial urease, if present, liberates tagged CO_2, which can readily be detected in breath samples within 10–15 minutes. The test has a high sensitivity and specificity, and has been validated for use after eradication therapy has been completed. Importantly, since carbon-13 is a stable isotope, there is no exposure of the patient to ionizing radiation; the carbon-13 is detected by mass spectrometry.

Nice guidelines [CG17]. Dyspepsia: managing dyspepsia in adults in primary care, August 2004. http://www.nice.org.uk/guidance/CG17

52. B. Vitamin C

The fat-soluble vitamins are vitamins A, D, E, and K. Inflammatory bowel disease such as Crohn's, cystic fibrosis, pancreatic insufficiency, and coeliac diseasse can also lead to fat and hence fat-soluble vitamin malabsorption, as can drugs which bind bile acids such as cholestyramine. Vitamin A deficiency results in night blindness, complete blindness, and xerophthalmia; vitamin D deficiency in osteomalacia (in adults) and rickets (in children); vitamin E in neuromuscular symptoms, visual symptoms, and haemolysis (although clinical deficiency is rare), and vitamin K deficiency in coagulopathy.

Warrell DA et al., *Oxford Textbook of Medicine*, Fifth Edition, Oxford University Press, 2010, Section 11.2, Vitamins and trace elements.

53. D. Night blindness

This question requires knowledge of which vitamins are fat soluble, namely A, D, E, and K. Night blindness is caused by vitamin A deficiency. The other answers are all associated with deficiencies of the B vitamins, with anaemia and neurological disorders resulting from B12 deficiency, peripheral neuropathy from pyridoxine (vitamin B6) deficiency, and thiamine deficiency leading to cardiomyopathy and encephalopathy in the form of Wernicke–Korsakoff syndrome.

Warrell DA et al., *Oxford Textbook of Medicine*, Fifth Edition, Oxford University Press, 2010, Section 11.2, Vitamins and trace elements.

54. C. The most common clinical features are periodic facial flushing, diarrhoea, and wheezing

Carcinoid syndrome is typically caused by a slow-growing gastrointestinal primary neuroendocrine tumour with liver metastases. The symptoms are due to vasoactive substances entering the systemic circulation (escaping first-pass metabolism) and typically facial flushing, diarrhoea, and wheezing may be seen. 5-Hydroxytryptamine (serotonin) is metabolized to 5-HIAA, which undergoes urinary excretion. False positives can be caused by tyramine intake and certain foods are best avoided during the 24-hour collection period. Despite having metastatic disease, patients often do well for long periods with a combination of interferon alpha therapy, somatostatin analogues, chemotherapy, radiolabelled therapy, and surgery. Indeed the five-year survival rate can be up to 50%.

Detterbeck FC, Management of carcinoid tumors, *Annals of Thoracic Surgery* 2010;89(3):998–1005.

55. A. Adenocarcinoma of the colon and rectum is the third commonest cause of cancer in the UK

Adenocarcinoma of the colon is the second commonest cause of cancer death in the UK and the third commonest UK cancer with an incidence of 30 to 50 per hundred thousand of the UK population. The only screening tests that have been proven to reduce the mortality from colorectal cancer are faecal occult blood testing and flexible sigmoidoscopy. Although widely employed, colonoscopy has never been proven in a randomized controlled manner to reduce mortality. The inflammatory, fibrotic condition of the biliary tree, primary sclerosing cholangitis increases the risk of colon cancer. The risk appears to persist in those who undergo a liver transplantation and surveillance strategies should thus be continued. HNPCC is an autosomal dominant condition from a mutation in the mismatch repair gene. It accounts for around 3.5% of all colorectal cancers and is associated with an increased risk of proximal colonic adenocarcinoma (often with synchronous and metachronous carcinomas) in the fourth decade. Extra colonic neoplasms are also common. The diagnostic criteria in clinical use include the Amsterdam and Bethesda scores. FAP is an autosomal dominant condition associated with a mutation in the APC tumour suppressor gene. It accounts for under 1% of all cases of colon cancer. Polyps develop from teenage years onwards and there is an inevitable progression to colonic cancer. Prophylactic colectomy and ileoanal pouch formation is the treatment of choice before the age of 20. Duodenal adenomas are frequently found and surveillance upper GI endoscopy recommended.

MacKay GJ et al., *Oxford Specialist Handbook in Colorectal Surgery*, Oxford University Press, 2010, pp. 285–335.

56. A. They are all pro drugs requiring activation by the parietal cells in the stomach

PPI are all pro drugs requiring activation by gastric parietal cells in the stomach to form the active sulfenamide moiety. After systemic absorption, the latter binds irreversibly to the hydrogen potassium ATPase on the parietal cells, inhibiting their ability to produce hydrochloric acid.

Rabeprazole, not omeprazole, appears to require the least metabolism by the hepatic cytochrome P450 system, thereby making interactions with other drugs, including warfarin, less common. The vegetative form of *Clostridium difficile* can survive in the non-acidic environment of a 'PPI-treated' stomach. As a consequence there is a two to three-fold linkage risk of *Clostridium difficile*-associated diarrhoea in PPI users.

Shin JM, Sachs G, Pharmacology of proton pump inhibitors, *Current Gastroenterology Reports* 2008;10(6):528–534.

57. C. Patients with widespread metastatic disease should not be undergoing radical surgical resection

There is no place for palliative oesophagectomies in those with advanced cancer as effective options such as endo-laser therapy and stenting are available and incur significantly less morbidity. The incidence of oesophageal adenocarcinoma and proximal gastric adenocarcinoma is increasing in Western countries. Risk factors include obesity, male sex, and Caucasian race. Endoscopic ultrasound has become the central technology to accurately judge the tumour (T) stage of the TMN classification and is generally superior to CT in this regard. Furthermore, fine needle aspiration cytology of suspicious lymph nodes can also help with diagnosis and staging Endoscopic mucosal resection can be curative for early gastric cancers, but the following criteria suggests a high risk of lymph node metastases; lesions greater than 2 cm in size, poorly differentiated histology, and surface ulceration. The management of upper GI malignancy now centres around discussions made by the multi-disciplinary team consisting of surgeons, physicians, radiologists, oncologists, palliative care, and specialist nurses. Complex management decisions made in clinical isolation are thus best avoided.

Guidelines for the Management of Oesophageal and Gastric Cancer

Allum WH, Blazeby JM, Griffin SM, Cunningham D, Jankowski JA, Wong R, On behalf of the Association of Upper Gastrointestinal Surgeons of Great Britain and Ireland, the British Society of Gastroenterology and the British Association of Surgical Oncology, *Gut* 2011;60:1449–1472.

58. A. It is the commonest cause of what is often termed cryptogenic cirrhosis

NAFLD is fast becoming the major liver condition seen in the Western world. It is associated with increasing levels of obesity and frequently seen in the setting of type 2 diabetes mellitus, hypertension, insulin resistance, and hyperlipidemia. It is now thought to account for the majority of cases for what was previously termed cryptogenic cirrhosis. With increasing fat deposition, the disease progresses in a significant proportion of patients through a steatohepatitis and then on to fibrosis and eventually cirrhosis. Perhaps unsurprisingly, the disease does indeed recur post orthotopic liver transplant although survival rates are comparable with other disease indications for liver transplant.

Ahmed MH, Abu EO, Byrne CD, Non-alcoholic fatty liver disease (NAFLD): new challenge for general practitioners and important burden for health authorities? *Primary Care Diabetes* 2010;4(3):129–137.

59. D. Oesophageal candidiasis

Oesophageal candidiasis typically presents with odynophagia and retrosternal discomfort; dysphagia may also be a presenting feature. Frailty and immunosuppression predispose. This lady is on inhaled steroids and will almost certainly have had a number of courses of oral steroids during exacerbations of her disease, particularly those necessitating admission to hospital. The Adcal-D3 and osteopenia on the chest X-ray both also point towards repeated oral corticosteroid use. Oral nystatin is insufficient to treat oesophageal candidiasis and is another pointer to upper

GI tract candida. Oesophagitis (without candida) may give similar symptoms but there are no precipitants identifiable in the history. Achalasia and oesophageal cancer would typically present with progressive dysphagia. Classically in motility disorders swallowing of liquids and solids is simultaneously impaired, whilst in mechanical obstruction (including malignancy) dysphagia is progressive from solids to liquids. In achalasia there may also be associated regurgitation and a widened mediastinum with a fluid level visible on the chest X-ray. Malignancy is often associated with systemic symptoms (anorexia, weight loss), which are not present in this case. Pharyngeal pouches present with oropharyngeal level dysphagia, neck swelling on eating, and regurgitation of food.

Longmore M et al., *Oxford Handbook of Clinical Medicine*, Eighth Edition, Oxford University Press, 2010, Chapter 6, Gastroenterology, Dysphagia.

60. B. Paracetamol

Paracetamol, at doses of 3 g/day or less, is the safest analgesic agent to use in chronic liver disease. NSAIDs may worsen both hepatic and renal dysfunction and risk precipitating gastrointestinal bleeding, especially in those with a previous history. Opiate-based analgesic agents may worsen hepatic encephalopathy, particularly if they cause constipation to develop.

Benson G et al., The therapeutic use of acetaminophen in patients with liver disease, *American Journal of Therapeutics* 2005;2:133–141.

61. B. Pancreatic carcinoma

This patient's liver function tests demonstrate a cholestatic picture with the alkaline phosphatase raised in excess of the transaminases. This makes a diagnosis of acute alcoholic hepatitis unlikely (transaminases elevated in excess of ALP would be expected with an AST:ALT ratio in excess of 2:1), especially in the absence of pain in the right upper quadrant, despite the excess alcohol consumption. The lack of pain also makes gallstone disease less likely; this diagnosis is also unlikely in the context of the patient's demographic and would not adequately explain the weight loss. A diagnosis of alcoholic cirrhosis would be unlikely in the absence of signs of chronic liver disease. Both pancreatic carcinoma and cholangiocarcinoma may present as a painless, obstructive jaundice; however, the significantly higher incidence of pancreatic carcinoma in comparison to cholangiocarcinoma makes this the most likely diagnosis.

Green RM, Flamm S, AGA technical review on the evaluation of liver chemistry tests, *Gastroenterology* 2002;123:1367–1384.

62. E. Sodium valproate

Sodium valproate is known to be associated with acute pancreatitis. Other drugs thought to be definitely associated with acute pancreatitis include azathioprine, doxycycline, HIV drugs such as didanosine, methyldopa, estrogens, furosemide, pentamidine, 5-aminosalicylic acid compounds, corticosteroids, and octreotide. Metronidazole and hydrochlorthiazide may also be associated with the condition.

emc+, Epilim 500 Gastro-resistant tablets. http://www.medicines.org.uk/emc/medicine/6781

63. A. Cotrimoxazole for 12 months

The history and findings here are consistent with Whipple's disease, which leads to villous atrophy and the presence of PAS positive macrophages on small bowel biopsy. Prolonged treatment is necessary with 12 months or more of co-trimoxazole. Despite the fact that co-trimoxazole may be associated with blood dyscrasias, it remains the treatment of choice for Whipple's. A prolonged course of ampicillin is an appropriate alternative.

Schneider T et al., Whipple's disease: new aspects of pathogenesis and treatment, *Lancet* 2008;8: 179–190. http://www.sciencedirect.com/science?_ob=ArticleURL&_udi=B6W8X-4RVX3BP-T&_ user=10&_coverDate=03%2F31%2F2008&_rdoc=1&_fmt=high&_orig=search&_origin=search&_ sort=d&_docanchor=&view=c&_searchStrId=1490513176&_rerunOrigin=scholar.google&_ acct=C000050221&_vers

64. E. Liver transplantation is curative in appropriately selected patients

Treatment with ursodeoxycholic acid may improve liver enzymes, help pruritis, and improve liver histology. There are no other proven effective pharmacological therapies. However, liver transplantation is curative in appropriately selected patients.

Pyrsopoulos NT, Primary Biliary Cirrhosis, *Medscape*. http://emedicine.medscape.com/article/ 171117-overview

65. E. Prednisolone

Presenting with this constellation of symptoms on a background of alcohol excess is suggestive of alcoholic hepatitis. The rapid onset of jaundice is a key feature. The blood parameters are also in keeping with this diagnosis: raised inflammatory markers, raised transaminases (with AST:ALT ratio of >2:1), markedly elevated bilirubin and coagulopathy. In this question stem it is also apparent that biliary obstruction has been excluded, as has intercurrent sepsis. A commonly used scoring system in grading the severity of alcoholic hepatitis is the Maddrey's discriminant function. It is calculated using the patient's prothrombin time and their serum bilirubin level (see weblink in further reading). Current evidence suggests that if a patient's Maddrey's score is greater than 32, administration of oral prednisolone (40 mg for 28 days) does improve the patient's 30-day mortality. It is important to bear in mind that intercurrent sepsis must be excluded prior to commencement of steroids. Lactulose will be important in this patient's management to help treat the encephalopathy but will confer no survival benefit. Pabrinex is also important in this patient to replace stores of vitamin B1 but again confers no survival benefit. Rifaximin is a minimally absorbed oral antimicrobial agent that is concentrated in the gastrointestinal tract and leads to decreased absorption of ammonia. It may be used to treat encephalopathy but not as a first-line agent; it will not impact on mortality outcomes. AntiTNF agents such as infliximab have been evaluated in the context of alcoholic hepatitis but trials suggest that they were associated with an increased incidence of severe infections and subsequent mortality. Current guidance appears to be that their use in this context is not appropriate.

On-line calculator for Maddrey's discriminant function. http://www.mdcalc.com/ maddreys-discriminant-function-for-alcoholic-hepatitis

66. A. Oesophageal squamous cell carcinoma

This patient is almost certainly suffering from oesophageal carcinoma. He has recent onset of dysphagia, worse with solids than liquids, and has also lost weight recently, despite having been trying for a long time. Broadly speaking there are two types of oesophageal carcinoma: squamous cell carcinoma and adenocarcinoma. It has been shown that alcohol and extra-hot drinks increase the risk of squamous cell carcinoma. This type of cancer occurs in the upper part of the oesophagus because the upper part is lined with squamous cells. On the other hand, the lower part of the oesophagus is prone to developing adenocarcinoma. The risk factors for this are acid reflux, leading to Barrett's oesophagus, which is a pre-cancerous condition, requiring regular follow-up endoscopy. Achalasia can present with dysphagia and weight loss, but the history is more in keeping with cancer here given the risk factors. In addition, pain is more of a feature in achalasia. Lung cancer itself very rarely causes mass effect large enough to cause dysphagia and the history is more in keeping with an oesophageal primary. Severe oesphagitis can cause feelings of dysphagia but should not cause weight loss. The patient requires urgent OGD.

Colledge NR et al., *Davidson's Principles and Practice of Medicine*, Twenty-first Edition, Churchill Livingstone Elsevier, Tumours of the oesophagus, p. 869.

67. A. Propranolol

This patient requires primary prophylaxis to reduce the risk of variceal bleeding. Studies have shown that propranolol, at the highest tolerated dose (according to symptoms, BP, and HR) will reduce the risk of bleeding in patients with varices. Terlipressin is used during acute variceal bleeding. Variceal banding is used during acute variceal bleeding and for secondary prophylaxis after a bleeding episode. Repeat endoscopy is not the correct option here as the patient needs active management to reduce his risk of variceal bleeding.

Colledge NR et al., *Davidson's Principles and Practice of Medicine*, Twenty-first Edition, Churchill Livingstone Elsevier, Liver and biliary tract disease—Portal hypertension, p. 945.

68. C. Achalasia

The most likely diagnosis here is achalasia. It results from inadequate relaxation of the lower oesophageal sphincter. This results from degeneration of the inhibitory ganglionic cells. The cause is unknown but infections such as varicella-zoster virus or autoimmune causes have been suggested. The other causes are less likely: oesophageal cancer and Barrett's oesophagus will be evident in endoscopy; the weight loss makes GORD less likely, and his symptoms are suggestive of a GI pathology and not cardiac. He needs to undergo a barium swallow test which will show the classic bird's beak appearance, and oesophageal manometery studies which will confirm failure of the relaxation of the lower oesophageal sphincter.

UptToDate. Patient information: achalasia (beyond the basics). http://www.uptodate.com/contents/patient-information-achalasia

69. C. Carcinoid syndrome

The most likely cause of the patient's symptoms is carcinoid syndrome. Carcinoid tumours produce 5HT amongst other hormones, which is the cause of the symptoms. However, those tumours arising in the GI tract are not symptomatic unless they metastasize to the liver. This is because the liver will destroy the 5HT produced by the GI tumour, but will not be able destroy the 5HT produced by the metastasis in the liver itself before the systemic effect is produced. The symtoms include bronchoconstriction, flushing, tricuspid incompetence, and pulmonary stenosis (caused by 5HT-induced fibrosis). Diagnosis is by measuring serum chromogranin A or urinary 24-hour urine 5-hydroxyindoleacetic acid, both of which are raised. Treatment is with octereotide (somatostatin analogue) or loperamide for diarrhoea.

Longmore M et al., *Oxford Handbook of Clinical Medicine*, Eighth Edition, Oxford University Press, 2010, Chapter 6, Gastroenterology, Carcinoid tumours.

70. D. Advise her to start eating normal bread for 4–6 weeks prior to investigations

The most likely diagnosis for this patient is coeliac, especially given that her symptoms have improved since she has adopted a gluten-free diet and also her strong family history. Coeliac disease is a sensitivity to gluten and can be diagnosed by performing D2 biopsies which will show flattened villi and also the anti-TTG antibodies will be raised. However, both of these will become normal once gluten is removed from the diet. Hence, the likelihood of getting a diagnosis in this patient whilst she is continuing with her gluten-free diet is very low. She needs to eat two pieces of toast per day for the next 4–6 weeks before the results can be relied upon. Most patients do not like the idea of this because it also means that their symptoms recur.

Colledge NR et al., *Davidson's Principles and Practice of Medicine*, Twenty-first Edition, Churchill Livingstone Elsevier, Diseases of the small intestine, Disorders causing malabsorption, Coeliac disease, p. 879.

71. C. Faecal elastase

This patient is likely to be suffering from chronic pancreatic insufficiency secondary to alcohol abuse. This is diagnosed by performing faecal elastase levels, which would be very low. The treatment involves oral replacement of pancreatic enzymes. Serum amylase will not help in this instance but is useful in the diagnosis of acute pancreatitis. Stool culture and microscopy are useful if an infectious cause of diarrhoea is suspected. Cholestyramine is a bile salt sequesterant. Bile salt is a major and under-appreciated cause of diarrhoea in patients with disease (or resection) of their ileum, such as those with Crohn's disease. The formal diagnosis of bile salt malabsorption is with SeHCAT study.

Colledge NR et al., *Davidson's Principles and Practice of Medicine*, Twenty-first Edition, Churchill Livingstone Elsevier, Chronic pancreatic insufficiency (p. 892), Bile salt malabsorption (Ileal resection, p. 882).

72. E. None of the above

The most likely diagnosis here is Gilbert's syndrome, which is an autosomal recessive disorder. These patients do not have any underlying liver disease and the bilirubin increases mildly during times of physiological stress. Bilirubin and liver function tests should be rechecked once he has recovered from the lower respiratory tract infection. If at that point he still has deranged LFTs, then it is reasonable to consider other causes and perform further investigations.

Nazer H, Unconjugated hyperbilirubinemia, *Mesdcape*, 2016. http://emedicine.medscape.com/article/176822-overview

73. A. Isolated portal vein thrombosis

Lone portal vein thrombosis does not cause ascites because the obstruction is presinusoidal. The others are all established causes of ascites.

Moore KP, Aithal GP, BSG 2005 guideline—management of acsites in cirrhosis. http://www.bsg.org.uk/images/stories/docs/clinical/guidelines/liver/ascites_cirrhosis.pdf

74. E. The pathophysiology of HRS is related to splanchnic vasodilatation

Hepatorenal syndrome is a type of renal failure that occurs in patients with advanced cirrhosis. It is defined by the absence of parenchymal kidney disease. The underlying cause relates to portal hypertension and complex haemodynamic changes occurring in chronic liver disease, including splanchnic arterial vasodilation, renal vasoconstriction, and reduced cardiac output. It is differentiated from other causes of renal dysfunction, in part, by the failure to improve with intravenous fluid administration

Baraldi O, Valentini C, Donati G, Comai G, Cuna V, Capelli I, Angelini ML, Moretti MI, Angeletti A, Piscaglia F, La Manna G, Hepatorenal syndrome: update on diagnosis and treatment, *World Journal of Nephrology* 2015 Nov 6;4(5):511–520.

75. B. Ascending cholangitis

Gas in the biliary tree may occur following surgical procedures to the distal biliary tree including sphincterotomy of the ampulla of Vater and biliary stunting. Biliary gas is also part of 'Rigler's Triad' of plain radiograph signs indicating gallstone ileus (gas in the biliary tree, small bowel obstruction, stone in the right iliac fossa). In gallstone ileus, a cholecysto-duodenal fistula is formed with resultant passage of a gallstone into the small bowel and small bowel obstruction due to stone impaction at the ileo-caecal junction. However, the toxic condition of this patient is suggestive of ascending cholangitis.

Warrell DA et al., *Oxford Textbook of Medicine*, Fifth Edition, Oxford University Press, 2010, Section 15.23, Diseases of the gallbladder and biliary tree.

76. A. HFE gene testing

Given that no other causes of iron overload are given in this question such as excess alcohol consumption, this patient is suffering from iron overload, almost certainly secondary to hereditary haemochromatosis (HH) resulting in diabetes and arthralgia. The *HFE* gene is located on chromosome 6 and is a recessive disorder. Other causes of iron overload, such as repeated blood transfusion (e.g. in sickle cell disease, myelodysplasia) result in raised ferritin. Ferritin is also an acute phase protein and is raised in alcoholic liver disease. Ferritin levels below 1000 are not associated with liver fibrosis. A high transferrin saturation level is unreliable in diagnosing haemochromatosis in the presence of cirrhosis as transferrin (produced by the liver) level is low. Liver biopsy will show liver cirrhosis and damage caused by elevation of iron levels, but again, it is not diagnostic of HH unless a dry weight liver iron is measured. MRI scanning can suggest liver iron but is not diagnostic of genetic HH. Liver ultrasound can show liver cirrhosis but is not diagnostic of HH.

AASLD practice guidelines, Haemochromatosis. http://www.aasld.org/practiceguidelines

77. A. Alcoholic liver disease

This patient has clinical evidence of chronic liver disease. An AST:ALT ratio of 2:1 or greater is very suggestive of alcoholic liver disease. Malnutrition may well suggest chronic excess alcohol consumption. Dupytren's contracture is associated with liver cirrhosis; associations with chronic alcohol consumption and diabetes are often cited but unproven. The previous admissions to hospital with abdominal pain may well represent recurrent episodes of pancreatitis secondary to alcohol with diabetes the result of recurrent pancreatic damage. The wide-based gait can also be explained by cerebellar dysfunction secondary to alcohol. A low normal serum caeruloplasmin does not support a diagnosis of Wilson's disease. The ferritin is just above the upper limit of normal, is difficult to interpret in the context of a raised CRP (ferritin is an acute phase reactant), and can also be elevated with chronic excess alcohol consumption. Measurement of transferrin saturations would help in the diagnosis of iron overload; however, in haemochromatosis serum ferritin may well be elevated to around 1000. Neither hepatocellular carcinoma nor autoimmune polyglandular syndrome would adequately explain all the features of the case above.

Green RM, Flamm S, AGA technical review on the evaluation of liver chemistry tests, *Gastroenterology* 2002;123:1367–1384.

78. C. Anti-mitochondrial

This patient's symptoms and biochemistry are classical for primary biliary cirrhosis. Itching is frequently the first symptom and an elevated alkaline phosphatase often the only abnormal finding on routine biochemistry. Anti-mitochondrial antibodies are found in around 95% of cases of primary biliary cirrhosis. Anti-scl-70 is an autoantibody directed against topoisomerase I, and is seen most frequently in scleroderma, more so in diffuse systemic sclerosis than limited scleroderma. Anti-centromere antibodies are also associated with scleroderma, but much more so limited scleroderma than systemic sclerosis. Anti-smooth muscle and anti-liver kidney microsomal antibodies are both associated with chronic autoimmune hepatitis. Whilst the symptoms described above might be compatible with a diagnosis of autommimune hepatitis, the biochemistry is not— aminotranferases are elevated in all cases of autoimmune hepatitis.

Longmore M et al., *Oxford Handbook of Clinical Medicine*, Eighth Edition, Oxford University Press, 2010, Chapter 12, Rheumatology, Polymyositis and dermatomyositis.

79. D. Previous hepatitis B infection, chronic hepatitis C infection

The presence of HBsAg in the serum is indicative of active HBV infection, either acute or chronic. Antibodies against hepatitis B surface antigen (anti-HBs) indicate a vaccinated individual (the vaccine is based upon the HBsAg protein) or previous infection with HBV (seroconversion to produce anti-HBs in the setting of HBV infection indicates the infection has been cleared). Antibodies against hepatitis B core antigen (anti-HBc) are only detected in individuals who have been infected with HBV. As with other antibodies generated in response to infection, IgM is present during the initial immune response; this is replaced over time by IgG antibodies. Anti-HBc IgM is detectable 6–32 weeks after exposure and indicates acute HBV infection. Anti-HBc IgG is produced from around 14 weeks after exposure; in the absence of anti-HBc IgM it may indicate cleared or chronic HBV infection. Presence of hepatitis C antibodies indicates exposure to the virus; if detected, a viral RNA load is required to determine whether there is active infection. Persistence of viral RNA in the bloodstream more than six months after exposure (or acute illness if symptoms develop) indicates chronic infection. Acute hepatitis C infection is asymptomatic in 60–70% of cases; infection is chronic in around 85% of individuals.

Longmore M et al., *Oxford Handbook of Clinical Medicine*, Eighth Edition, Oxford University Press, 2010, Chapter 9, Infectious Diseases, Viral hepatitis.

80. B. Primary sclerosing cholangitis

The clinical picture here, with the development of itching and lethargy against the background of a long history of inflammatory bowel disease, is consistent with the development of primary sclerosing cholangitis. Around 60% of patients with PSC have co-existent positive ANCA, and this is associated with potentially more rapid progression of disease. IgM and IgG are also usually elevated in association with PSC. Alkaline phosphatase is elevated; there may be a lesser, or no rise in transaminases. A hallmark of the disease is bile duct dilatation and stricture, and this has a characteristic appearance on MRCP/ERCP. Liver biopsy may be of value in initial staging, but because of patchy disease is not very useful with respect to monitoring changes over time.

Dancygier H, *Clinical Hepatology*, Springer, 2010, Chapter 75, Primary Sclerosing Cholangitis. http://www.springerlink.com/content/tp172t077897331x/

81. A. Autoimmune hepatitis type 1

This clinical picture is most consistent with autoimmune hepatitis type 1. Type 2 autoimmune hepatitis tends to be associated with anti-LKM antibodies. The rise in transaminases which is greater than the rise in alkaline phosphatase is more consistent with autoimmune hepatitis than alternative conditions where obstruction is more apparent such as primary sclerosing cholangitis or primary biliary cirrhosis. Liver biopsy is the diagnostic modality of choice, and corticosteroids +/ – azathioprine are the mainstay of therapy. Twenty-year life expectancy is 80% in those who are managed with immune-modifying therapies.

Decock S et al., Autoimmune liver disease for the non-specialist, *British Medical Journal* 2009;Sep 8;339:b3305. http://www.ncbi.nlm.nih.gov/pubmed/19737821?dopt=Abstract

82. E. Type 1 autoimmune hepatitis typically affects elderly or immunosuppressed individuals

E is false: type 1 autoimmune hepatitis is classically said to have a bimodal age distribution, most commonly affecting those aged 10–30 and 40–50 years. In practice, almost any age group can be affected from infants to the elderly. Autoimmune hepatitis is a chronic hepatitis, characterized by hepatocellular inflammation and necrosis which, untreated, frequently progresses to cirrhosis. Liver damage must not be attributable to chronic viral hepatitis (B or C), or to alcohol or drug-induced hepatitis. Based upon serological testing, two main types are recognized: (1) type 1 is associated with a homogeneous pattern of anti-nuclear antibody staining, and anti-smooth muscle antibodies directed against p-actin. Although typically a disease of young and middle aged adults, any age group may be affected. (2) Type 2 is associated with anti–liver-kidney microsomal antibodies (anti-LKM) and tends to affect a younger age group, including children and adolescents. Additionally, type 3 autoimmune hepatitis, though less common, may be recognized by antibodies to soluble liver-kidney antigens. All types of autoimmune hepatitis are more common in females, with a female:male ratio of around 4:1. There are multiple associations with other autoimmune diseases, including rheumatoid arthritis, autoimmune haemolytic anaemia, ITP, inflammatory bowel disease, and type 1 diabetes mellitus. Patients may present with acute hepatitis (fever, right upper quadrant pain, and jaundice), or with features of chronic liver disease or cirrhosis. Diagnosis requires evidence of liver disease with elevated aminotransferases, alongside a typical autoantibody profile. Viral and toxic/metabolic causes of liver disease should be excluded. Liver biopsy allows histological confirmation and assessment of cirrhosis. Treatment requires prolonged immunosuppression with oral steroids. Azathioprine may be introduced at the start of treatment, or after initial stabilization with high-dose steroids.

Czaja AJ, Freese DK, Diagnosis and treatment of autoimmune hepatitis, *Hepatology* 2002;36:479–497.

83. B. Arrange measurement of hepatitis B viral DNA load

This is important to help differentiate the inactive HBsAg carrier state from chronic hepatitis B infection with active viral replication. Hepatitis B virus is a DNA virus composed of an outer lipid envelope around a core of viral protein and nucleic acid. Key proteins encoded by the viral genome include the surface antigen (HBsAg), as well as the core antigen HBcAg. The so-called 'e-antigen' (HBeAg) is generated from a RNA splice variant of the gene encoding the core antigen. During initial infection with the hepatitis B virus, viral DNA load is high, and HBeAg is expressed, along with HBcAg and HBsAg. Infection in adulthood is typically associated with viral clearance, reflected by the presence of antibodies to both surface and core antigens (anti-HBs and anti-HBc) without the presence of HBsAg. This differs from those who have not been exposed to the intact virus but who have received vaccination, who will have anti-HBs but not anti-HBc. Those infected at a young age, or who are immunosuppressed, are at higher risk of chronic hepatitis B infection, reflected by the persistence of HBsAg for >6 months. In these individuals HBeAg typically becomes undetectable over time, as seroconversion occurs and antibodies develop (anti-HBe). Seroconversion is more likely to occur in older individuals and those with elevated ALT levels. HBsAg+, anti-HBe+, HBeAg− represents the inactive carrier state with little residual viral replication and essentially normal liver histology. However, a number of individuals with serology suggestive of the inactive carrier state will in fact have higher levels of viral replication and detectable serum viral DNA levels. In these cases, viral mutation has occured within the promoter region of the gene encoding HBcAg or within the 'pre-core' region of the same gene. This leads to a virus that is unable to produce HBeAg, but that is competent to replicate and cause liver inflammation and damage. Individuals with HBeAg- chronic hepatitis thus have more advanced liver disease and a higher risk of complications than those in the inactive carrier state. Unlike the latter group, these patients require more active monitoring and may require biopsy and consideration for treatment.

Lok ASF, McMahon BJ, American Association for the Study of Liver Disease practice guidelines: chronic hepatitis B: update 2009. http://www.aasld.org/practiceguidelines/Documents/Bookmarked%20Practice%20Guidelines/Chronic_Hep_B_UPDAte_2009%208_24_2009.pdf

84. B. The *HFE C282Y* mutation accounts for over 80% of cases among persons of northern European descent

Haemochromatosis is the abnormal accumulation of iron in organs, including the heart, liver, pancreas, pituitary, skin, and joints. It is the most common inherited liver disease in whites and the most common autosomal recessive genetic disorder. The gene responsible for the disease is *HFE*, located on chromosome 6. A full model of how mutant *HFE* leads to pathological iron accumulation remains unclear, but the product of *HFE* interacts with the transferrin receptor decreasing the affinity for transferrin and modulating cellular iron uptake. When mutant *HFE* is present, ferritin levels are not regulated, leading to the accumulation of iron in peripheral tissues. There is no mechanism of iron excretion, renal or otherwise. Hereditary haemochromatosis is most common in white populations, particularly those of celtic descent. Homozygosity for one particular missense *HFE* mutation, *C282Y*, accounts for 82–90% of cases in white populations. A less common mutation *H63D* may play a role in iron overload in *C282Y/H63D* in compound heterozygotes. Transferrin saturation is a measurement of the ratio of serum iron to total iron-binding capacity. Persistently elevated transferrin saturation is a useful screening test for hereditary haemochromatosis in the absence of other causes of iron overload (e.g. multiple blood transfusions or alcoholic liver disease with consumption of iron-fortified wines). A value greater than 60% in men and 50% in women is highly specific. Lower levels of iron overload in women may be related to recurrent menstrual blood loss. This approach is not without flaws, since values are not always raised in younger individuals with haemochromatosis, especially females. An appropriate screening threshold would be a fasting transferrin saturation of 45–50%. In white patients with clinical evidence of iron overload and persistently elevated transferrin saturations, demonstration of the genetic mutations described above would usually be considered sufficient to make the diagnosis. However, in black patients, causative genetic mutations are less predictable. Where diagnostic uncertainty remains, liver biopsy allows for assessment of iron overload as well as the degree of fibrosis or cirrhosis.

European Association for the Study of the Liver: EASL Clinical Practice Guidelines for HFE Hemochromatosis, *Journal of Hepatology* 2010. doi: 10.1016/j.jhep.2010.03.001. http://www.easl.eu/assets/application/files/03d32880931aac9_file.pdf

85. D. Pruritis is a common symptom

PBC affects predominantly females and onset is usually age 40–60 years. Positivity for AMA is diagnostically specific (98%). Both pruritis and fatigue are common, but are notoriously difficult to treat satisfactorily.

Pyrsopoulos NT, Primary Biliary Cirrhosis, *Medscape*. http://emedicine.medscape.com/article/171117-overview

86. E. Patient age over 60

In patients aged over 60, looser and/or more frequent stools lasting for more than six weeks is a 'red flag' symptom for referral to secondary care for further investigation. Irritable bowel syndrome causes chronic, recurrent abdominal pain or discomfort associated with altered bowel habit in the absence of structural gastrointestinal abnormalities to account for these symptoms. The diagnostic criteria have been refined in a series of international symposia meeting in Rome ('The Rome Criteria'); Rome III, the most recent definitions from 2006, define irritable bowel syndrome as: recurrent abdominal pain or discomfort at least three days a month in the past three months, associated with two or more of the following: improvement with defaecation; onset associated with a change in frequency of stool; onset associated with a change in form (appearance) of stool. Criteria should be fulfilled for the past three months, with symptom onset at least six months before diagnosis. Other well-recognized features of irritable bowel syndrome include the passage of mucus with stool, and the sensation of abdominal bloating or visible distension (more common in women than men). Symptoms may be made worse by eating. Prevalence in the developed world is between 5–15%. Frequency peaks in the third and fourth decades of life, with a female preponderance of 2:1 in this age range. Although any age group may be affected, a new presentation of these symptoms in anyone over the age of 60* or with a family history of bowel or ovarian cancer should prompt a higher level of suspicion for colorectal cancer. Likewise, any abdominal or rectal mass should prompt further investigation. In those meeting the diagnostic criteria and who do not have any of these 'red flags', check full blood count, inflammatory markers, and coeliac serology.

*There is some disagreement as to what age should be regarded as suspicious for a first presentation. NICE IBS guidelines define age at presentation over 60 as a red flag; British Society of Gastroenterology guidelines list age over 50.

NICE guidelines, Irritable bowel syndrome in adults: diagnosis and management of irritable bowel syndrome in primary care. Issued February 2008. http://www.nice.org.uk/CG061

87. D. Entamoeba histolytica

Bacillus cereus causes a toxin-mediated gastroenteritis that is characterized by the onset of profuse vomiting within 6–12 hours of eating contaminated food; diarrhoea is not usually a feature. Giardia is a cause of both acute and chronic diarrhoea, usually with features of malabsorption. Flatulence and bloating are common. Campylobacter, Salmonella and Entamoeba are all infective causes of bloody diarrhoea. Campylobacter dysentery typically has an onset 5–7 days after exposure and a duration of 1 week. Salmonella has a shorter incubation period (12–72 hours) and duration (4–7 days). This is most likely to be a case of amoebic dysentery. It has a longer incubation period of 2–4 weeks (exposure was most likely whilst abroad). It is common in developing countries, such as India, and occurs most frequently in those in the area for a month or longer. The infection can cause a spectrum of disease from asymptomatic infection to necrotizing colitis. Spontaneous resolution of invasive disease is uncommon. Adequate therapy for amoebic colitis is necessary to reduce the severity of illness, prevent the development of complicated disease and extraintestinal spread, and decrease infectiousness and transmission to others.

Amoebic dysentery.

Marie C, Petri WA Jr., *BMJ Clinical Evidence* 2013 Aug 30;2013.

88. A. The bacterium may be detected in the bowel flora of 15% of the adult population

The bacterium may be readily detected in the bowel flora of up to 50% of infants, but this colonization falls to around 2% of the adult population. *C. difficile* is a motile, Gram-positive spore-forming rod which is the commonest cause of hospital-acquired infectious diarrhoea. Although small numbers of the adult population (1–2%) may demonstrate chronic intestinal carriage without any symptoms, the use of broad spectrum antibiotics, particularly in an inpatient setting, may allow the acquisition and germination of spores, and the overgrowth of toxin-producing strains of *C. difficile*. *C. difficile*-associated disease is characterized by watery or mucoid diarrhoea, abdominal pain, and low-grade fever. Occasionally, traces of blood may appear in the stool. More severe manifestations include fulminant colitis or toxic megacolon. All antibiotics are associated with increased risk of development of *C. difficile*-associated diarrhoea, typically 3–9 days after starting therapy. However, broad spectrum antibiotics, particularly fluroquinolones and third- generation cephalosporins are associated with highest risk. *C. difficile* should be tested for wherever clinical suspicion exists. Cytotoxicity assays are based upon demonstration of cytopathic effects of stool filtrates on cultured cells. These assays are sensitive and specific, but labour intensive. Enzyme-linked immunosorbent assays (ELISA) for *C. difficile* toxin A or B (or both) are faster and less expensive, and are used in most clinical settings. However, the lower sensitivity of most commercially available tests necessitates testing two to three separate stools. Alternative diagnostic tests include PCR, which is increasingly used in many centres. Standard treatment is with oral metronidazole or oral vancomycin. Both have comparable response and relapse rates.

Because oral vancomycin is poorly absorbed, high stool concentrations can be achieved without systemic side effects. There is no role for intravenous vancomycin; where the oral route is not possible, intravenous metronidazole may be useful. After resolution of diarrhoeal symptoms, patients' stools may remain positive for C. *difficile* toxin for some weeks/months. Up to 25% of adult patients will experience disease recurrence, which necessitate pulsed or tapering courses of vancomycin.

Heinlen L, Ballard JD, Clostridium difficile infection, *American Journal of the Medical Sciences* 2010;340(3):247–252.

89. A. Metabolic acidosis

Cyclic vomiting syndrome is a disorder characterized by recurrent episodes of severe nausea and vomiting separated by symptom-free periods. The syndrome is linked to migraine headaches, and is more common in those with either a personal or family history of migraine. Other associations include cannabis use, food allergy, and occurrence during menstrual periods. Recurrent vomiting is usually associated with metabolic alkalosis.

Fleisher DR et al., Cyclic vomiting syndrome in 41 adults: the illness, the patients, and problems of management, *BMC Medicine* 2005;3:20. http://www.biomedcentral.com/1741-7015/3/20

90. B. Prucalopride

NICE recommends prucalopride as a possible treatment for women with chronic constipation. It is indicated in women who have tried at least two different types of laxatives at the highest possible recommended doses without benefit. Prucalopride is a selective, high affinity 5-HT4 receptor agonist. Pelvic floor exercises are useful in incontinence, rather than in constipation. Dietary advice should be given to all patients with constipation, but is unlikely to improve provide full symptom relief at this stage.

Surgical management of constipation, although useful in highly selected patient groups, should be regarded as a last resort.

NICE guidelines [TA211], Prucalopride for the treatment of chronic constipation in women. http://guidance.nice.org.uk/TA211

91. D. Cyclical vomiting syndrome

Cyclic vomiting syndrome is a disorder characterized by recurrent episodes of severe nausea and vomiting, separated by symptom-free periods. The syndrome is linked to migraine headaches, and is more common in those with either a personal or family history of migraine. Other associations include cannabis use, food allergy, and occurrence during menstrual periods.

Fleisher DR et al., Cyclic vomiting syndrome in 41 adults: the illness, the patients, and problems of management. *BMC Medicine* 2005;3:20. http://www.biomedcentral.com/1741-7015/3/20

92. E. Selenium-homocholic acid taurine (SeHCAT) test

The onset of diarrhoea following cholecystectomy is a clue to the diagnoisis of bile salt malabsorption. This characteristically causes watery diarrhoea, but is not usually associated with sinister features such as weight loss. There are no historical features to suggest pancreatic disease or thyroid dysfunction. A SeHCAT test allows diagnosis of bile salt malabsorption: the Se-labelled bile acid is given orally and the total body retention is measured with a gamma camera after seven days—a value of less than 15% is considered abnormal and indicates bile acid malabsorption. This test is often poorly available, and a widely used alternative would be a therapeutic trial of bile salt sequestrants.

Pattni S, Walters JRF, Recent advances in the understanding of bile acid malabsorption, *British Medical Bulletin* 2009;92:79–93. http://bmb.oxfordjournals.org/content/92/1/79.full

93. C. Is metabolized to mercaptopurine in vivo

Azathioprine is commonly used as a steroid-sparing immunosuppressant in inflammatory bowel disease. It belongs to the thiopurine family and is non-enzymatically metabolized in vivo to mercaptopurine (6-MP). Further metabolism by the enzyme thiopurine-methyltransferase (TPMT) inactivates 6-MP, producing 6-MMP. A minority of individuals have reduced activity of TPMT, rendering them at greater risk of azathioprine toxicity (bone marrow suppression, myelotoxicity). The drug has a delayed onset of therapeutic action in IBD, usually taking 8–12 weeks for full onset of effect. Although it is not usually recommended that azathioprine be commenced during pregnancy, it is generally regarded as a safe treatment that can be continued during pregnancy. It belongs to US FDA category D, which means that evidence indicates foetal harm may occur, but the benefits of treatment may outweigh this risk. British Society for Gastroenterology guidelines for the management of IBD support the use of azathioprine during pregnancy, in order to maintain disease remission.

Torkamani A, Azathioprine metabolism and TPMT, *Medscape*, 2011. http://emedicine.medscape.com/article/1829596-overview

94. E. It is a monoclonal antibody against tumour necrosis factor alpha

Infliximab is a chimeric monoclonal antibody against TNF alpha. It consists of both mouse and human components; hence it is chimeric. This is is contrast to adalimumab, which is a fully human anti-TNF antibody, which is administered as a subcutaneous injection. Infliximab is given as an intravenous infusion. Anti-TNF therapies are reserved for IBD that has not responded to conventional first-line therapies such as corticosteroids and azathioprine or methotrexate.

NICE guidelines [TA187], Infliximab and adalimumab for the treatment of Crohn's disease. http://guidance.nice.org.uk/TA187

95. B. Plan cisplatin-based chemotherapy pre- and post-oesophagectomy

Adenocarcinoma of the oesophagus is poorly responsive to radiotherapy; the combined chemoradiotherapy approach is usually reserved for squamous cell carcinoma of the oesophagus. Extensive trials have examined the timing of chemotherapy, and in those patients who have a good functional status pre-operatively, both pre and post-oesophagectomy platinum-based chemotherapy is associated with the greatest improvement in survival. Clearly due to the association with smoking and obesity, many patients who present with oesophageal carcinoma may be unsuitable for surgical intervention. In these individuals alternatives such as stenting for symptoms of obstruction are considered. Five-year survival of early tumours which are resectable approaches 80–90%; for late-presenting tumours survival is depressingly poor, at only around 10%.

Chikwe J et al., *Oxford Specialist Handbook of Cardiothoracic Surgery*, Oxford University Press, 2006.

96. D. Co-amoxiclav

Until recently, cephalosporins were thought to be most strongly implicated in *C. difficile* infection (CDI), but with more restricted use of these agents, co-amoxiclav and piperacillin-tazobactam have emerged as the agents most commonly associated with CDI. Diagnosis is now based on microbiology alone, apart from those patients who have diarrhoea which is resistant to intervention, where flexible sigmoidoscopy may be considered. Both oral metronidazole and oral vancomycin are highly effective in treating the condition.

Shannon-Lowe J et al., Prevention and medical management of *Clostridium difficile* infection, *British Medical Journal* 2010;340:c1296. http://www.bmj.com/content/340/bmj.c1296

97. E. >12

The Blatchford score is used to predict the need for urgent endoscopy, a score of <4 indicating a low need for urgent procedure. Urea, haemoglobin, systolic BP, and other markers including pulse, presence of melaena, presence of syncope, pre-existing hepatic disease and pre-existing cardiac disease are all taken into account. In this case the patient scores 4 for her urea, 6 for her haemoglobin, and 2 for her blood pressure. An additional 2 points are added for pre-existing cardiac failure.

Blatchford O et al., A risk score to predict need for treatment for upper-gastrointestinal haemorrhage. *Lancet* 2000;356:1318–1321. http://europepmc.org/abstract/MED/11073021/reload=0;jsessionid=aR6 5i7ctPL4E0YNHw4I4.10

98. A. Ursodeoxycholic acid

The clinical picture seen here fits best with intra-hepatic cholestasis of pregnancy, the incidence of which varies widely across the world, from 10% in some parts of Chile, to 0.1% in Canada. Treatment is symptomatic: with ursodeoxycholic acid, increased fetal complications are seen in pregnancies where intrahepatic cholestasis occurs, particularly after 38 weeks gestation. Therefore elective delivery normally takes place at this point. Acute fatty liver of pregnancy is a much rarer condition, and progression of symptoms is more rapid, with headache, nausea, and vomiting which can progress to severe jaundice within 14 days. Immunomodulation does not impact on progression of intra-hepatic cholestasis, so azathioprine or steroids are not indicated, nor is anti-coagulation.

Warrell DA et al., *Oxford Textbook of Medicine*, Fifth Edition, Oxford University Press, 2010, Chapter 14.9, Liver and gastrointestinal diseases in pregnancy.

99. D. Peginterferon alpha-2a, ribavirin and boceprevir

Triple anti-viral therapy including either boceprevir or teleprevir is now recommended as an option by NICE for patients who are treatment naive or in whom previous therapies have failed to achieve viral clearance, who have compensated liver disease and the type 1 genotype. The 'previrs' inhibit NS3/4A serine protease which is essential for hepatitis C viral replication and which may also help it to evade clearance by the host immune system. Dual therapy is only thought to achieve viral clearance in 40–50% of individuals with genotype 1 hepatitis C, and triple therapy represents a significant improvement on this (up to 66% viral clearance).

emc+, Boceprevir: pharmacodynamic properties. http://www.medicines.org.uk/emc/medicine/24768/ spc#PHARMACODYNAMIC_PROPS

100. D. Admit, IV hydrocortisone 100 mg QDS

This patient has acute severe colitis according to the Truelove and Witts' criteria (>6 bloody stools per day + any 1 of: Haemoglobin <10.5g/dL, ESR>30mm/hr, pulse rate >90 beats/min, temp >37.5°C). He should be admitted and commenced on parenteral steroids at a high dose (usually hydrocortisone 100mg QDS). Other important management points include abdominal X-ray, thromboprophylaxis, daily monitoring of U+E and CRP, and early review by a gastroenterologist. The surgical team should also be involved at an early stage, in case medical therapy fails and surgical management is required.

Jakobovits SL, Travis SPL, Management of acute severe colitis, *British Medical Bulletin* 2006;75 and 76:131–144. http://bmb.oxfordjournals.org/content/75-76/1/131.full.pdf

101. D. Phosphate

This patient has the typical symptoms associated with re-feeding syndrome, with hypotension, muscle weakness, and evidence of cardiac failure. It occurs because of a rise in insulin secretion associated with re-feeding, which drives phosphate from the extra-cellular to the intra-cellular compartment. Patients with anorexia and alcoholism are phosphate depleted, and re-feeding thus leads to even lower levels of extra-cellular phosphate and the symptoms of muscle weakness seen. It can be avoided by adequately replacing phosphate.

Semple D, Smyth R, *Oxford Handbook of Psychiatry*, Second Edition, Oxford University Press, 2009, Chapter 10, Eating and impulse-control disorders.

102. C. 5HT4 receptor agonist

Prucalopride is a selective 5-HT4 receptor agonist that targets the impaired motility associated with chronic constipation. It is an alternative treatment to laxative drugs, and is licensed in women who have tried laxatives without benefit for six months. Bile acid sequestration is the mechanism of action of cholestyramine and colesevelam, drugs used in bile acid malabsorption, which is associated with diarrhoea.

NICE guidelines [TA211], Constipation (women)—prucalopride. http://guidance.nice.org.uk/TA211

103. D. Radiation proctitis

Lymphocytic colitis and bile acid malabsorption do not typically cause rectal bleeding. Inflammatory bowel disease, especially ulcerative colitis, usually involves diarrhoea and CRP is often elevated, making this diagnosis less likely. Colorectal carcinoma is possible, but the lack of weight loss and normal PR exam are against this. His past history and symptoms are suggestive of radiation proctitis.

Pal N, Radiation enteritis and proctitis, *Medscape*, 2011. http://emedicine.medscape.com/article/197483-overview

104. D. Faecal calprotectin

When faced with a young person with abdominal pain and possible weight loss, it is important to consider both organic and functional causes. In this case, there are some clues as to a possible organic aetiology, including a borderline low haemoglobin, although in a female of reproductive age this could well be related to menstrual loss. Proceeding straight to a trial of anti-spasmodic medication without further consideration of organic disease would be inappropriate. The differential diagnosis must include Crohn's disease (the absence of rectal bleeding makes ulcerative colitis less likely). Evidence of terminal ileal inflammation on colonoscopy would be the useful in this regard, but this is an invasive test, particularly for such a young adult. Barium enema is unlikely to provide useful information. Calprotectin, released from degranulating neutrophils, is a non-specific marker of inflammation within the GI tract and would provide a non-invasive test for inflammatory bowel disease which would be useful in this scenario. A raised faecal calprotectin would then provide good justification for a full colonoscopy. Although not presented as an option in this question, measuring blood markers of inflammation, including CRP or ESR, as well as measuring B12, folate, and iron levels would be sensible. Although coeliac disease can cause weight loss and anaemia through malabsorption, it does not usually cause significant pain. Duodenal biopsies are the investigation of choice for coeliac disease, although tissue transglutaminase antibodies can help to exclude coeliac disease where the index of suspicion is low.

Ghazi LJ, Crohn disease, *Medscape*, 2013. http://emedicine.medscape.com/article/172940-overview

105. C. Pellagra

Pellagra is characterized by extensive dermatitis which may be the only sign in 3% of patients who suffer from it. This occurs predominantly on sun-exposed skin, and fades to leave red-brown pigmentation. It occurs due to a chronic lack niacin (vitamin B3), in this case most likely due to the extensive small bowel resection. Over the long term it leads to dementia if left untreated. Zinc deficiency is associated with diarrhoea, but not with the rash seen here. Given the history of type 1 diabetes, coeliac disease is a possibility, although the rash associated with coeliac is dermatitis herpetformis which is blistering and itchy, not consistent with the picture seen here. Treatment of pellagra is usually with nicotinamide supplementation.

Burge S, Wallis D, *Oxford Handbook of Medical Dermatology*, Oxford University Press, 2010, Chapter 24, Skin and gastroenterology.

1. **A 72-year-old man had begun to mobilize four days after admission with a left lower lobe pneumonia, complicated by renal impairment. His renal function was improving and his chest X-ray, on day 4, showed only a small left pleural effusion. However, the nurses were concerned because he had a persistent low-grade fever and some suprapubic pain. He had a catheter in situ. Investigations: catheter specimen of urine— multi-resistant *E. coli*. Creatinine now 132 micromol/l. Which of the following is the best course of action?**

    A. Instil chlorhexidine wash within the catheter tubing each morning
    B. No specific action need be taken
    C. Regular bladder washouts
    D. Remove catheter
    E. Three days of trimethoprim

2. **An 84-year-old woman presents to A&E following a fall. She has a past medical history of dementia, hypertension, mild aortic stenosis, and polymyalgia rheumatica. Her medications are 5 mg prednisolone, 2.5 mg bendroflumethiazide, and aspirin 75 mg, each taken once daily. The patient has no recollection of events, but her husband reports that she tripped on a loose rug and was unable to mobilize afterwards owing to severe pain in her left hip. He called an ambulance and she was given 5 mg intramuscular morphine for pain relief. X-ray confirmed a fractured left neck of femur. Owing to her confusion, a medical opinion is sought. Which of the following is consistent with best practice?**

    A. Delay surgery until a formal echocardiogram can determine the degree of aortic stenosis
    B. Initiate osteoporosis treatment with intravenous bisphosphonate within 24 hours of fracture
    C. Referral to on-call anaesthetist to consider performing a regional nerve block
    D. Urgent review by the psychogeriatric liaison team to assess capacity to consent for surgery
    E. Withhold steroid medication to promote bone and wound healing post-operatively

3. **A frail 90-year-old woman is referred to the falls clinic having experienced numerous falls in the previous two months. Her most recent fall occurred on going to the kitchen to make a cup of tea. She recalls reaching up into the cupboard and then feeling extremely 'dizzy'. She describes falling backwards to the floor but not losing consciousness. Her previous falls had all been similar in nature.She also reported feeling 'dizzy' around bed-time and occasionally waking up in the night with episodes of dizziness and nausea. Which of the following is the most appropriate initial investigation?**

   A. Active stand
   B. CT head scan
   C. Dix–Hallpike test
   D. Tilt table testing with carotid sinus massage
   E. 24-hour blood pressure and electrocardiograph monitoring

4. **You are asked to advise on the care of a 75-year-old woman who has undergone a right hemi-arthroplasty for hip fracture some two days earlier. She has become confused and aggressive and has told the nurses they are 'trying to poison her'. There is a past history of hypertension and osteoporosis, and you suspect she drinks a small amount of alcohol each evening at home. Which of the following is the most appropriate next step?**

   A. Diazepam
   B. Haloperidol
   C. Chlordiazepoxide
   D. Reassurance and 1:1 nursing
   E. Risperidone

5. **Mrs Driver is a 75-year-old woman who has been admitted to hospital with new onset atrial fibrillation and an infective exacerbation of COPD. Her past medical history also includes hypertension. After 48 hours she begins to complain of nausea and vomiting. Which new medication is most likely to be causing her symptoms?**

   A Doxycycline True
   B Paracetamol False
   C Prednisolone False
   D Salbutamol False
   E Verapamil False

6. **Which of the following would give a negative result on urine dipstick for proteins?**

    A. Radio contrast agents
    B. Light chain immunoglobulins in the urine
    C. Highly alkaline urine (pH>8)
    D. Urinary infection
    E. Exercise

7. **A 76-year-old woman who is being treated for giant cell arteritis has acute onset of back pain and urinary retention. Which is the single most discriminating investigation?**

    A. Bone scan
    B. CT scan of spine
    C. MRI scan of spine
    D. Myelogram
    E. X-ray of spine

8. **A 70-year-old man has vomiting, anorexia, and polyuria. He is an ex-smoker of 25 pack-years. The following are his blood results: Na 141 mmol/l (137–144), K 3.6 mmol/l (3.5–4.9), U 10 mmol/l (2.5–7.5), Cr 159 micromol/l (60–110), bilirubin 20 micromol/l (2–17), ALP 90 U/l (30–130), ALT 28 U/l (5–30), albumin 30 g/l (35–55), total protein 85 g/l (60–85), corrected Ca 3.3 mmol/l (2.12–2.65), phosphate 1.52 mmol/l (0.7–1.4). Which is the most appropriate next investigation?**

    A. CT scan of the chest
    B. Chest X-ray
    C. Ultrasound of neck
    D. Skeletal survey
    E. Serum ACE

9. **A 70-year-old man presents with difficulty in breathing which started the night before. His lower jaw is so painful that he is unable to speak. On examination, he is dyspnoeic and anxious. He has a temperature of 38.1°C. His lower jaw is swollen, inflamed, and tender. What would be your first step in the management of this patient?**

    A. Seek anaesthetic support
    B. Examine his throat with a tongue depressor
    C. Get a portable chest X-ray
    D. Do blood cultures
    E. Give IV antibiotics

10. **You are called by the technician operating the MRI scanner. An elderly outpatient has attended for an MRI brain, but his medical records are unavailable. You are asked to speak to him to ascertain if he is safe to enter the scanner. Which detail in his past medical history is concerning for an absolute contraindication to undergoing an MRI?**

    A. Fracture of the femur requiring internal fixation five years earlier

    B. Angioplasty of the coronary arteries

    C. Childhood rheumatic fever, with subsequent carciac surgery as an adult, and life-long anti-coagulation

    D. Laparoscopic removal of the gallbladder four months earlier, with dislodgment of a surgical clip at time of surgery

    E. Severe allergic reaction to iodine contrast

11. **A 76-year-old woman with a six-year history of Parkinson's disease complains of watery diarrhoea (x8 motions per day) of three weeks duration. She has lost 3 kg in weight in the last 6 months. She has not noticed any blood in her motions and has no difficulty flushing it down the toilet. There is no recent history of travel and her husband, her only carer, is well. She is normally mobile with a frame around the house and needs assistance from her husband for dressing. In the last week she has become increasingly weak, lost her appetite, and her abdomen has become more distended. Over the last two days she had been unable to mobilize even with assistance. Two weeks ago she was treated by her GP for a urinary tract infection with ciprofloxacin. What is the most likely cause of her diarrhoea?**

    A. *Clostridium difficile* enteritis

    B. Colon cancer

    C. Constipation with overflow

    D. Small bowel bacterial overgrowth

    E. Ulcerative colitis

12. **A 69-year-old woman is referred to the medical admissions unit with a two-week history of bilateral redness of the legs. She says that her legs often swell towards the end of the day, but this has become worse in the last month. The skin on her legs has been dry for a couple of years, but lately it has begun to itch. She had a deep vein thrombosis in the left leg 24 years ago following an operation to remove an ovarian cyst and received anti-coagulation for 6 months. She has been generally well since and takes no regular medication. However, she finished a five-day course of trimethoprim for a urinary tract infection ten days ago. Examination reveals moderate pitting oedema bilaterally, but more marked on the left. Between the knees and ankles, there is erythema and scaling and there are a few excoriations. Select the most appropriate management plan.**

    A. Advise her that she is allergic to trimethoprim
    B. Anti-coagulate with low molecular weight heparin pending venous ultrasound
    C. Commence treatment with an emollient and potent topical steroid
    D. Commence furosemide 40 mg daily and monitor the urea and electrolytes
    E. Obtain blood cultures and commence oral flucloxacillin

13. **Which of the following is not an absolute contraindication to stress testing?**

    A. Acute myocarditis.
    B. Significant systemic infection.
    C. Asymptomatic severe aortic stenosis.
    D. Uncontrolled heart failure.
    E. Unstable angina.

14. **A 72-year old patient is referred to cardiology outpatients with a suspected diagnosis of heart failure. They have no history of previous ischaemic heart disease. The GP has checked the level of serum b-type natriuretic peptide (BNP) and is requesting advice regarding the interpretation of this blood result. Which one of the following may lead to a reduction in serum BNP levels?**

    A. Renal dysfunction (Glomerular filtration rate (GFR) of <60 ml/min)
    B. Chronic obstructive pulmonary disease (COPD)
    C. Angiotensin converting enzyme (ACE) inhibitors
    D. Pulmonary embolism (PE)
    E. Sinus tachycardia

15. **A 71-year-old woman comes in with a swollen left leg, and you suspect a deep vein thrombosis (DVT). Which of these features is least likely to add to her risk of DVT?**

    A. Previous DVT five years ago
    B. Dental surgery under local anaesthetic one week ago
    C. Diagnosis of breast cancer one month ago
    D. Knee replacement three weeks ago.
    E. Bedridden for the past week with influenza

16. **Which of the following is not true concerning neuroradiological investigations?**

    A. MR imaging is preferable for visualizing the posterior fossa
    B. CT scanning is preferable for visualizing the orbits
    C. MR imaging avoids exposure to ionizing radiation
    D. MR imaging has poor visualization of white matter tracts
    E. CT scanning is preferable for the investigation of acute stroke

17. **An 80-year-old woman presents to the medical assessment unit with a week's history of productive cough and pyrexia. She was started on oral amoxicillin by her GP five days ago but she feels worse. She has no known drug allergies. On examination, her pulse was 104 bpm, BP 86/60, respiratory rate of 32/min. CXR revealed a right lower lobe consolidation. ABG on air: pH 7.38, pCO_2 5.6 kPa, pO_2 9.9 kPa. Which is the most appropriate treatment for her?**

    A. Continue amoxicillin and add erythromycin
    B. Switch to intravenous tazocin and clarithromycin
    C. Switch to intravenous vancomycin and clarithromycin
    D. Switch to oral co-amoxiclav and erythromycin
    E. Switch to intravenous benzylpenicillin and clarithromycin

18. **An 89-year-old woman is admitted to the medical assessment unit severely unwell. She is pyrexial with a temperature of 39°C, pulse rate of 120 bpm and blood pressure of 78/40 mmHg. She is tachypnoeic; SpO_2 is 92%. On examination she has bronchial breathing at the right base, a chest X-ray confirms the presence of consolidation. Her urine output is only 25 ml/hour. In response to 2 litres of intravenous 0.9% saline the blood pressure improves to 108/40 mmHg and the urine output over the next hour is 28 ml. Which of the following most accurately describes her condition?**

    A. Sepsis
    B. Systemic inflammatory response syndrome
    C. Severe sepsis
    D. Septic shock
    E. Multiple organ dysfunction syndrome

19. **A 67-year-old woman presents with shortness of breath, orthopnoea, and paroxysmal nocturnal dyspnoea. She has a history of rheumatoid arthritis which began at the age of 24 and she has had multiple drugs for this but at present is taking sulfasalazine, methotrexate, and NSAID. On examination her rheumatoid arthritis is relatively quiescent. Her pulse was 88 sinus rhythm and blood pressure 140/85 mmHg. Jugular venous pressure was elevated 5 cm and she had bilateral basal crepitations. Investigations showed: serum globulin 43 g/l, serum albumin 27 g/l, routine urinalysis, blood –ve, protein 3+. Renal biopsy showed congo red staining positive in the glomeruli. What is the best way to assess response to treatment?**

    A. Atrial natriuretic factor
    B. C-reactive protein
    C. Erythrocyte sedimentation rate
    D. Serum amyloid P scan
    E. Serum globulin levels

20. **A 66-year-old man comes to the radiology department for a PET scan. He has had a transbronchial biopsy which confirmed a squamous cell carcinoma of the bronchus. There is a group of suspicious lymph nodes at the right hilum, and the PET scan is planned to look for tumour activity. Which of the following is the most likely tracer to be used?**

    A. Fluorodopa
    B. Metomidate
    C. Fluoroethyltyrosine
    D. Fluorodexoyglucose
    E. L-methylmethionine

21. **A 65-year-old male non-smoker is referred for investigation of breathlessness and wheeze. He had been previously well until he was admitted four months previously with respiratory failure secondary to severe community acquired pneumonia, and required intubation and ventilation for 12 days. Since discharge he has complained of persistent cough, dyspnoea, wheeze, and difficulty clearing secretions. The lung fields are normal on chest X-ray, with full resolution of the pneumonia. At spirometry, which one of the following flow-volume loops is he most likely to produce (see Figure 4.1)?**

   A. Variable upper (extrathoracic) airway obstruction
   B. Peripheral airway obstruction (reduced mid-expiratory flows)
   C. Normal flow-volume loop
   D. Fixed upper or lower airways obstruction
   E. Variable lower (intrathoracic) airway obstruction

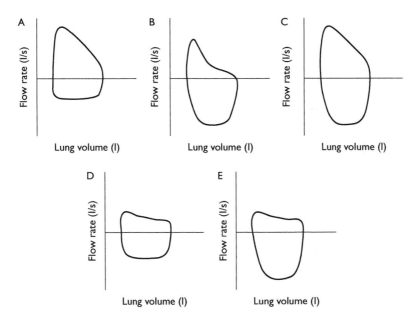

Figure 4.1 Flow-volume loops

GERIATRIC MEDICINE

ANSWERS

1. D. Remove catheter.

This man is improving from the point of view of his pneumonia, and it is virtually impossible to eradicate bacterial colonization from a catheter. Given that the *E. coli* that has grown is multi-resistant, the best course of action is removal of the catheter, and re-testing of the urine. In all likelihood, removal of the catheter will lead to resolution of the infection.

Bowker LK et al., *Oxford Handbook of Geriatric Medicine*, Second Edition, Oxford University Press, 2012, Chapter 24, Infection and immunity, Recurrent urinary tract infection.

2. C. Referral to on-call anaesthetist to consider performing a regional nerve block

Neck of femur repair constitutes emergency surgery. Delayed surgery is associated with increased peri-operatively morbidity and prolonged recovery. Delaying surgery for a patient with known pre-existing mild aortic valve disease for repeat echocardiography is inappropriate. In patients with clinically significant valvular heart disease, echocardiography may aid with planning an anaesthetic (general versus spinal); however, unless it is readily available, decisions to delay should only be taken after discussion between senior anaesthetic, orthopaedic, and orthogeriatric clinicians. Consideration of secondary osteoporosis prevention is essential after any fragility fracture. However, controversy persists regarding the timing, with concern that treatment too early may impair callus formation and bone healing. Capacity should be assessed by clinicians responsible for an intervention. In cases of uncertainty, assessment should be escalated to more senior clinicians. Expert psychiatric assessment may be required in borderline cases. Sudden withdrawal of steroids might precipitate an adrenal crisis in a patient on long-term prednisolone. The dose may need increasing to cover the stress of surgery and their use should be highlighted to the anaesthetist as intravenous doses may be needed peri-operatively.

Nice guidelines [CG103], Delirium: diagnosis, prevention and management, 2010. http://www.nice.org.uk/nicemedia/live/13060/49909/49909.pdf

3. C. Dix–Hallpike test

This patient's symptoms are suggestive of an underlying diagnosis of benign paroxysmal positional vertigo. This classically causes episodes of true vertiginous dizziness, most commonly precipitated by: rolling over in bed, bending over, looking upward (in this case into the cupboard). Whilst the condition is called benign it can carry serious consequences in elderly, frail patients who run the risk of fragility fractures with recurrent falls. This condition can be diagnosed with a simple bedside test called the Dix–Hallpike test (see further reading). The importance of making the diagnosis is that it can be easily cured by performing Epley's manoeuvre (>90% patients cured after two Epley's). The other tests all may have a role to play in investigation of the falling patient but the history here suggests Dix–Hallpike is the most appropriate initial test.

Bromstein A, Benign paroxysmal positional vertigo (BPPV): diagnosis and physical treatment, *ANCR* 2005;5(3):12–14. http://www.acnr.co.uk/pdfs/volume5issue3/v5i3revbbpv.pdf

4. D. Reassurance and 1:1 nursing

Use of sedatives, traditional or atypical anti-psychotics is not recommended with respect to the management of delirium. Instead, the patient should be nursed in a suitable low-risk environment, with adequate lighting and provision of any visual or auditory aids. Use of benzodiazepines or anti-psychotic medication significantly increases the risk of falling or may reduce airway protection, worsening the risk of subsequent lower respiratory tract infection.

Sheehan B et al., *Oxford Specialist Handbook of Old Age Psychiatry*, Oxford University Press, 2009, Chapter 3, Delirium. http://oxfordmedicine.com/view/10.1093/med/9780199216529.001.0001/med-9780199216529-chapter-3#med-9780199216529-div1-56

5. A. Doxycycline

Doxycycline is a tetracycline antibiotic frequently prescribed for exacerbations of chronic bronchitis, with particular effectiveness against *H. influenzae*. Gastrointestinal disturbance, including nausea, vomiting, and diarrhoea are common side effects of tetracyclines. Side effects of paracetamol are rare. Prednisolone has a range of important side effects but nausea and vomiting are not among them. Important side effects of salbutamol include tremor, headache, muscle cramps, and palpitations. Verapamil can cause GI disturbance, but this is predominantly constipation.

https://www.medicines.org.uk/emc/medicine/26378

6. B. Light chain immunoglobulins in the urine

Most of the routine dipstick methods for measuring albumin and protein do not detect other urinary proteins. Light chains are not usually detected by urine dipstick methods. Urine that is highly alkaline may react with the dipstick to cause a false positive reaction. Radio contrast material will cause a false positive test by dipstick and by sulphosalicylic acid. Urinary infection and exercise may cause an increase in urinary albumin/protein and give a positive test.

FPIN's Clinical Inquiries, Urine dipstick for diagnosing urinary tract infection, *American Family Physician* 2006;73(1):129–132.

7. C. MRI scan of spine

This patient gives a history suggestive of acute cord compression due to prolonged use of corticosteroids resulting in a wedge fracture of a vertebra causing cord compression. MRI scan of the spine is the investigation of choice.

Longmore M et al., *Oxford Handbook of Clinical Medicine*, Eighth Edition, Oxford University Press, 2010, Chapter 10, Neurology, Weak legs and cord compression.

8. B. Chest X-ray

This man has hypercalcaemia and hypophosphataemia. In a man of his age, malignancy must be considered. Therefore, the most appropriate next investigation is a chest X-ray to assess for any primary lung lesion with secondary hypercalcaemia or sarcoidosis. A skeletal survey, along with investigations for myeloma, would be the next to look for any lytic lesions due to myeloma or metastatic disease.

Longmore M et al., *Oxford Handbook of Clinical Medicine*, Eighth Edition, Oxford University Press, 2010, Chapter 15, Clinical chemistry, Calcium and phosphate physiology.

9. A. Seek anaesthetic support

This is Ludwig's angina which is an infection of the submandibular space. It usually occurs as a result of dental infection. It is more common in adults than in children. Treatment involves ensuring the airway is secure, giving high flow oxygen, gaining IV access with blood samples and administering IV co-amoxiclav and antipyretics.

Corbridge R, Steventon N, *Oxford Handbook of ENT and Head and Neck Surgery*, Second Edition, Oxford University Press, 2009, Chapter 14, The neck, Neck infections.

10. C. Childhood rheumatic fever, with subsequent carciac surgery as an adult, and life-long anti-coagulation

Absolute contraindications to MRI include insertion of a pacemaker, intracranial ferromagnetic material (e.g. aneurysm clipping), cochlear implant, metal in the orbit, and a prosthetic heart valve. Childhood rheumatic fever and surgery strongly suggest a valve replacement has occurred, and it is likely to be metallic if anti-coagulation is required. Iodine allergy is not a contraindication to receiving MRI contrast agents (which contain gadolinium).

MRIsafety.com. http://www.mrisafety.com/

11. C. Constipation with overflow

Almost all Parkinson's patients suffer from constipation. The loss of appetite may reflect high constipation and the weakness leading to loss of mobility is due to hypokalaemia. The diarrhoea began before the patient was treated with antibiotics and so *Clostridium difficile* is unlikely. Mild weight loss is common in Parkinson's patients and precedes the diarrhoea by such a long lead-in time that if these were due to colonic cancer one would expect more significant weight loss. The abdominal distension might lead one to suspect bacterial overgrowth as could the loss of appetite and mild weight loss but the patient has no predisposing risk facors, such as previous bowel surgery. Whilst there is a bimodal distribution to age of onset of inflammatory bowel disease there is no history of recurrent bowel symptoms, mucus or blood so ulcerative colitis is also unlikely.

Leung FW, Rao SS, Approach to fecal incontinence and constipation in older hospitalized patients. *Hospital Practice* (1995) 2011 Feb;39(1):97–104.

12. C. Commence treatment with an emollient and potent topical steroid

The diagnosis is gravitational (also known as venous, varicose, or stasis) eczema. Her leg swelling is likely to be due to chronic venous insufficiency. The itching is an important pointer towards eczema. The examination lends further evidence, with scaling and excoriation. Bilateral cellulitis or deep vein thrombosis are both very rare and do not give rise to scaling or pruritus. The timing of the presentation in relation to her course of trimethoprim is compatible with a drug eruption; however, eczematous drug eruptions are very unusual and would not be confined to the legs. Gravitational eczema is a common problem affecting the gaiter area. Other signs of chronic venous insufficiency are often found in association. These include oedema, varicose veins, haemosiderin deposition causing macular red-brown discoloration, lipodermatosclerosis—fibrosis of the subcutaneous tissues and induration of the skin leading to an 'inverted champagne bottle' appearance—ulceration, and atrophie blanche manifesting as white scar-like areas. The eczema usually responds well to an emollient (not aqueous cream, which is a soap substitute) and potent topical steroid ointment. Compression stockings can also be helpful, though are not always well tolerated.

Varicose Veins in the Legs: The Diagnosis and Management of Varicose Veins. Editors National Clinical Guideline Centre (UK). London: National Institute for Health and Care Excellence (UK); 2013 Jul.

13. C. Asymptomatic severe aortic stenosis

Traditionally, it was felt that a patient with severe aortic stenosis should not be stressed. It is now recognized that exercise in experienced centres in a controlled environment can be useful in the management of a patient with asymptomatic severe aortic stenosis, for example to guide timing of intervention. This does not apply to a patient who already meets criteria for treatment, as exercise in symptomatic aortic stenosis is absolutely contraindicated. Exercise in acute myocarditis can provoke arrhythmia and should be avoided. A patient with significant systemic pyrexial illness should not be exercised until resolved. Heart failure should be treated and controlled before stress testing. Patients with stable chest pains can be exercised, but if a diagnosis of unstable angina has been made, this is contraindicated.

Guidelines on the management of valvular heart disease (version 2012), *European Heart Journal* 2012;33:2451–2496.

14. C. Angiotensin converting enzyme (ACE) inhibitors

B-type natriuretic peptide (BNP) is a cardiac neurohormone secreted from the cardiac ventricles in response to ventricular volume expansion and pressure overload, the result being arterial and venous dilatation. Essentially, this peptide can be thought of as the polar opposite to the renin-angiotensin system in terms of maintenance of arterial pressure. In heart failure the serum level of BNP is elevated. There is evidence suggesting that the degree of elevation is related to the severity of the underlying cardiac dysfunction. The test is, however, affected by a variety of factors. The level can be reduced in patients on treatment with diuretics, ACE inhibitors, angiotensin II receptor antagonists, and aldosterone antagonists. Conversely, the level can be elevated in patients with cardiac ischaemia, left ventricular hypertrophy, right ventricular overload (can be secondary to pulmonary pathology, e.g. PE, COPD) or renal dysfunction. Recently published NICE guidelines on the management of chronic heart failure suggest that BNP measurement should have a role in diagnosis of suspected heart failure. They advise checking serum BNP levels in patients with suspected heart failure without previous myocardial infarction (MI). If the level is <400 pg/ml, they advise urgent referral for trans-thoracic echocardiography and assessment by a specialist within two weeks. In patients with a serum BNP <100 pg/ml their guidance suggests that in an untreated patient this makes a diagnosis of heart failure unlikely.

NICE guidelines [CG108], Management of chronic heart failure in adults in primary and secondary care, August 2010. http://www.nice.org.uk/nicemedia/live/13099/50517/50517.pdf

15. B. Dental surgery under local anaesthetic one week ago

When assessing a patient with a potential DVT, the risk factors should be taken into account to weigh up the probability that this is the diagnosis. A commonly used system is the Wells' criteria (see Box 4.1). A score is calculated out of a possible 9 points, depending on the risk factors and certain clinical features that are present. This can help the clinician to decide whether to treat the patient on clinical suspicion, wait for a scan, or look for an alternative diagnosis. For further information, see further reading. This includes a table of the Well's scoring system. D-dimers are also used to assess the risk, and are useful in helping to rule out a DVT if negative. However, they may increase for a variety of reasons including recent surgery. They are therefore not always useful and if positive do not confirm the diagnosis.

Page P, Skinner G, *Emergencies in Clinical Medicine*, Oxford University Press, 2007, Chapter 3, Cardiology, Deep vein thrombosis.

Box 4.1 Wells' score for DVT probability

Active cancer (treatment ongoing, or within 6 months or palliative)	+1
Paralysis or recent plaster immobilization of the lower extremities	+1
Recently bedridden for >3 days or major surgery <4 weeks ago	+1
Localized tenderness along the distribution of the deep venous system	+1
Entire leg swelling	+1
Calf swelling >3 cm compared to the asymptomatic leg	+1
	+1
Pitting oedema (greater in the symptomatic leg)	+1
Previous documented DVT	+1
Collateral superficial veins (non-varicose)	+1
Alternative diagnosis as likely or greater than that of DVT	−2

- Score ≥3—high probability (75%)
- Score 1–2—intermediate probability (17%)
- Score ≤0—low probability (3%)

Reproduced from Page P, Skinne G, *Emergencies in Clinical Medicine*, 2008 with permission from Oxford University Press.

16. D. MR imaging has poor visualization of white matter tracts

Posterior fossa lesions are better visualized with magnetic resonance imaging. The resolution on MR scanners can now be used to visualize white matter tracts and tractography is beginning to have more of a clinical role. It also has the benefit of having no ionizing radiation exposure. CT scanning is preferable for the investigation of acute stroke (it is quick and might pick up middle cerebral artery occlusions—the 'dense MCA sign') and for visualizing the orbits.

Manji H et al., *Oxford Handbook of Neurology*, Oxford University Press, 2007, Chapter 7, Neuroradiology.

17. B. Switch to intravenous tazocin and clarithromycin

Her CURB 65 score is 3. Hence, she should be switched to intravenous tazocin and clarithromycin. In view of the severity, it would be well worth getting a set of blood cultures and sending urine to test for pneumococcal and legionella urinary antigen. It is always advisable to check with one's local hospital microbiological guidelines because microbiological data, flora, and resistance patterns vary from place to place.

Longmore M et al., *Oxford Handbook of Clinical Medicine*, Eighth Edition, Oxford University Press, 2010, Chapter 4, Chest medicine, Pneumonia, British Thoracic Society Guidelines for Community-Acquired Pneumonia 2009.

18. C. Severe sepsis

Although the terms listed are often used interchangeably, in medical practice they have distinct definitions. The systemic inflammatory response syndrome is defined as the presence of two or more of temperature disturbance (pyrexia or hypothermia), tachycardia, tachypnoea (or hypocapnia due to hyperventilation), and an abnormal white cell count (leucopenia or leucocytosis). Sepsis is SIRS but in the presence of a confirmed infective process. Severe sepsis is sepsis associated with hypotension, hypoperfusion (demonstrated, for example, by a low urine output), or organ dysfunction. Septic shock is sepsis with persistent arterial hypotension desite adequate, aggressive fluid resuscitation. Multiple organ dysfunction syndrome is the presence of altered organ function in acutely ill patients such that homoeostasis cannot be maintained without intervention. It usually involves two or more organ systems and in many patients represents the end of a continuum from sepsis to severe sepsis. This patient has severe sepsis—there are sufficient criteria present for the diagnosis of SIRS, a clear infective process, and oliguria (indicative of renal dysfunction/hypoperfusion). Improvement in the blood pressure in response to filling excludes the possibility of septic shock. The criteria are not met for diagnosis of multiple organ dysfunction syndrome.

Singer M, Webb A, *Oxford Handbook of Critical Care*, Third Edition, Oxford University Press, 2009, Chapter 31, Infection and inflammation, Systemic inflammation/multi-organ failure—causes.

19. D. Serum amyloid P scan

Secondary amyloidosis is the result of the deposition of serum amyloid A (SAA), which is one of the acute phase proteins. Secondary amyloidosis in the UK was historically associated with chronic infections (e.g. osteomyelitis, tuberculosis, and bronchiectasis), but it is now more commonly seen in association with chronic inflammatory conditions (e.g. rheumatoid arthritis, ankylosing spondylitis, psoriatic arthropathy, and inflammatory bowel disease). Detection of amyloid is by congo red staining with apple green birefringence in polarized light. Scintigraphy using 123I-labelled amyloid P component is beneficial in identifying the extent of the amyloid deposition and the response to treatment. However, it is not widely available. Resolution of proteinuria in patients with renal involvement only may be helpful in assessing response to treatment, as may measurement of free light chains.

Provan D et al., *Oxford Handbook of Clinical Haematology*, Third Edition, Oxford University Press, 2009, Chapter 8, Paraproteinaemias.

20. D. Fluorodexoyglucose

Fluorodeoxyglucose is commonly used in the imaging of bronchial tumours. Metomidate and fluorodopa are tracers used in the imaging of adrenal tumours. Fluoroethyltyrosine and L-methylmethionine are tracers used in the imaging of brain tumours. The field of PET scanning is rapidly expanding, with both this and functional MRI both now widely used in specialist centres for evaluation of malignant disease.

Darby MJ et al., *Oxford Handbook of Medical Imaging*, Oxford University Press, 2011, Chapter 1, Techniques. http://oxfordmedicine.com/view/10.1093/med/9780199216369.001.0001/med-9780199216369-chapter-0001

21. D. Fixed upper or lower airways obstruction

The patient presents several weeks after a period of intubation with symptoms of upper airways obstruction (although he does not complain of stridor, patients will often describe this symptom as wheeze, and the clinician should be able to differentiate this on history and examination). The most likely cause is laryngeal or tracheal stenosis, an important late complication of intubation that can occur in up to 10% of patients. The classic spirometric finding is one of a fixed obstruction to airflow, during both inspiration (causing stridor) and expiration, though spirometry may not be able to detect mild cases, particularly if underlying lung disease complicates the picture. Further investigation includes bronchoscopy and CT of the entire tracheal length. Laryngeal and tracheal injury from artificial airways is the most common cause of upper airway obstruction; alternative diagnoses to consider include goitre, bronchial stenosis, and endo-bronchial tumours. Variable upper airway obstruction may be found in unilateral or bilateral vocal cord paralysis (the cords are pushed apart on expiration, relieving the obstruction). Reduced mid-expiratory flows are seen in conditions of small airway collapse or obstruction, such as COPD, asthma, or cystic fibrosis. There is relative preservation of the peak expiratory flow, but collapse of the middle portion of the expiratory flow-volume loop. Variable intra-thoracic obstruction may be caused by tumours of the lower airways or main bronchus.

Maskell N, Millar A, *Oxford Desk Reference: Respiratory Medicine*, Oxford University Press, 2009, Chapter 2, Respiratory physiology. http://oxfordmedicine.com/view/10.1093/med/9780199239122.001.0001/med-9780199239122-chapter-002

1. **Regarding onchocerciasis, which of the following statement are incorrect?**
   A. Most cases occur in tropical Africa
   B. Subcutaneous nodules are common
   C. Chronic onchodermatitis causes skin atrophy and a change in pigmentation which resembles a leopard skin
   D. Chronic onchocerciasis causes elephantitis
   E. Blindness is caused by migration of microfilaria to the ocular tissues and the body's subsequent inflammatory response to it

2. **A 23-year-old woman who admits to unprotected sexual intercourse with a number of partners is diagnosed with syphillis. She is treated by the infectious disease nurses with a 14-day course of doxycycline, but they ask you to review her care as they are concerned about her serology results. Pre-treatment: VDRL positive; TPHA titre 1:256. Post-treatment: VDRL negative; TPHA titre 1:16. What would you recommend?**
   A. Repeat doxycycline
   B. Give azithromycin
   C. Do nothing
   D. Give ceftriaxone IM
   E. Give ciprofloxacin

3. **A 53-year-old abattoir worker presents with two months of fevers
    and night sweats. On examination he has splenomegaly and
    finger clubbing. There is a loud pansystolic murmur, and trans-
    oesophageal echocardiography demonstrates thickening of the
    mitral valve with a discrete vegetation on the anterior leaflet.
    Multiple sets of blood cultures drawn prior to the administration
    of antibiotics are sterile and the patient fails to improve with
    intravenous antibiotic therapy. What is the most likely cause of
    this presentation?**

    A. *Coxiella burnetti*
    B. *Mycobacterium bovis*
    C. *Neisseria gonorrhoea*
    D. *Staphylococcus aureus*
    E. *Streptococcus viridans*

4. **A 21-year-old female schoolteacher presents with a four-
    day history of fever and a rash. The rash is maculopapular. It
    began around the ears and spread to the rest of the body. On
    examination she is febrile with a temperature of 38°C. She has
    red eyes and a runny nose. She has a dry cough. There are small,
    white spots visible on her buccal mucosa. Which of the following
    is the most likely diagnosis?**

    A. Measles
    B. Meningococcal meningitis
    C. Mumps
    D. Syphilis
    E. Typhoid

5. **A 35-year-old man is due to be commenced on treatment for
    hepatitis C virus with pegylated interferon alpha and ribavirin.
    He is keen to discuss adverse effects of treatment. Which of the
    following are NOT recognized adverse effects/concerns regarding
    treatment of this patient?**

    A. Alopecia
    B. Depressed mood
    C. Erythema multiforme
    D. Haemolytic anaemia
    E. Need to avoid conception for at least six months after therapy

6. **A 17-year-old woman presents with headache and neck stiffness of two days' duration. Lumbar puncture results are as follows: WCC 380 x 10^6/ l (80% lymphocytes) RCC 27 x 10^6/l, protein 0.64 g/l, Glu 4.1 mmol/l (serum 5.6 mmol/l). Gram stain reveals no organisms. What is the most likely diagnosis?**

    A. Enterovirus
    B. Haemophilus influenzae
    C. Mycobacterium tuberculosis
    D. Neisseria meningitidis
    E. Streptococcus pneumoniae

7. **A 45-year-old man is seen urgently at the hepatitis clinic having defaulted from follow-up for several years. He has asked for review because of rapidly worsening ascites. He has a 20-year history of hepatitis C infection and cirrhosis. On examination he has jaundice and ascites. A tender liver edge is palpable 4 cm below the costal margin. His GP has checked routine bloods prior to his attendance at clinic and finds anaemia, thrombocytopaenia, and deranged liver function tests as shown in Table 5.1. Which of the following investigations is most important to establish the cause of his deterioration?**

    Table 5.1 Liver function test results

Bilirubin	125	(0–19 istmol/l)
AST	65	(19–40 iu/l)
ALT	42	(10–40 iu/l)
ALP	467	(30–120 iu/l)
GGT	345	(<51 mg/l)

    A. Alpha-fetoprotein
    B. Hepatitis B surface antigen
    C. Hepatitis C PCR
    D. Hepatitis D (Delta) antibody
    E. Serum ethanol level

8. **Regarding the life cycle of the malarial parasite, which of the following statements is correct?**

    A. For the parasite to propagate, a female and male sporozoite must be ingested by the mosquito in a blood meal
    B. After maturation within the mosquito gut wall, the oocyst bursts to release merozoites which are stored in the mosquito salivary glands
    C. The malaria parasite is transmitted by the female Aedes mosquito
    D. The trophozoites of the malaria parasite are responsible for infecting the human host
    E. The part of the parasite life cycle that occurs in the human host is the asexual cycle

9. **A 32-year-old woman with recurrent genital herpes simplex comes to see you for advice. She takes regular aciclovir as prophylaxis against recurrent attacks, and she is three months pregnant. She asks you what the risks of neonatal infection are if she delivers vaginally during a recurrence. Which of the following percentages fits best with the risks of infection of the neonate?**

   A. 80%
   B. 60%
   C. 40%
   D. 15%
   E. <5%

10. **A 22-year-old nursery nurse comes to the clinic with headache, confusion, and a stiff neck. She also has suffered from severe nausea over the past few days and has had episodes of diarrhoea. Apparently a number of children at the nursery where she works have also become unwell. On examination her BP is 149/84, pulse is 90 and regular, she has a temperature of 38°C. Her abdomen is soft but generally tender, bowel sounds are present. There is meningism and left-sided sensory inattention on neurological examination. There is extensive bruising. Investigations: Hb 8.9 (fragmented red cells), WCC 13.1, PLT 64, Na 137, K 5.9, Cr 195. Which of the following is the most likely diagnosis?**

   A. Thrombotic thrombocytopaenic purpura (TTP)
   B. Salmonellosis
   C. Viral meningitis
   D. Herpes encephalitis
   E. Idiopathic thrombocytopaenic purpura

11. **A 24-year-old woman presents to A&E with a three-day history of progressive left-sided weakness and headaches. She is noted to be febrile with a temperature of 38°C. She is known to be HIV-positive and the most recent CD4 count was 80/mm^3. A CT scan of her head reveals multiple ring-enhancing lesions. Which of the following is the most likely diagnosis?**

   A. Tuberculoma
   B. Lymphoma
   C. Pneumococcal meningitis
   D. Toxoplasmosis
   E. Viral encephalitis

12. **A 21-year-old student comes to the emergency department complaining of exquisitely painful genital ulceration and problems passing urine. She admits to unprotected sexual intercourse with a casual partner. On examination there are multiple small vulval ulcers with obvious surrounding erythema. Some of the lesions are beginning to crust over. Which of the following is the most appropriate treatment?**

    A. Doxycycline 100 mg daily for seven days
    B. Famcyclovir 250 mg TDS for five days
    C. Ciprofloxacin 500 mg BD for seven days
    D. Topical acyclovir BD for five days.
    E. Cephalexin 500 mg BD for seven days

13. **A 34-year-old sheep farmer presents with a small painful nodule at the base of the index finger dorsally. He first noticed the lesion a week earlier. It is red and painful. He otherwise remains stable. Two of his children had similar lesions on the hand four weeks earlier that resolved spontaneously. What is the most likely diagnosis?**

    A. Orf
    B. Lichen planus
    C. Impetigo
    D. Psoriasis
    E. Paronychia

14. **A 56-year-old Welsh farmer attends the medical admission unit with headaches, myalgia, nausea and vomiting, and jaundice. He had been previously well without medical problems and took no medication. On examination he was slightly confused, jaundiced with conjunctival haemorrhage. Bloods revealed deranged liver and renal function. What is the most likely cause of this patient's presentation?**

    A. Bartonella
    B. Malaria
    C. Hepatitis B
    D. Leptospirosis
    E. Brucellosis

15. In cutaneous leishmaniasis which of the following statements is correct?

A. An amastigote is transferred to the human vector
B. The parasite is transferred through the bite of a sandfly
C. Parasites multiply in the extracellular space in the dermis of the skin
D. Raised red nodules appear within hours to days after the initial inoculation
E. CL classically exhibits symmetrical lesions

16. Regarding infection with *E. histolytica*, which one of the following statements is incorrect?

A. Transmission is usually faecal–oral
B. Most carriers are asymptomatic
C. Symptoms are due to pathogenic amoebae penetrating the mucous barrier of the gut causing diarrhoeal illness and/or extra-intestinal disease
D. With dysentery resolution, an amoebic liver abscess is formed
E. Treatment is with tinidazole

17. Regarding the life cycle of the malarial parasite, which of the following statements is correct?

A. For the parasite to propagate, a female and male sporozoite must be ingested by the mosquito in a blood meal
B. After maturation within the mosquito gut wall, the oocyst bursts to release merozoites which are stored in the mosquito salivary glands
C. The malaria parasite is transmitted by the female *Aedes* mosquito
D. The trophozoites of the malaria parasite are responsible for infecting the human host
E. The part of the parasite lifecycle that occurs in the human host is the asexual cycle

18. Which of the following statements is about infection with the dengue virus?

A. It is transmitted by the female Anopheles mosquito
B. Incubation time is approximately 21 days
C. Symptoms can include rash, fever, myalgia, and shock
D. Treatment includes fluids and aspirin
E. Travellers going to dengue-affected areas should be vaccinated

19. **A 28-year-old Indian man presents with shortness of breath and night sweats. He is HIV-positive and had TB as a child for which he cannot recall if he had any treatment or not. On examination his respiratory rate is 30. The right base is stony dull to percussion with reduced air entry. CXR reveals a right-sided pleural effusion. Three sputum samples do not stain for acid-fast bacilli on Ziehl–Neelsen stain. Which of the following would be the most useful in order to obtain the highest yield for the diagnosis of TB?**

A. Heaf test
B. CD4 count
C. Pleural fluid microscopy, culture, and sensitivity
D. Pleural biopsy microscopy, culture, and sensitivity
E. Pleural biopsy histology

20. **A 32-year-old woman is six months pregnant with her third child. She has been suffering from dysuria and frequency over the past three days. On examination she is pyrexial 37.9°C and has suprapubic tenderness. Her urine is positive for blood and protein, routine bloods are normal. She is allergic to penicillin. Which of the following antibiotics is the most appropriate choice for her?**

A. Trimethoprim
B. Ciprofloxacin
C. Doxycycline
D. Erythromycin
E. Cephalexin

21. **A 62-year-old man who has a history of recurrent cholecystitis comes to the emergency department complaining of recurrent lethargy and night sweats over the past few weeks. The only other past history of note is some recent dental work. On examination his BP is 135/75, his pulse is 78 and regular. There is a systolic murmur on auscultation of the heart and he has a mild pyrexia of 37.8°C. Investigations: Hb 10.9, WCC 10.1, PLT 183, Na 138, K 4.4, Cr 123, ESR 88; Blood cultures: S. bovis. Where is the most likely source of infection?**

A. Skin
B. Oral cavity
C. Biliary tree
D. Large bowel
E. Urinary tract

22. **A 17-year-old sixth-form student comes to the clinic with a dry cough and a rash. Her mother apparently refused childhood vaccinations on her behalf. She has a temperature of 40°C, a dry cough and a rash over her face neck and upper chest. There are small red spots on examing her buccal mucosa. Which of the following is the most likely diagnosis?**

    A. German measles
    B. Measles
    C. Mumps
    D. Meningococcal meningitis
    E. Streptococcal meningitis

23. **Which of the following condition is associated with hepatitis B. infection?**

    A. Microscopic polyangitis
    B. Polyarteritis nodosa
    C. Psoriatic arthritis
    D. Rheumatoid arthritis
    E. Systemic lupus erythematosus

24. **A 25-year-old man attends A&E feeling unwell. He complains of malaise, fever, pharyngitis, and arthralgia. He had asthma as a child and did not take any regular medications. He returned from a business trip to Malawi four weeks previously and admits to skipping doses of his anti-malarial medication, particularly if he was out entertaining clients. On examination he has a widespread maculopapular rash and generalized lymphadenopathy. He is not anaemic, and has normal cardiovascular, respiratory, and abdominal examinations. Examination of the affected joints does not reveal any swelling or deficit in function. What is the most likely diagnosis?**

    A. Typhoid
    B. Plasmodium ovale malaria
    C. Infectious mononucleosis
    D. Acute HIV infection
    E. Dengue fever

25. **A 21-year-old student presents with symptoms of haematuria and dull bladder pain above his symphysis pubis. On further question he tells you that he has been travelling as a backpacker accross Africa and the Far East, stayed on local camp sites, and swam in a number of local areas of open water. On examination he has dull tenderness across his lower abdomen. Investigations: Hb 10.9, WCC 11.2 (raised eosinophils), PLT 178, Na 138, K 4.3, Cr 122, urine blood +++. Which of the following has he most likely been colonized with?**

    A. *S. japonicum*
    B. *S. mansoni*
    C. *S. mekongi*
    D. *S. intercalatum*
    E. *S. haematobium*

26. **Treatment of *Mycobacterium tuberculosis* infection at which of the following sites requires routine extension of antimycobacterial therapy beyond six months?**

    A. Caecum
    B. Central nervous system
    C. Cervical lymphadenitis
    D. Disseminated (milliary) disease
    E. Pericardium

27. **A 35-year-old man presents with headache and left arm weakness. An MRI brain shows a solitary mass lesion within the right basal ganglia which enhances on administration of gadolinium contrast and demonstrates mass effect. A presumptive diagnosis of neoplastic disease is made and a brain biopsy planned. However, as part of the diagnostic evaluation, an HIV test is positive with a CD4 count of 34 cells/microlitre. Along with CNS malignancy, which infectious diagnosis should also be strongly considered?**

    A. Cryptococcus neoformans
    B. Cytomegalovirus
    C. JC virus
    D. Mycobacterium tuberculosis
    E. *Toxoplasmosis gondii*

28. **Which of the following regarding management of needlestick injury is true?**

A. Bleeding should not be encouraged

B. If HIV post-exposure prophylaxis is given, adverse effects of medication are a common problem

C. Risk of transmission of hepatitis C can be reduced with specific immunoglobulin

D. The patient who is the source of the injury can be tested regardless of their ability to consent

E. Transmission of hepatitis B should be prevented by administration of a single dose of hepatitis B vaccine

29. **Which of the following is an RNA virus?**

A. Epstein–Barr virus

B. Hepatitis B virus

C. Hepatitis C virus

D. Herpes simplex virus

E. Varicella zoster virus

30. **Which of the following diseases is NOT correctly matched with its vector?**

A. African trypanosomiasis—Tsetse fly

B. Leishmaniasis—*Aedes* mosquito

C. Lyme disease—*Ixodes* ticks

D. Malaria—*Anopheles* mosquito

E. Schistosomiasis—Freshwater snails

31. **A 45-year-old man presents with weight loss and chronic diarrhoea. He complains of odynophagia. On examination he has oral candida. An HIV test is positive with a CD4 count of 12 cells/mm^3 and a viral load of 124,000 copies/ml. His family report that he has been mildly confused for several months and a mini-mental state examination reveals a score of 25/30. On examination he has brisk reflexes in the right leg with an upgoing plantar reflex on both sides. Coordination is mildly impaired on the right. MRI of the brain shows multiple non-enhancing lesions within the white matter on both sides. The lesions are not causing a mass effect. Which infectious agent is most likely to be directly responsible for these findings?**

A. Cryptococcus neoformans

B. Cytomegalovirus

C. Human immunodeficiency virus

D. JC virus

E. *Toxoplasmosis gondii*

32. **A 21-year-old male student comes to the university health service. He has spent his summer holidays travelling in Thailand and has eaten very cheaply, often from street vendors. His major symptoms are abdominal pain, bloating, and intermittent foul-smelling diarrhoea. On examination his BP is 112/82, his temperature is 37.8°C. He has a mildly distended abdomen with mild tenderness and active bowel sounds. Blood results are entirely normal. Which of the following fits best with this clinical picture?**

    A. Campylobacter
    B. Shigella
    C. Salmonella
    D. Yersnia
    E. Giardia

33. **A 19-year-old gap year traveller is admitted directly from the airport after returning from a backpacking trip to Central America. Apparently he had an open jaw ticket and had been travelling the world. His vaccination history is unavailable. There had been a flu-like illness 7–10 days earlier, and now he is deeply jaundiced with extensive bruising and blood loss around his gum line. Which of the following is the most likely diagnosis?**

    A. Dengue fever
    B. Malaria
    C. Weil's disease
    D. Yellow fever
    E. Influenza

34. **A 47-year-old farmer is admitted with fever, cough, bruising, and jaundice. He has hepatomegaly and is oliguric. Investigations show: haemoglobin 11.5 mg/l, urea 41 mmol/l, serum creatinine 653 micromol/l, serum potassium 6.3 mmol/l, bilirubin 68 micromol/l, alkaline phosphatase 391 IU/l, ALT 154 IU/l, GGT 184 IU/l. What is the likely cause of his illness?**

    A. Acute viral hepatitis
    B. Hepato-renal syndrome
    C. Legionnaire's disease
    D. Mycoplasma pneumonia
    E. Weil's disease

35. **A 22-year-old homosexual male presents to clinic complaining of a painless lesion on his penis. His last sexual contact was three weeks ago with a man. He has not been feeling otherwise unwell. On examination there is a small rubbery painless ulcer and some associated inguinal lymphadenopathy. What is the most appropriate treatment?**

    A. A single dose of intramuscular penicillin G benzathine 2.4 mU
    B. Oral aciclovir 200 mg five times a day for five days
    C. Oral aciclovir 800 mg five times a day for ten days
    D. Oral metronidazole 800 mg three times a day for five days
    E. Topical acyclovir cream as required

36. **An elderly Jamaican man presents to the GP with confusion. As part of his confusion screen syphilis serology is sent. He is unable to recall if he was previously treated for syphilis. The results are as follows: IgG positive, TPPA positive, RPR 1 in 4. Which of the following is NOT a possible interpretation of these serology results?**

    A. He has an alternative diagnosis such as TB or lupus and was previously treated for syphilis
    B. He has been previously treated for syphilis but has persistent infection and will therefore require further treatment
    C. He has had yaws in the past
    D. He has Lyme disease and has no evidence of past or current syphilis
    E. He has untreated syphilis infection

37. **A 19-year-old military recruit complains of recurrent skin abscesses. He has a current abscess on his arm causing swelling and fever. A nasal swab reveals MRSA, sensitive to tetracyclines. The most appropriate management would be:**

    A. Apply topical fusidic acid to the lesion and surrounding area for five days
    B. Chlorhexidine 4% bodywash daily from neck to feet and mupirocin nasal ointment for five days followed by a combination of oral doxycycline and rifampicin for five days
    C. Chlorhexidine 4% bodywash daily from neck to feet and mupirocin nasal ointment for five days followed by oral flucloxacillin for five days
    D. Chlorhexidine 4% bodywash daily from neck to feet and mupirocin nasal ointment for 5 days. There is no need for antibiotics
    E. Oral flucloxacillin for 5 days followed by chlorhexidine 4% bodywash daily from neck to feet and mupirocin nasal ointment.

38. **A doctor visits A&E as they have just had a needle-stick injury from a patient on the ward. The patient was from Zimbabwe and their HIV status was not known. The donor patient has agreed to have an HIV test but the result will not be available for 36 hours. The doctor is known to have an hep B sAb level of >100 IU. What action is most appropriate?**

    A. HIV post-exposure prophylaxis should be started immediately. The donor patient should be tested for HIV, hep B, and hep C, and the duration of prophylaxis can be reviewed with these results

    B. The doctor needs a hepatitis B. booster immunization but no HIV prophylaxis

    C. The doctor needs HIV prophylaxis immediately and a booster for hepatitis B

    D. The donor should be tested for HIV, hep B, and hep C, and a decision can be made regarding prophylaxis for HIV once these results are available

    E. There is no risk to the doctor and they can be reassured

39. **A 26-year-old woman presents to A&E with coryzal symptoms, cough, and fever of two days' duration. Her 2-year-old child was unwell prior to the onset of her illness. On examination she has a respiratory rate of 22/min, temperature of 39°C, and bronchial breath sounds at the left base. A CXR shows a small area of consolidation obscuring the left hemidiaphragm. Blood tests show a CRP of 97, Hb 11.8, WCC 2.2, Plt 230, urea 3.6, Cr 86, Na 133, K 4.5. She is sent home with oral amoxicillin but presents a few hours later severely unwell with multilobar consolidation and hypotension. What is the appropriate management at this stage?**

    A. Call ITU and administer IV augmentin and clarithromycin

    B. Call ITU and administer IV clindamycin, linezolid, and rifampicin

    C. Call ITU and administer IV rifampicin

    D. Continue oral amoxicillin

    E. This pneumonia is likely to be caused by *Staphylococcus aureus* and flucloxacillin should therefore be administered in combination with other agents

40. **A 68-year-old man presents with a two-week history of progressive decline in general health, malaise, and confusion. Three days prior to his admission to the hospital he became short of breath and was febrile. While he is in hospital, the echocardiogram confirms the presence of vegetations. The blood culture grew *Streptococcus bovis* from repeated samples. Which one of the following statements is true?**

    A. *Streptococcus bovis* is part of the normal oral flora

    B. *Streptococcus bovis* is a Gram-negative bacillus

    C. Intravenous vancomycin is the treatment of choice

    D. Mortality is estimated as 50% of cases

    E. Colonoscopy would be advised to exclude bowel malignancy

41. **A 76-year-old man is admitted with abdominal pain, rigors, and pyrexia. He is normally wheelchair-bound due to a combination of Parkinson's disease and fixed flexion deformities after bilateral knee replacements. He undertakes intermittent self-catheterization due to benign prostatic hypertrophy and also had Raynaud's disease and Barrett's oesophagus. He lives with his wife. He is taking furosemide, candesartan, ropinirole, senna, trimethoprim, esomeprazole, tamsulosin, meloxicam, co-beneldopa, and simvastatin. He has not been compliant with his medication for three days prior to admission to hospital. On examination he is confused, pulse 105/min regular, BP 97/63, respiratory rate 28/min, oxygen saturations 97% on 5 litres of oxygen. He has decreased air entry in both lungs with no advential sounds. Heart sounds are normal. There is tenderness on palpation in the supra-pubic region and right upper quadrant with no guarding. Investigations: Hb11.3 g/dl(13–18), WBC 13.7 x10^9/l (4–11), Plt 584 x10^9/l (150–400); urea and electrolytes normal apart from creatine 256 micromol/l (60–110), CRP 110 mg/l (<10), ALP 125 U/l (45–105), ALT 89 U/l (5–35); urinalysis: leucocytes +ve, nitrites –ve; blood culture Gram –ve bacilli in all bottles, ABGs, HCO$_3$ 12.6 mmol/l (19–24), base excess –9.2 mmol/l (±2), lactate 8.9 mmol/l (0.6–1.8). He is treated initially with gentamicin and later switched to ciprofloxacin. On day 11 he becomes tachypnoeic with a respiratory rate of 40/min, fever of 38°C, his BP is 96/50 and heart rate 120 bpm, there is a pan-systolic murmur audible at the left sternal edge with no radiation. Jugular venous pressure is not raised and there are no splinter haemorrhages or haematuria. Oxygen saturation is 94% on air. The remainder of the physical examination is normal. Further investigations: CRP 226 mg/l (<10), WBC 16.5 x10^9/l (4–11), neutrophils 11.2 x10^9/l (1.5–7.0), blood cultures no growth, CTPA: raised R hemidiaphragm, R basal effusion, cyst in R lobe of liver, white cell scan slight concentration in R knee, transthoracic echo normal. What is the most likely diagnosis?**

    A. Infective endocarditis
    B. Liver abscess
    C. Pulmonary embolism
    D. Pyelonephritis
    E. Septic arthritis

42. **An 80-year-old patient who was treated with IV antibiotics for a chest infection developed severe diarrhoea. *C. difficile* toxins were identified from the stool specimen. Oral metronidazole was not successful and the patient's diarrhoea persisted. At this stage which one of the following treatments would be appropriate?**

    A. Intravenous metronidazole
    B. Oral vancomycin
    C. Intravenous immunoglobulin
    D. Intravenous vancomycin
    E. Intravenous gentamycin

43. **A 60-year-old diabetic woman is admitted to the emergency unit with high fever, rigors, and severe pain and swelling in the right knee. Her temperature is 39.2°C. Examination of the right knee reveals a red, hot, swollen, and tender joint. What is your next immediate action?**

    A. Swab and culture of the overlying skin
    B. Plain X-ray of the knee
    C. MRI of the knee
    D. Blood culture
    E. Synovial fluid aspiration and analysis

44. **You are working in the A&E department and regularly see patients with infectious diseases. Which of the following conditions, if suspected or diagnosed, does NOT require you to notify the Health Protection Agency?**

    A. Measles
    B. Mumps
    C. Rubella
    D. Malaria
    E. Shingles

45. **The following are all used to treat HIV infection. Which of the following is a non-nucleoside reverse transcriptase inhibitor (NNRTI)?**

    A. Emtricitabine
    B. Lamivudine
    C. Nevirapine
    D. Tenofovir
    E. Zidovudine

46. **A 32-year-old woman presents with a four-day history of fever, productive cough, and shortness of breath. Chest radiograph shows consolidation in the left lower zone. She is known to be HIV positive. A blood culture is taken on admission, and is positive for bacteria. Gram staining of the blood reveals Gram-positive cocci in pairs and chains. The organism likely to be causing her illness is:**

    A. *Enterococcus faecium*
    B. *Haemophilus influenzae*
    C. *Pseudomonas aeruginosa*
    D. *Staphylococcus aureus*
    E. *Streptococcus pneumoniae*

47. **A 22-year-old man presents to the sexual health clinic with a three-day history of purulent urethral discharge. Gram stain of the discharge reveals intracellular Gram-negative diplococci. The likeliest cause of the discharge is:**

    A. *Candida albicans*
    B. *Chlamydia trachomatis*
    C. *Neisseria gonorrhoeae*
    D. *Staphylococcus aureus*
    E. *Treponema pallidum* (syphilis)

48. **The following are all used to treat HIV infection. Which of the following is a nucleotide analogue reverse transcriptase inhibitor (NRTI)?**

    A. Atazanavir
    B. Lopinavir
    C. Ritonavir
    D. Saquinavir
    E. Tenofovir

49. **A 32-year-old woman presents to casualty with high fever, nausea, and joint pains. Her blood pressure is 110/70, heart rate is 122, and she has impaired consciousness, with a Glasgow Coma Score of 13 out of 15. She returned two weeks ago from a visit to her relatives in West Africa, where she was born and spent most of her life. She has not taken malaria chemoprophylaxis. Malaria is suspected and thin blood film confirms the presence of malaria parasites infecting red blood cells. Which of the following species is the likeliest cause of her illness?**

    A. *Plasmodium falciparum*
    B. *Plasmodium knowlesi*
    C. *Plasmodium malariae*
    D. *Plasmodium ovale*
    E. *Plasmodium vivax*

50. **The following are all used to treat HIV infection. Which of the following is a non-nucleoside reverse transcriptase inhibitor (NNRTI)?**

    A. Efavirenz
    B. Lopinavir
    C. Ritonavir
    D. Tenofovir
    E. Zidovudine

51. **A 21-year-old woman presents with a one-week history of high fevers, abdominal cramps, alternating constipation and diarrhoea, and malaise. She returned to the UK two weeks ago from a backpacking trip in India. On examination she has a temperature of 39°C; she has a normal pulse rate of 70 despite the fever. You notice several small pink macules on her abdomen and back. Full blood count reveals a neutrophilia, and LFTs are abnormal with ALT and alkaline phosphatase raised, although the bilirubin is normal. You take a blood culture and admit the patient. The next morning, the microbiology laboratory calls to inform you that Gram-negative rods are growing in the blood culture. What is the likeliest cause of her illness?**

    A. Typhoid fever
    B. Amoebiasis (*Entamoeba histolytica*)
    C. Cholera
    D. Bacillary dysentery (Shigellosis)
    E. Malaria

52. Regarding AIDS-related malignancy:

A. The proportion of deaths attributable to cancer in patients with HIV has fallen significantly in recent years

B. The diagnosis of Karposi's sarcoma confirms the onset of AIDS in patients with HIV

C. Development of Karposi's sarcoma is associated with infection with the human papilloma virus (HPV)

D. Treatment for non-Hodgkins lymphoma in HIV-positive patients is associated with higher response rates and a more optimistic prognosis than in seronegative patients

E. Non-AIDS-defining cancers in patients with HIV tend to follow a more indolent course than observed in the seronegative population

53. Regarding human papilloma virus:

A. It accounts for 25% of cervical cancers worldwide

B. Infection is most commonly via vertical transmission

C. Untreated, up to 15% of infections with HPV will progress to either cervical intraepithelial neoplasia (CIN) or cervical cancer

D. It is associated with anal, penile, vaginal, vulval, and uterine cancers

E. A quadrivalent vaccine is now offered to girls in the UK as part of the pre-school immunization programme

54. Haemolytic uraemic syndrome (microangiopathic haemolytic anaemia, thrombocytopenia, and acute renal failure) is most commonly associated with which infectious enteropathogen?

A. *Campylobacter jejuni*

B. *Escherichia coli*

C. *Salmonella enteritidis*

D. *Shigella flexneri*

E. *Giardia lamblia*

55. A 70-year-old woman under your care is diagnosed with *Clostridium difficile*-associated diarrhoea (CDAD). She has a fever of 39°C, with a pulse rate of 120, and a blood pressure of 120/80 mmHg. Her abdomen is soft but diffusely tender, and she has opened her bowels ten times in the last 12 hours. An abdominal X-ray shows widespread colonic mucosal oedema, but no dilatation, and she has a peripheral white cell count of 30 x 10⁹/l. She is tolerating oral fluids. What is the most appropriate antibiotic choice for this patient?

A. Intracolonic vancomycin

B. Intravenous metronidazole

C. Intravenous vancomycin

D. Oral metronidazole

E. Oral vancomycin

56. **A 79-year-old man hospitalized four days ago with a severe pneumonia and treated with co-amoxiclav and erythromycin, develops profuse diarrhoea on antibiotics. Faecal samples are sent and the patient is diagnosed with *Clostridium difficile*-associated diarrhoea (CDAD). What is the underlying pathophysiology of this illness attributed to?**
    A. Direct invasion of colonic epithelium
    B. Inhibition of glucose transport in the small intestine
    C. The production of toxins
    D. Trapping of magnesium ions in the colonic lumen
    E. Upregulation of intestinal motility

57. **With reference to appropriate infection control measures when managing cases of *Clostridium difficile*-associated diarrhoea, which of the following statements is true?**
    A. Patients should be isolated in side rooms until they have been diarrhoea-free for at least 48 hours and have passed a formed stool
    B. After patient contact, alcohol hand rub should be used to prevent the transmission of spores
    C. Gloves and aprons do not need to be worn for each patient contact
    D. Environmental cleaning of rooms of *C. difficile* patients should be carried out every 4fourdays using chlorine-containing cleaning agents
    E. Routine environmental screening is recommended

58. **A 21-year-old man is admitted to the medical service with a three-day history of profuse diarrhoea (>6 stools/day), which is intermittently bloody. He attended a friend's barbecue seven days prior to admission. On examination he has a fever of 40°C, and a soft, but diffusely tender abdomen. What is the most likely infectious cause of his diarrhoea?**
    A. *Campylobacter jejuni*
    B. *Cryptosporidium parvum*
    C. *Giardia lamblia*
    D. *Escherichia coli O157*
    E. *Shigella dysenteriae*

59. ***Campylobacter jejuni*-associated Guillain–Barré syndrome is thought to be associated with antibodies cross-reacting to:**
    A. Acetylcholine receptors
    B. GM1 ganglioside
    C. HLA-B27
    D. NMDA receptors
    E. Voltage-gated potassium channels

60. **A 24-year-old voluntary service worker in Nigeria collapses shortly after returning home to the UK to visit his mother. According to his friend who returned to the UK with him he has been deterioratiing with increasingly severe flu-like symptoms over the past few days. He had been taking malaria prophylaxis, but his compliance with medication is unknown. On examination he is very drowsy and his temperature is 38.8°C. His BP is 88/60, and his pulse is 102. Investigations: Hb 8.2 g/dl, WCC 15.3 x10^9/l, PLT 64 x10^9/l, Na$^+$ 132 mmol/l, K$^+$ 5.3 mmol/l, creatinine 181 micromol/l, *Falciparum parasitaemia* 11%. You start IV quinine immediately. Which other treatment may be of benefit?**

    A. Proguanil
    B. Intravenous mefloquine
    C. Intravenous chloroquine
    D. Intravenous artesunate
    E. Doxycycline

61. **A 19-year-old woman student is admitted from the airport after she collapsed on her return from an gap-year trip in Kenya. According to her friend she has been complaining of flu-like symptoms during the past few days, which worsened during the flight and were accompanied by a severe headache and neck stiffness. On examination in the emergency room she is pyrexial 38.9°C, her BP is 100/60, and her pulse is 95 and regular. Investigations: Hb 7.8 g/dl, WCC 14.2 x10^9/l, PLT 73 x10^9/l, Na$^+$ 134 mmol/l, K$^+$ 5.2 mmol/l, creatinine 185 micromol/l, *Falciparum parasitaemia* 8%. Which of the following is the most appropriate treatment?**

    A. Oral quinine
    B. Intravenous quinine
    C. Oral primaquine
    D. Intravenous primaquine
    E. Oral chloroquine

62. **A 19-year-old man returns from Thailand complaining of painful discharge and pus from his penis. He also has significant pain on passing urine. He admits to sex with local prostitutes during his visit. A penile swab reveals Gram-negative diplococci. Which of the following is the most appropriate treatment for him?**

    A. Cefuroxime 500 mg PO
    B. Ciprofloxacin 500 mg PO
    C. Olfloxacin 400 mg PO
    D. Amoxicillin 500 mg PO
    E. Cefixime 400 mg PO

63. **A 19-year-old university student is brought to the emergency unit by flatmates. She had been ill for 24 hours with severe headache, drowsiness, and flu-like symptoms. She is generally unwell, febrile, and has a purpuric rash over her arms. Her pulse is 119 bpm and blood pressure is 80/60 mmHg. The full blood count results are as follows: WBC 24 x 10⁹ with 90% neutrophils. Your immediate action is to:**

A. Order an urgent CT scan of her brain
B. Perform lumbar puncture and obtain CSF for analysis
C. Take blood cultures prior to any treatment given
D. Administer acyclovir 10 mg/kg intravenously
E. Start cefotaxime 2 g intravenously

64. **A 34-year-old woman of Indian ethnicity visits relatives in rural India. Prior to travel she attends a travel clinic and receives all the recommended vaccines. A few days after her return she develops mild gastrointestinal upset and notices pale stools with dark urine. Shortly after this she develops jaundice. Clinical examination reveals an enlarged tender liver. Liver biochemistry is shown in the Table 5.2. What is the most likely cause of her illness?**

A. *Entamoeba histolytica*
B. Hepatitis A
C. Hepatitis C
D. Hepatitis E
E. Leptospirosis

Table 5.2 Laboratory results

Bilirubin	132	(0–19 μmol/l)
AST	1834	(19–40 iu/l)
ALT	1260	(10–40 iu/l)
ALP	220	(30–120 iu/l)
GGT	174	(<51 mg/l)

65. **A 48-year-old HIV-positive man has progressive confusion, ataxia, and slurred speech. His cognition is also impaired. MRI brain shows diffuse inflammatory changes of the cerebellum with low signal changes on T1-weighted imaging which enhance on contrast. Which is the single most likely diagnosis?**

A. AIDS-related dementia complex
B. Cerebral toxoplasmosis
C. Cryptococcal meningitis
D. Herpes simplex encephalitis
E. Progressive multifocal leucoencephalopathy

66. **A 22-year-old male presents to hospital with a four-day history of sweating, headaches, and a dry cough. On examination he has a temperature of 38°C, hepatosplenomegaly, and lymphadenopathy. He was backpacking through Africa four weeks earlier, swimming in freshwater lakes. Full blood count reveals an eosinophilia. Which of the following is the most likely cause of his illness?**

A. Cholera
B. Filariasis
C. Schistosomiasis
D. Strongyloidiasis
E. Trypanosomiasis

67. **A 31-year-old HIV-positive female presents with a three-week history of increasing headache. On examination she is cachectic. Cranial nerve examination is normal. She has normal tone, power, and sensation in all limbs, but she appears confused and is not orientated in time or place. A full blood count reveals a lymphopenia, and a CD4 count of 20 cells/mm^3. Lumbar puncture is performed. The CSF has a white cell count of 150, of which 60% are lymphoctyes and 40% are polymorphs. Indian ink staining shows multiple budding yeast cells. What is the cause of this patient's illness?**

A. Cerebral tuberculosis
B. Cryptococcal meningitis
C. Herpes simplex encephalitis
D. Lymphoma
E. Toxoplasmosis

68. **Which of the following statements about infection with the ascaris is correct?**

A. Infection is not a cause of bowel obstruction
B. Infection is associated with neutropenia during larval migration
C. It is not related to deranged liver function
D. Children are affected more than adults
E. It is treated with tetracycline antibiotics

69. **A 43-year-old woman is seen in the general medical clinic with a one-month history of bloating, intermittent diarrhoea, and weight loss. She travelled to India four months ago, and three faecal samples are sent for microscopy. *Giardia lamblia* cysts are seen in all three samples. What would be the most appropriate treatment choice in this clinical context?**

    A. Azithromcyin
    B. Ciprofloxacin
    C. Metronidazole
    D. Vancomycin
    E. No antimicrobial treatment

70. **A 21-year-old man presents with profuse watery diarrhoea, malaise, low-grade fever, and crampy abdominal pain. He has no significant past medical history, but went swimming with a friend eight days ago, and mentions that his friend has similar symptoms, although much less severe. Microscopy of faeces confirms the diagnosis, which is most likely to be:**

    A. Ascariasis
    B. Campylobacteriosis
    C. Cryptosporidiosis
    D. Schistosomiasis
    E. Shigellosis

71. **A 28-year-old man presents with a three-day history of fevers, chills, and nausea. He had been travelling through Africa on an overland trek and returned to the UK six months ago. He had experienced similar symptoms one month earlier which had resolved after one week. He had taken chloroquine prophylaxis during his trip in Africa. Full blood count reveals a slight anaemia with haemoglobin of 11 g/dl and platelet count of 100 x 10⁹/l. A thin blood film reveals erythrocytes infected with ring-form parasites. What is the likeliest cause of his illness?**

    A. *Plasmodium falciparum*
    B. *Plasmodium vivax*
    C. Relapsing fever (Borrelia recurrentis)
    D. *Plasmodium malariae*
    E. Tuberculosis

72. **A 28-year-old man has visited his family in Uganda. During his stay he had intermittent fevers and rigors. He had no other symptoms. On his return he attends A&E and is found to have a fever of 39°C and bibasal crackles on examination. Otherwise examination is unremarkable. A CXR shows mild pulmonary oedema but no focal consolidation. Blood tests showed Hb 6.8g/dl, WCC 4.4 x 10⁹/l, PLT 77 x 10⁹/l, bilirubin 54 micromol/l, ALT 32 IU/l, ALP 86 U/l, CRP 87 mg/l, Ur 9.2 mmol/l, Cr 215 micromol/l, Na 133 mmol/l, K 4.5 mmol/l. What is the most likely diagnosis?**

A. Bacterial pneumonia

B. Mild malaria

C. Severe malaria

D. Schistosomiasis

E. Typhoid

73. **Which of the following causes of malaria has demonstrated widespread, worldwide chloroquine resistance?**

A. *Plasmodium falciparum*

B. *Plasmodium knowlesi*

C. *Plasmodium malariae*

D. *Plasmodium ovale*

E. *Plasmodium vivax*

74. **Which of the following is an AIDS-defining illness?**

A. Enterovirus meningitis

B. Listeria meningitis

C. Invasive cervical cancer

D. Oropharyngeal candida

E. Streptococcal pneumonia

75. **A 43-year-old Chinese man is tested for hepatitis B. His hepatitis B serology results are as follows: hepatitis B. surface Ag –ve, hepatitis B. surface Ab +ve, hepatitis B core IgG +ve, hepatitis B core IgM –ve. With which disease state is this serology most consistent?**

A. Acute hepatitis B infection

B. Chronic hepatitis B infection

C. Chronic hepatitis B infection with a virus expressing a pre-core mutation

D. Previous hepatitis B infection

E. Previous hepatitis B vaccination

76. **A 42-year-old woman flies to Bangkok, Thailand, for a business conference. She stays for a week, during which time she eats at a variety of venues, including one of the larger street markets. On the returning flight she develops diarrhoea, with nausea, mild abdominal cramps, and a fever. What is the most likely cause of her diarrhoeal illness?**

    A. *Campylobacter jejuni*
    B. *Escherichia coli*
    C. *Giardia lamblia*
    D. *Shigella flexneri*
    E. *Vibrio cholerae*

77. **A 60-year-old man presents to A&E with high fevers. On examination he has a hot, red, swollen left lower leg with a small area of pustular discharge. The discharge is swabbed and sent to microbiology for culture. The culture report states 'Heavy growth of Staphylococcus aureus'. The patient is treated with flucloxacillin and recovers quickly. Which of the following is true of *Staphylococcus aureus*?**

    A. It is always susceptible to flucloxacillin
    B. It is a cause of toxic shock syndrome
    C. It is a Gram-negative organism
    D. It is coagulase negative
    E. It is the commonest cause of community-acquired pneumonia

78. **Which of the following is the usual causative organism in meningitis epidemics?**

    A. *Haemophilus influenzae*
    B. *Neisseria meningitidis*
    C. *Listeria monocytogenes*
    D. *Staphylococcus aureus*
    E. *Streptococcus pneumoniae*

79. **A 25-year-old man with a history of recent *Campylobacter*-associated diarrhoea re-presents to the acute medical with a six-day history of progressive bilateral leg weakness. On examination he is tachycardic and hypertensive, with 2/5 power in all lower limb muscle groups, and absent lower limb tendon reflexes. Sensory function is preserved and there is no back pain or fever. What is the most likely diagnosis?**

    A. Acute motor axonal neuropathy (AMAN)
    B. Botulism
    C. Epidural abscess
    D. Miller–Fisher syndrome
    E. Mononeuritis multiplex

80. **A 25-year-old man presents to A&E with fever, headache, and profuse, intermittently bloody diarrhoea. He attended a barbecue four days ago. A faecal specimen has cultured *Campylobacter spp.* Which of the following statements about campylobacteriosis is true?**

    A. First-line antibiotic treatment would include a third-generation cephalosporin, such as ceftriaxone
    B. Antibiotic treatment is indicated in most cases
    C. 60–70% of infected individuals may experience a relapse
    D. *Campylobacter* infection is a trigger for Guillain–Barré syndrome
    E. Person-to-person transmission is common

81. **Antibiotics have been shown to predispose to the development of *Clostridium difficile*-associated diarrhoea (CDAD) by disrupting the normal enteric flora allowing colonization by potential pathogens. Which of the following antibiotics is considered to put patients most at risk of CDAD?**

    A. Clindamycin
    B. Doxycycline
    C. Gentamicin
    D. Trimethoprim
    E. Vancomycin

82. **A 50-year-old farmer presents with a six-month history of weight loss, diarrhoea, and arthralgia. His joint symptoms are migratory, and tend to affect his large joints. Over the last couple of weeks he has developed worsening shortness of breath on exercise, and a chest X-ray has demonstrated a moderate-sized pleural effusion. He has extensive investigations, which culminate in a small bowel biopsy. This stains positive for periodic acid-Schiff (PAS) granules. The most likely diagnosis is:**

    A. Coeliac disease
    B. Hyperthyroidism
    C. Rheumatoid arthritis
    D. Small bowel lymphoma
    E. Whipple's disease

83. **A 27-year-old man presents with a six-week history of a productive cough, weight loss, and night sweats. He is known to be HIV positive. On examination he is cachectic, with prominent crackles in the right upper zone on auscultation. Which of the following would be the most useful initial investigation to diagnose this patient's condition?**

    A. Bronchealveolar lavage
    B. CT of the chest
    C. Mantoux test
    D. Sputum smear for acid-fast bacilli
    E. Upper gastrointestinal endoscopy

84. **All of the following are recognized complications of infection with *Mycoplasma pneumoniae* except:**

    A. Encephalitis
    B. Erythema nodosum
    C. Haemolytic anaemia
    D. Necrotizing fasciitis
    E. Stevens–Johnson syndrome

85. **A 22-year-old student presents with a two-day history of fever and headache. Examination reveals neck stiffness and normal neurological examination. Her pulse is 110 bpm and regular, and her BP is 88/48. Examination of the skin reveals purpura. Fluid resuscitation is commenced and the ITU team are contacted to request urgent support. What is the most appropriate next step?**

    A. CT head
    B. Intravenous aciclovir 10 mg/kg
    C. Intravenous ceftraixone 1 g
    D. Intravenous ceftriaxone 2 g
    E. Lumbar puncture

86. **A 27-year-old woman complains of recurrent attacks of dysuria and frequency over the last 15 months. Blood tests show urea 4.5 mmol/l, serum creatinine 67 micromol/l and a serum calcium (corrected) of 2.34 mmol/l. She is advised to increase her fluid intake and regularly empty her bladder. A MSU following her consultation grew *Proteus*. What further investigations would you undertake?**

    A. Early morning urine for acid-fast bacilli
    B. Plain abdominal X-ray.
    C. Regular MSU after current infection eradicated
    D. Serum urate estimation
    E. 24-hour urinary calcium estimation

87. **An intravenous drug user presents with fever and a pan-systolic murmur at the lower left sternal edge. A blood culture is positive. What is the most likely Gram-stain appearance?**

    A. Gram-negative cocci mostly seen in pairs
    B. Gram-negative rod-shaped organisms
    C. Gram-positive cocci forming into clusters
    D. Gram-positive cocci forming short chains
    E. Gram-positive rod-shaped organisms

88. **A 43-year-old accountant visits A&E having returned from visiting his family in India. He was there for four weeks and had no travel advice prior to travel. He was well whilst there. One week after his return he developed a fever. This resolved with paracetamol but returned as the medication wore off. He has a mild cough and some mild abdominal discomfort but no other symptoms of note. On examination his chest is clear and his abdomen is soft and non-tender. His pulse is 80 bpm and regular and his blood pressure is 121/72. Blood tests were as follows: Hb 14.2 g/dl, WCC 6.4 x 10^9/l, lymphocytes 1.1 x 10^9/l, platelets 247 x 10^9/l, bilirubin 18 micromol/l, ALT 115 iU/l, ALP 86 U/l, albumin 41 g/l, CRP 87 mg/l, Ur 6.3 mmol/l, Cr 98 micromol/l, Na 135 mmol/l, K 4.4 mmol/l. The most likely diagnosis is:**

    A. Pneumonia
    B. Schistosomiasis
    C. Tuberculosis
    D. Typhoid
    E. Urinary tract infection

89. **An 89-year-old man is admitted to hospital with cough productive of green sputum. His temperature is 38.2°C. He has bronchial breathing and course crepitations at the right base and a right-sided consolidation is seen on his chest X-ray. The CURB-65 score is 1/5 but he requires admission as he is not able to manage at home. He is treated with oral amoxicillin and after 48 hours in hospital remains stable. His CRP is falling and he is apyrexial. The microbiology laboratory telephones the ward to report that his sputum culture is positive with a growth of methicillin-resistant *Staphylococcus aureus* (MRSA). A nasal swab is also positive for MRSA growth. What changes to his drug therapy should be made?**

    A. Continue oral amoxicillin and commence MRSA eradication therapy with mupirocin
    B. Discontinue amoxicillin and commence fucidic acid and rifampicin
    C. Discontinue amoxicillin and commence linezolid
    D. Discontinue amoxicillin and commence piperacillin/tazobactam (Tazocin®)
    E. Discontinue amoxicillin and commence vancomycin

90. **A 27-week pregnant woman presents to hospital with fever and rigors. There are no focal signs to indicate a source of sepsis. The following day, her blood cultures are positive for a Gram-positive rod which demonstrates characteristic tumbling motility. Which of the following would be the antibiotic treatment of choice for this condition?**

    A. Amoxicillin
    B. Cefotaxime
    C. Ciprofloxacin
    D. Gentamicin
    E. Vancomycin

91. **A 45-year-old smoker attends the A&E department with a history of cough productive of green sputum and right-sided chest discomfort. He is not confused. His heart rate is 88, blood pressure 118/76, and respiratory rate 21. His oxygen saturations are 97% on room air and he has a temperature of 38.1°C. He has course crackles in the right lower zone and a chest X-ray confirms a right-sided consolidation. Which of the following would be appropriate antibiotic therapy?**

    A. Intravenous amoxicillin and gentamicin
    B. Intravenous co-amoxiclav and clarithromycin
    C. Oral amoxicillin and clarithromycin
    D. Oral ciprofloxacin
    E. Oral clarithromycin

92. A 23-year-old student returns from a summer trip which involved building a school on the shores of Lake Malawi. Four weeks after his return he develops low-grade fever, cough, and an urticarial rash. On examination he has splenomegaly. Full blood count shows an eosinophil count of 3.46 (normal range 0–0.4). What is the most likely diagnosis?

A. Asthma
B. *Burkholderia pseudomallei*
C. Dengue fever
D. *Plasmodium falciparum*
E. *Schistosoma mansoni*

93. A 60-year-old man with Karposi's sarcoma and HIV presents with a dry cough and a fever. He has been unwell for some days and is now finding it impossible to walk more than a few metres before he becomes exhausted. On examination his BP is 105/70, pulse is 85 and regular. There are scattered crackles and wheeze on auscultation of his chest. You notice his oxygen saturation falls by 3% on walking across the room. Which of the following would you expect to find on further investigation?

A. Elevated LDH
B. Normal chest X-ray
C. Elevated transfer factor
D. Normal CD4 count
E. Identification of the organism on routine culture

94. Which of the following bacterial infections is caused by a species of Salmonella?

A. Murine typhus
B. Epidemic typhus
C. Rocky Mountain spotted fever
D. Scrub typhus
E. Typhoid (enteric fever)

95. Which of the following is about human papillomavirus?

A. It is an RNA virus
B. It may be auto-inoculated from non-genital to genital sites
C. Most cross-sectional studies show prevalence of type specific serum antibodies against HPV are same in both sexes
D. Genital and common skin warts are both morphologically and antigenically distinct
E. All of the above

96. The **BHIVA** (British HIV Association) guideline recommends therapy-naive patients start **ART** (antiretroviral therapy) on a combination of two nucleos(t)ide reverse transcriptase inhibitors (NRTIs) and which one of the following number(s) of drug classes?

    A. One
    B. Two
    C. Three
    D. Four
    E. Five

97. A 42-year-old hiker comes to the emergency department complaining of extreme lethargy and drooping of the left side of his face, some ten days after returning from a two-week trip to the Alps. There is also a history of flitting joint pains. During his time away he remembers being bitten on his leg by a tick, but he removed this with a pair of tweezers after soaking the area in alcohol. On examination his BP is 105/60, pulse is 48 and regular. He has a left Bell's palsy. Investigations reveal a mildly elevated white count and a CRP of 75. Which of the following therapies is most likely to be of value in this case?

    A. Doxycycline
    B. Cefuroxime
    C. Penicillin V
    D. Clarithromycin
    E. Ciprofloxacin

98. A 42-year-old woman is taking oral corticosteroids and methotrexate for the treatment of rheumatoid arthritis. She comes to the emergency department as she has been exposed to her niece some three days earlier, and the child has now developed chicken pox. She looks well and has no significant symptoms of acute illness. As far as she knows she never developed chicken pox as a child. Which of the following is the most appropriate course of action?

    A. Check VZV IgG
    B. Prescribe oral acyclovir
    C. Prescribe IV acyclovir
    D. Prescribe varicella zoster immunoglobulin
    E. Prescribe a live attenuated vaccine

99. **A 68-year-old woman has received a course of clindamycin for osteomyelitis from the orthopaedic surgeons, as she is penicillin allergic. Unfortunately, she develops severe diarrhoea, which is mixed with blood and mucus. On examination she is hypotensive at 100/60, her pulse is 85 and regular. Her abdomen is generally tender but soft, and her stool is positive for *C. difficile* toxin. Which of the following is the most appropriate therapy?**

A. Metronidazole
B. Amoxycillin
C. Ciprofloxacin
D. Rifampicin
E. Teicoplanin

100. **A 26-year-old man returns from a trip to Zambia, where he has been teaching English in a school for the past six months. He has had problems with increasing lethargy over the past few months, and has had pain on passing urine. He has no past medical history of note. On examination he looks pale. His BP is 105/70, pulse is 85 and regular. There are no significant abnormal findings. Investigations: Hb 9.4, WCC 9.5 (raised eosinophils), PLT 203, Na 139, K 4.1, Cr 129, ESR 67, urine dipstick blood +++, protein ++. Which of the following is the most likely diagnosis?**

A. Schistosomiasis
B. Gonorrhoea
C. *Proteus* urinary tract infection
D. IgA nephropathy
E. Minimal change glomerulonephritis

101. **A 22-year-old man presents with an extremely itchy interdigital rash between his fingers and toes, He has a history of mild eczema, but nil else of note. Three to four weeks earlier he returned from a 'boys' holiday in Spain. On examination there are small red papules around the web spaces of his fingers and toes, hands and feet and around his thighs, buttocks and lower abdomen. Which of the following treatments is most likely to be effective?**

A. Permethrin
B. Hydrocortisone cream
C. Oral prednisolone
D. Oral penicillin
E. Oral doxycycline

102. **Persistence of HPV infection for more than six months in women is correlated with:**

   A. Younger age
   B. Infection with single type of HPV
   C. Infection with high-risk HPV type
   D. Development of immunity to HPV
   E. Smoking

103. **Which one of the following is about HIV treatment recommendations from the UK national guideline?**

   A. Patients with chronic infection should start treatment when CD4 lymphocyte count is ≤ 350 cells/μl
   B. Late diagnosis of HIV has no significant impact on longevity
   C. The main reason for starting treatment is to prevent sexual transmission
   D. Treatment should always commence as soon as HIV is diagnosed
   E. Antiretroviral treatment is not cost effective as it outweighs all benefits in the long term

104. **Which of the following types of human papillomavirus is commonly associated with carcinomas in the ano-genital region of men and women?**

   A. 27
   B. 16
   C. 2
   D. 11
   E. None of the above

105. **Which of the following pairs of human papillomavirus are commonly associated with all of the following conditions—condylomata acuminate, squamous intraepithelial lesions (SIL) in male and female ano-genitalia, and laryngeal papillomata?**

   A. 6 and 11
   B. 3 and 10
   C. 27 and 2
   D. 13 and 32
   E. None of the above

INFECTIOUS DISEASES AND GUM

ANSWERS

1. D. Chronic onchocerciasis causes elephantitis

Onchocerciasis is a parasitic infection caused by the nematode Onchocerca volvulus. It is transmitted to humans through the bite of a simulium blackfly, a fly which lives near fast-flowing rivers. While the majority of infections occur in tropical Africa, there have been cases documented in Central and South America. The adult worms form subcutaneous nodules over bony prominences. Other skin manifestations include itching, vesicles, papules, oedema, skin atrophy, hyperpigmentation, and hypopigmentation (C). Microfilaria can migrate to the ocular tissue where disease is caused, not by the worm itself, but after the worm dies, with the release of the endosymbiont bacteria, *Wolbachia*, which triggers an inflammatory reaction which can lead to blindness. Since the induction of the onchocerciasis eradication programme in 1974 the rate of onchocerciasis has dramatically decreased. Elephantitis is caused by lymphatic filariasis.

World Health Organization, Onchocerciasis. http://www.who.int/topics/onchocerciasis/en/

2. C. Do nothing

The VDRL test becoming negative is an indication of successful treatment of syphillis, although a small percentage of patients remain VDRL positive after eradication. The reduction in titre for TPHA from 1 in 256 to 1 in 16 is also a pointer towards successful therapy. Whilst doxycycline is the third option after IM benzylpenicillin and azithromycin it remains effective for syphilis eradication.

Eddleston M et al., *Oxford Handbook of Tropical Medicine*, Third Edition, Oxford University Press, 2008.

3. A. *Coxiella burnetti*

Culture-negative infective endocarditis is a significant diagnostic problem. In this case, the consistent finding of sterile blood cultures despite these being drawn prior to the administration of empirical antibiotic therapy means that *Staphylococcus aureus* and *Streptococcus viridans* are now unlikely—despite these generally being the most common causes of infective endocarditis. Where several sets of blood cultures are not drawn until after the administration of antibiotics, these common causes cannot be excluded as they will be covered by empirical therapy. This case therefore represents true culture-negative endocarditis. In more recent case series, fastidious organisms which resist culture are the cause in around 2–5% of cases. These organisms include anaerobes and slow-growing Gram negatives such as those of the HACEK group. *Bartonella sp.* (the cause of cat scratch fever) have also been identified as a cause. Finally, obligate intracellular organisms must be considered, and these organisms are often impossible to culture from peripheral blood. Causes in this category include *Coxiella burnetti* (the cause of Q fever), *rickettsiae*, and *T. whippelii* (the cause of Whipple's disease). *Neisseria gonorrhoea* used to be a common cause of infective endocarditis but is now rarely seen. Infection with *Coxiella burnetti* is most commonly seen in those who find themselves in close contact with cattle. Acute Q fever causes self-limiting febrile illness in the majority of patients, which is rarely successfully diagnosed. Some of those with acute Q fever may present with pneumonia. Chronic infection with *C. burnetti* can present as endocarditis, hepatitis, or a wide range of other rare manifestations including osteomyelitis. It is a cause of first trimester abortion.

Parker NR et al., Q fever, *Lancet* 2006;367:679–688.

4. A. Measles

Measles is caused by a morbillivirus. It is highly contagious and easily spread by coughing and close contact. A prodrome consists of fever, malaise, and Koplik spots, with the three 'Cs'— cough, coryza, and conjunctivitis. This is followed by the appearance of a characteristic rash, often appearing around the fourth day of illness, which frequently starts from behind the ears and spreads to the rest of the body. The rash usually persists for four or five days followed by resolution of symptoms. Measles is prevented by vaccination. It usually causes a mild, self-limiting illness, but can lead to secondary pneumonia, xerophthalmia, and encephalitis. It continues to be a major problem in the developing world, where it remains a major cause of morbidity and mortality.

Mandell G et al., *Prinicples and Practice of Infectious Diseases*, Seventh Edition, Volume 2, Churchill Livingstone Elsevier, 2010, Chapter 160, Measles virus (Rubeola), pp. 2229–2236.

5. C. *Erythema multiforme*

Current treatment for hepatitis C consists of combination therapy with ribavirin and interferon alpha. Most patients are now treated with pegylated interferons which facilitate more convenient drug delivery and have been shown to be superior. Treatment duration depends on a range of prognostic indicators but in most cases is between six months and one year. The most important pre-treatment factors influencing treatment success are virus genotype and the extent of any chronic liver disease. Unfortunately, side effects of therapy are common and most patients are affected by at least one significant side effect. The most frequently experienced adverse effects are: fatigue, influenza-like symptoms, depressed mood, haemolytic anaemia, neutropaenia, thrombocytopaenia, and alopecia. In addition, ribavirin is teratogenic and persists in the body for many months after treatment is completed. It is also excreted in semen. Therefore, both men and women on treatment must be very careful to avoid pregnancy both during treatment and for at least six months after its completion.

Hepatits C Trust, patient information website. http://HepCTrust.org.uk

6. A. Enterovirus

Streptococcus pneumonia, *Neisseria meningitidis*, and *Haemophilus influenza* are all potential causes of bacterial meningitis (although *N. meningitidis* would be most common in this age goup). However, the presence of a predominance of lymphocytes in the CSF makes these causes less likely. Furthermore, the normal CSF glucose makes bacterial causes of meningitis much less likely. Lymphocytic meningitis is most commonly caused by viral infection, such as that caused by enteroviruses. Acute HIV infection is another important cause. The CSF glucose is usually normal in viral infection. Of non-viral causes, tuberculosis characteristically causes a lymphocytic pleocytosis as does *Listeria monocytogenes*. Other less common causes include Lyme disease and syphilis. In this case, the combination of a lymphocytic pleocytosis and normal CSF glucose makes viral meningitis the most likely cause.

Logan S, MacMahon E, Viral meningitis, *British Medical Journal* 2008;336:36–40.

7. A. Alpha-fetoprotein

There are many reasons for a patient with cirrhosis to develop decompensated liver disease. Chronic hepatitis C can progress to decompensated cirrhosis without the need for other exacerbating factors. Secondary infection with other hepatitis viruses can also lead to decompensation and should be considered. However, hepatitis D can only infect patients who already carry hepatitis B, and is therefore extremely unlikely in this case. Alcohol consumption accelerates the progression of liver disease in chronic hepatitis C and can lead to decompensation. For this reason, all patients with hepatitis C are advised to abstain from alcohol. However, the presence of an enlarged, tender liver is unusual in cirrhosis, as the liver is usually small. This suggests that the most likely cause of decompensation in this patient is hepatocellular carcinoma, which is likely to result in a significantly elevated alpha-fetoprotein. Further imaging will also be important and is likely to take the form of an ultrasound scan in the first instance.

Schuppan D, Afdhal N, Liver cirrhosis, *Lancet* 2008;371:838–851.

8. E. The part of the parasite life cycle that occurs in the human host is the asexual cycle

The life cycle of the malarial parasite is made up of two parts. It has the asexual cycle in the human host followed by the sexual cycle in the female mosquito. When a female mosquito bites a human, sporozoites are transferred from her salivary glands to the human blood, where they work their way to the liver. The sporozoites develop in the liver into schizonts, which will eventually rupture, releasing many merozoites into the bloodstream. (Schizonts may also become hypnozoites, which is a dormant form of the parasite responsible for latent infection.) Merozoites released from schizonts enter red blood cells and develop into trophozoites. Some will go on to develop into gametocytes which may be ingested by the mosquito. Both male and female gametes must be ingested in order to produce the zygote. The zygote undergoes further maturation and eventually forms an oocyst within the mosquito gut wall. When this bursts, the sporozoites released migrate to the salivary glands to commence a new cycle.

Herchline TE, Malaria: practice essentials, *Medscape*. http://emedicine.medscape.com/article/221134-overview

9. E. <5%

The transmission rate for vaginal delivery during primary maternal herpes infection is thought to be as high as 50%. In contrast, the rate of neonatal infection is thought to be less than 5% where recurrent maternal herpes simplex is concerned. As such the risks of operative delivery by caesarean section should be weighed against the risks of infection. If neonatal infection does occur then 25% is restricted to eyes and mouth only, although infection is widely disseminated in the other 75% of neonates. Acyclovir has been shown in a meta-analysis to reduce recurrence of herpes during pregnancy by around 75%.

Collins S et al., *Oxford Handbook of Obstetrics and Gynaecology*, Second Edition, Oxford University Press, 2008, Chapter 4, Infectious diseases in pregnancy, Herpes simplex.

10. A. Thrombotic thrombocytopaenic purpura (TTP)

The clinical picture here is consistent with *E. coli 157* infection, outbreaks having been known to occur in the nursery setting. The evidence of haemolytic anaemia and renal failure adds to the likelihood of the underlying diagnosis. Whilst rapid progression to renal failure occurs in children, worsening of creatinine may occur more slowly in adults. Antibiotics do not usually have a role in the treatment of the condition.

Ramrakha PS et al., *Oxford Handbook of Acute Medicine*, Third Edition, Oxford University Press, 2010, Chapter 10, Haematological emergencies, Thrombotic thrombocytopenic purpura (TTP) and haemolytic-uraemic syndrome (HUS).

11. D. Toxoplasmosis

Toxoplasmosis is caused by the parasite *Toxoplasma gondii*. The definitive host is cats but infection in humans is common. Infection is most often through contaminated food or water and ingestion of undercooked meat. Infection is usually asymptomatic but can cause serious illness in the immunocompromised, such as patients with HIV, particularly those with a CD4 count of less than 100/mm^3. Cerebral toxoplasmosis can result in formation of toxoplasma abscesses which typically are multiple and ring-enhancing after administration of contrast on CT scanning. Presentation is with focal neurological deficit depending on the site of the lesions. Presentation can also be with fever, headaches, and seizures. Treatment is with sulphadiazine and pyrimethamine. Tuberculosis of the central nervous system can occasionally cause intracerebral mass lesions known as tuberculomas, but it more commonly presents with an altered level of consciousness and focal neurological deficits. HIV infection greatly increases the risk of tuberculosis. Cerebral lymphoma can present as intracerebral mass lesions, causing focal neurological deficits, and, whilst rare in the general population, is more common in patients with HIV. Bacterial meningitis such as *Streptococcus pneumoniae* (pneumococcus) or *Neisseria meningitidis* (meningococcus) usually causes a syndrome of high fever, neck stiffness, and photophobia. Imaging of the brain is often normal. Viral encephalitis such as HSV or CMV presents with seizures, decreased consciousness or focal neurological deficit. Temporal lobe enhancement is often seen on imaging but viral encephalitis does not cause discrete ring-enhancing lesions.

Török E et al., *Oxford Handbook of Infectious Diseases and Microbiology*, Oxford University Press, 2009, Chapter 4, Systematic microbiology, pp. 567–570.

12. B. Famcyclovir 250 mg TDS for five days

This clinical picture is consistent with a diagnosis of genital herpes. It is most likely that the patient acquired her infection from an asymptomatic viral shedder. Anti-virals should be started within five days of the onset of the ulcers; famciclovir and valacyclovir require less frequent doses, and as such they are preferred for convenience reasons. Long-term anti-viral therapy is usually considered when there are greater than six recurrences in any one year. This is not intended to be a treatment course, but is intended to suppress episodes of recurrent clinically overt herpes.

Pattman R et al., *Oxford Handbook of Genitourinary Medicine, HIV and AIDS*, Second Edition, Oxford University Press, 2010, Chapter 21, Anogenital herpes.

13. A. Orf

Orf is a highly contagious disease of sheep and goats caused by a parapoxvirus. Orf can be transmitted to humans by contact with an infected animal or contaminated fomites. Orf is most frequently diagnosed in those directly handling sheep, in particular those bottle-feeding lambs in the spring, and those involved in shearing and slaughtering sheep. Orf appears as a solitary lesion or as a few lesions, most commonly on the fingers, hands, or forearms. The lesion starts as a small, firm, red-to-blue papule that becomes haemorrhagic and flat-topped. The fully developed lesion is typically 2–3 cm in diameter. The dorsal aspect of the index finger at the MCP is a common site of infection. Orf lesions heal spontaneously in approximately 5–7 weeks. Classical lichen planus is characterized by purple shiny, flat-topped, firm papules, often crossed by fine white lines (called 'Wickham's striae'). It is often very itchy. Impetigo is a simple infection of the skin that manifests as a small crusted ulcer that is very contagious. Adults can acquire the disease from contact with infected children. Paronychia is an infection of the skin just next to a nail (the nail fold). The infected nail fold looks swollen and inflamed, and may be tender. Abscesses that form in the area may require drainage.

Paiba GA et al., Orf (contagious pustular dermatitis) in farmworkers: prevalence and risk factors in three areas of England, *Veterinary Record* 1999;145(1):7–11.

14. D. Leptospirosis

The diagnosis that fits the best with this presentation is leptospirosis. Leptospirosis is primarily a zoonosis but affects humans when the spirochaetes enter the human body via cuts in the skin and spread to multiple organ sites. The clinical picture is due to the leptospirochaetes themselves and/or the human host's immune response to them. The disease is most commonly seen in farmers and drain workers who are in contact with contaminated water. Symptoms range from subclinical to multi-organ failure and can include fever, headache, myalgia, nausea and vomiting, and conjunctival suffusion or haemorrhage. In severe infection symptoms may include breathlessness, and haemoptysis, as well as respiratory or renal failure. Diagnosis is made on clinical suspicion and subsequent testing for leptospires in blood or CSF in the first 7–10 days and from urine during the second to third week of illness. Treatment depends on disease severity with oral or intravenous antibiotics. However in severe cases haemodialysis and respiratory support on intensive care may be required.

Leptospirosis information centre. http://www.leptospirosis.org/

15. B. The parasite is transferred through the bite of a sandfly

Cutaneous leishmaniasis (CL) is a multi-system disease that presents in a variety of ways and is caused by a number of different species of the leishmania parasite. The promastigotes are transmitted from the bite of the Phlebotomus or Lutzomyia sand flies; the parasite then multiplies intracellularly within the skin macrophages at the site of the bite, causing tissue damage. This can be seen as a slow-growing raised red nodule which may present weeks to years after the initial bite. The lesion can ulcerate and become secondarily infected by bacteria. The lesion will either spontaneously heal, heal with scarring, or reappear elsewhere. There are three main subgroups of cutaneous leishmaniasis. (1) Mucocutaneous leishmaniasis (MCL), which only occurs in New World CL. Mucocutaneous lesions may appear months to years after the primary lesion has healed. MCL is a destructive process and eventually destroys the tissue it is invading. (2) Diffuse cutaneous leishmaniasis (DCL) is a slow growing subtype that is usually caused by *L. mexicana* or *L. aethiopica*. The nodule tends not to ulcerate and spreads symmetrically. This type of leishmania is mainly seen in immunocompromised individuals. It is important to distinguish this subtype of leishmaniasis from leprosy, as they can look similar. Individuals do not respond well to chemotherapy. (3) Recidivans leishmaniasis (also called lupoid leishmaniasis) is a relapsing form of CL which only ever partially heals. The lesions can be confused with tuberculosis of the skin; however, the causative parasite is *L. tropica*.

Broek I et al., Clinical guidelines, Diagnosis and treatment manual, Médecins Sans Frontiers, 2010. http://apps.who.int/medicinedocs/documents/s17078e/s17078e.pdf

16. D. With dysentery resolution, an amoebic liver abscess is formed

Amoebiasis is the infection with the intestinal protozoa *Entamoeba histolytica*. From the cyst ingested, usually non-pathogenic amoeba are released; thus, not all cases where cysts detected in stool samples need treatment. Approximately 90% of patients are asymptomatic. Where symptoms occur, they usually include abdominal cramps, bloating, watery or bloody diarrhoea, and fever. Amoebic liver abscesses are caused by migration of the amoeba to hepatic tissue. Symptoms of a liver abscess include right upper quadrant pain, shoulder tip pain, sweats (particularly nocturnally), tender hepatomegaly with or without vomiting, and intermittent fevers. Treatment is with tinidazole. If the abscess fails to respond to antibiotics often aspiration is performed, particularly if there is a high risk of rupture.

Broek I et al., Clinical guidelines, Diagnosis and treatment manual, Médecins Sans Frontiers, 2010. http://apps.who.int/medicinedocs/documents/s17078e/s17078e.pdf

17. B. The part of the parasite life cycle that occurs in the human host is the asexual cycle

The life cycle of the malarial parasite is made up of two parts. It has the asexual cycle in the human host followed by the sexual cycle in the female mosquito. When a female mosquito bites a human, sporozoites are transferred from her salivary glands to the human blood, where they work their way to the liver. The sporozoites develop in the liver into schizonts which will eventually rupture, releasing many merozoites into the blood stream. (Schizonts may also become hypnozoites, which is a dormant form of the parasite responsible for latent infection.) Merozoites released from schizonts enter red blood cells and develop into trophozoites. Some will go on to develop into gametocytes which may be ingested by the mosquito; both male and female gametes must be ingested in order to produce the zygote. The zygote undergoes further maturation and eventually forms an oocyst within the mosquito gut wall. When this bursts, the sporozoites released migrate to the salivary glands to commence a new cycle.

Palmer SR et al., *Oxford Textbook of Zoonoses*, Second Edition, Oxford University Press, 2013, Chapter 48, Babesiosis and malaria. http://otzoon.oxfordmedicine.com/cgi/content/full/2/1/med-9780198570028-chapter-048

18. C. Symptoms can include rash, fever, myalgia, and shock

Dengue fever, also known as break-bone fever, is transmitted by the *Aedes* mosquito, typically *Aedes aegypti*, which is a day-biting mosquito. *Aedes* breed in small man-made containers such as pots, buckets, or old tyres; hence its habitat is entwined with that of humans which put those people living in temperate areas at risk. Incubation time ranges from 3–15 days but is usually between 5–8 days in most cases. Symptoms include fever, rashes, headaches, myalgia, and arthralgia. Complications of dengue fever include progression to dengue haemorrhagic fever (due to vascular leak) or dengue shock syndrome. Diagnosis is based on the clinical syndrome in a person residing in a susceptible area. The presence of the virus can be shown using PCR or viral antigen detection, both of which are limited in the resource-poor setting. Treatment is supportive but aspirin should be avoided due to risk of bleeding and DIC. In those with DHF or DSS, volume resuscitation remains the cornerstone of treatment. A vaccine is not currently available.

Eddleston M et al., *Oxford Handbook of Tropical Medicine*, Third Edition, Oxford University Press, 2008, Chapter 18, Multi-system diseases and infections, Arboviruses.

19. D. Pleural biopsy microscopy, culture, and sensitivity

This patient may have a positive Heaf test from his previous TB. A low CD4 count does not predispose to TB and CD4 < 200 cells/mm³ may be related to a lower risk of tuberculous pleural effusion. Ziehl–Neelsen stains of pleural fluid are positive in about 20% of tuberculous effusions, culture is positive in about 40%, and pleural biopsy culture is positive in about 75%. Pleural histology may demonstrate granulomas, but has a lower sensitivity than pleural biopsy cultures.

Chapman S et al., *Oxford Handbook of Respiratory Medicine*, Second Edition, Oxford University Press, 2009, Chapter 42, Respiratory infection: mycobacterial.

20. E. Cephalexin

Doxycycline and ciprofloxacin are contraindicated for use in pregnancy, tetracyclines are recognized to lead to permanent tooth staining, and quinolones are thought to lead to increased risk of tendon rupture. Whilst erythromycin may be used, coverage is unlikely to be appropriate for the majority of urinary pathogens. Trimethoprim may interfere with folate metabolism and as such it is not recommended. This leaves cephalexin, which appears relatively safe in pregnancy and has broad coverage against a wide range of urinary pathogens.

emc+, Cefalexin 500mg capsules. http://www.medicines.org.uk/EMC/medicine/23096/SPC/Cefalexin+500mg+Capsules/

21. C. Biliary tree

S. bovis is usually associated either with colonic pathology or infection via the biliary tree. Given his previous history of cholecystitis, the biliary tree is therefore the likeliest source of infection. Imaging of both the biliary tree and the colon to rule out an underlying large bowel tumour is advised.

S. bovis is highly susceptible to penicillin, although studies suggest mortality from S. bovis endocarditis is higher than that for non-S. bovis disease.

Török E et al., *Oxford Handbook of Infectious Diseases and Microbiology*, Oxford University Press, 2009, Chapter 4, Systematic microbiology, Streptococcus bovis.

22. B. Measles

The clinical picture here is consistent with measles. Typically after an incubation period of 14 days, presentation is with a dry cough, severe fever, and photophobia. Rash initially begins on the head and neck, but later spreads to involve the upper body. German measles is associated with a rash which begins on the face and then spreads across the trunk lasting for approximately three days. The most prominent other symptom is marked post-auricular and cervical lymphadenopathy. Mumps is primarily associated with parotid swelling. We are not given any history of headache or meningism so this does not really fit with meningitis.

Török E et al., *Oxford Handbook of Infectious Diseases and Microbiology*, Oxford University Press, 2009, Chapter 4, Systematic microbiology, Measles. http://oxfordmedicine.com/view/10.1093/med/9780198569251.001.0001/med-9780198569251-chapter-4#med-9780198569251-div1-236

23. B. Polyarteritis nodosa

Polyarteritis nodosa (a vasculitis affecting medium-sized vessels) is a rare complication of hepatitis B. It presents in the first six months of acute hepatitis B, and presents with arthralgia, myalgia, and large joint oligo-arthritis (rarely). Treatment is with anti-virals and immunosuppressive agents.

A small proportion of patients in the pre-icteric phase of acute hepatitis B develop symmetric polyarthropathy resembling rheumatoid arthritis—with involvement of the proximal inter-phalangeal joints, knees, and ankles. Rheumatoid factor may be present in a quarter of instances, and complements are low—suggesting immune complex deposition disease. There are extremely high AST and ALT levels. The arthritis generally resolves in 2–3 weeks, and no specific treatment is necessary.

Colledge NR et al., *Davidson's Principles and Practice of Medicine*, Elsevier, 2006, pp. 1065–1144.

24. D. Acute HIV infection

With this history the most important diagnosis not to miss is HIV seroconversion. This can mimic infectious mononucleosis. However, with a history of travel to an HIV-endemic country a full sexual history should be taken and the patient risk assessed. Acute seroconversion presents 2–12 weeks post infection in 50–70% of individuals who develop a viral syndrome with a widespread maculopapular rash and generalized lymphadenopathy. In acute seroconversion initial HIV testing is usually negative; however PCR for HIV RNA will be positive due to high viral load. If PCR is unavailable the patient should be recalled three months later for repeat testing.

Gill GV, Beeching N, *Tropical Medicine (Lecture Notes)*, Sixth Edition, Blackwell Publishing, 2009.

25. E. *S. haematobium*

S. haematobium migrates to the venous plexus around the bladder; this precipitates an intense inflammatory response leading to granuloma formation and haematuria. The parasites migrate through the bladder wall, leading to shedding in the urine. Praziquantel is the drug of choice for the treatment of schistasomiasis. The other shistosoma migrate to the portal vein and lead to hepatic fibrosis and scarring.

Torok E et al., *Oxford Handbook of Infectious Diseases and Microbiology*, Oxford University Press, 2009.

26. B. Central nervous system

A series of clinical trials has established the efficacy of short-course combination therapy in the treatment of the vast majority of cases of tuberculosis. Short-course treatment consists of two months of intensive therapy with isoniazid, rifampicin, pyrazinamide, and ethambutol followed by four months of consolidative therapy with isoniazid and rifampicin only. Treatment of tuberculosis at extrapulmonary sites can be more complex because of the potentially serious effects of local complications at some sites. Corticosteroids have historically been advocated in a wide range of tuberculous syndromes but their use remains controversial. Most authorities currently advocate their routine use in meningeal and pericardial disease only. Extension of the duration of therapy beyond six months can be undertaken in several clinical scenarios. Twelve months of therapy is usually recommended in disease involving the central nervous system while tuberculosis at any site caused by drug-resistant organisms may require much longer therapy, particularly in cases of multi-drug resistance.

Golden M, Vikram H, Extrapulmonary tuberculosis: an overview, *American Family Physician* 2005;72: 1761–1769. http://www.aafp.org/afp/2005/1101/p1761.html

27. E. *Toxoplasmosis gondii*

Patients with HIV infection and low CD4 counts are at risk of opportunistic infections which can frequently involve the CNS. They are also at risk of the development of primary CNS lymphoma. The options listed can all cause infection of the central nervous system. Tuberculosis causes meningitis and can also lead to tuberculoma and abscess formation. Cryptococcal meningitis usually presents with an insidious onset of headache and low-grade meningism. Intra-cranial pressure is often significantly elevated and should be aggressively managed with serial lumbar puncture. Toxoplasmosis typically causes space-occupying lesions, which can be single or multiple. The basal ganglia are a frequently affected site. JC virus causes progressive multifocal leukoencephalopathy, a cause of cognitive decline and focal neurological signs associated with deep white matter change on MRI but no mass effect. HIV itself can cause an encephalopathy which presents as a sub-cortical dementia associated with atrophy on CNS imaging. Cytomegalovirus is a relatively unusual cause of central nervous system disease. Its more usual clinical features are retinopathy, colitis, and peripheral neuropathy. Toxoplasmosis is the most common cause of a solitary space-occupying lesion in a patient with advanced HIV-related immunosuppression. Patients with imaging suggestive of cerebral toxoplasmosis are usually treated empirically for several weeks with brain biopsy being reserved for those who fail to improve.

Longmore M et al., *Oxford Handbook of Clinical Medicine*, Eighth Edition, Oxford University Press, 2010, Chapter 9, Infectious diseases, complications of HIV infection.

28. B. If HIV post-exposure prophylaxis is given, adverse effects of medication are a common problem

Needlestick injury is a common incident affecting healthcare workers and those in related fields. Understandably, it is a source of considerable anxiety for those involved, although transmission of blood-borne viruses is actually relatively low. First aid is effective in reducing the risk of transmission and involves cleaning the affected area and encouraging bleeding. Splashes onto mucous membranes or wounds should be irrigated but not scrubbed to the extent that barrier integrity might be compromised. Hepatitis B infection can be effectively prevented by vaccinating those at risk of infection before they are exposed. Those who have not been vaccinated can be protected by the administration of hepatitis B immunoglobulin and beginning a course of vaccination to offer long-term protection. The accelerated course of vaccination offers some protection against acute infection and can be offered alone in low-risk cases. Hepatitis C cannot be prevented by any means other than the first aid measures outlined above since there is no effective vaccination or immunoglobulin therapy. Hepatitis C can, however, be treated and therefore those exposed to hepatitis C should be closely followed so that treatment can be offered in the event of seroconversion. HIV transmission can be reduced by the administration of Antiretrovirals. These are normally given for four weeks in a combination that is known to be effective in the management of established HIV infection. Unfortunately, adverse effects of the Antiretrovirals are common (they seem to be more common than among patients taking the same drugs for treatment of HIV). If begun within a few hours of the injury and continued for four weeks, Antiretrovirals probably reduce the risk of HIV transmission by around two-thirds. In order to provide the best advice and treatment to those affected, it is important to try to test the source of the injury if their blood-borne virus status is not known. However, testing can only be carried out with consent.

Riddell A, Kennedy I, Tong CY, Management of sharps injuries in the healthcare setting, *British Medical Journal*. 2015 Jul 29;351:h3733. http://webarchive.nationalarchives.gov.uk/20140714084352/ http://www.hpa.org.uk/Topics/InfectiousDiseases/InfectionsAZ/BloodborneVirusesAnd OccupationalExposure/

29. C. Hepatitis C virus

Viruses have varied life cycles and utilize many different mechanisms to circumvent the immune response. However, all of them ultimately have to replicate their genetic material in order to cause infection. Viruses can be divided based on the way their nucleic acid is constituted. Herpes viruses (one of the largest groups of viruses commonly causing disease in humans) are double-stranded DNA viruses which tend to cause persistent dormant infection by integrating their DNA with that of the host. The most common examples of herpes viruses are herpes simplex virus (HSV) 1 and 2, and varicella zoster virus. Less common examples include cytomegalovirus and human herpes virus-8 (the cause of Kaposi's sarcoma). HIV is a retrovirus which generates DNA from RNA within the host cell through the expression of reverse transcriptase. Hepatitis viruses come from different classes and therefore do not fall simply into one group. Hepatitis A and C are RNA viruses while hepatitis B is a DNA virus which incorporates a reverse transcriptase step in its life cycle (hence why some Antiretrovirals such as lamivudine are also active against it). Finally, the common childhood diseases measles, mumps, rubella, and enteroviruses (which include poliovirus) are all RNA viruses.

Wilkins R et al., *Oxford Handbook of Medical Sciences*, Second Edition, Oxford University Press, 2011, Chapter 12, Infection and immunity, Viral structure and classification.

30. B. Leishmaniasis—*Aedes* mosquito

Zoonoses are relatively uncommon in the United Kingdom but are a major cause of morbidity and mortality elsewhere in the world, particularly the tropics. The life cycles of these organisms are often complex, involving multiple animal hosts, but an understanding of the animals that transmit them to humans is important to understand the epidemiology and presentation of the disease. The most important zoonosis worldwide is malaria, which is transmitted by infected *Anopheles* mosquitoes. However, the presence of the mosquito is not sufficient to allow the disease to become endemic since various other environmental and climatic factors are at work. It also means that if infected mosquitoes are transported elsewhere in the world, they can cause localized cases of malaria anywhere (for example sporadic cases have been reported around airports). The *Aedes* mosquito is responsible for the transmission of several viral illnesses including yellow fever and dengue. It does not transmit leishmaniasis, however. Leishmaniasis is transmitted by sandflies, while African trypanosomiasis is transmitted by the bite of the Tsetse fly. Ticks can transmit a range of diseases of which the disease receiving the most attention in the developed countries is Lyme disease. This causes a characteristic rash (erythema chronicum migrans) with a clearing centre. If untreated, it can go on to cause joint, cardiac, and neurological disease. Other tick-borne diseases include rickettsial diseases and tick typhus. Finally, schistosomiasis is a parasitic infection with a complex life cycle involving freshwater snails. Snails shed motile larvae which invade through the skin of those exposed to the water source. Acute infection causes fever and eosinophilia (Katayama fever) while chronic infection can lead to a range of symptoms depending on the infecting species including haematuria and portal hypertension.

Török E et al., *Oxford Handbook of Infectious Diseases and Microbiology*, Oxford University Press, 2009, Chapter 4, Systematic microbiology, Borrelia species.

31. D. JC virus

All of the above pathogens can cause neurological disease in the context of HIV infection with a low CD4 count. This patient has a very low CD4 count which leaves him vulnerable to multiple CNS infections, which can often co-exist with other opportunistic infections. CNS lymphoma is another important cause of neurological symptoms and signs in patients such as this one. Toxoplasmosis causes contrast-enhancing lesions which have a predilection for the basal ganglia but can occur throughout the CNS. Patients present with focal neurological signs and sometimes evidence of raised intracranial pressure. Diagnosis can be facilitated by the finding of IgG to toxoplamosis but this has low specificity and so the diagnosis is usually made on the basis of a clinical and radiological response to appropriate therapy. The most frequent differential diagnosis is CNS lymphoma. Cryptococcus causes insidious onset of headache and meningism. Diagnosis is based on the finding of cryptococcal antigen in cerebrospinal fluid and the organism can frequently be cultured from CSF and blood in affected patients. Treatment is with combination antifungal therapy and control of raised intracranial pressure (if present) with serial lumbar puncture, which is vitally important to prevent death and disability. Cytomegalovirus causes CNS disease relatively infrequently, with other sites such as the GI tract, eyes, and peripheral nerves being much more commonly affected. If the CNS is affected then this usually manifests as polyradiculopathy although meningoencephalitis and myelitis can also occur. In this case, the patient has slowly progressive, diffuse neurological signs and MRI shows bilateral white matter change. HIV encephalopathy causes progressive neurological decline and partially responds to Antiretrovirals. The presence of discrete white matter lesions on MRI, however, suggests progressive, multifocal leukoencephalopathy caused by JC virus, which can usually be detected by PCR of CSF. There is no specific treatment for either HIV encephalopathy or PML except treatment with HAART. Recently, PML has also been associated with the use of certain biological therapies for inflammatory conditions. Natalizumab is used in multiple sclerosis and Crohn's disease and rituximab in B-cell lymphomas. Both have been associated with a small but significant risk of PML (around 1 in 500–1000 patients per year treated).

CDC, Guidelines for Prevention and Treatment of Opportunistic Infections in HIV-Infected Adults and Adolescents, *Morbidity and Mortality Weekly Report*, 2009;58:RR4. http://www.cdc.gov/mmwr/pdf/rr/rr5804.pdf

32. E. Giardia

This clinical picture fits best with giardiasis. Giardia infection is transmitted by the faecal–oral route and the patient is likely to have been infected during his trip to Thailand. Intermittent symptoms similar to those of irritable bowel syndrome can be seen for a number of weeks. Antigen testing to confirm the diagnosis is now routinely available. Metronidazole or tinidazole are treatments of choice, and one course of therapy is usually sufficient to prevent recurrence. Long-term lactose intolerance may be seen. Campylobacter is associated with acute gastroenteritis and symptoms usually begin within 2–5 days of eating infected food. It is characterized by severe abdominal cramps, nausea, vomiting, and diarrhoea. Shigella causes bacillary dysentery with profuse bloody/mucous diarrhoea, and has an incubation period which may be as short as one day. It occurs in outbreaks, often in children's day care centres. Salmonellosis has an incubation period of 12–24 hours, occurs usually through infected poultry or dairy products, and results in vomiting, diarrhoea, and abdominal cramps. It is usually self-limiting. Yersinia pestis is spread by fleas and is associated with plague infection.

Bloom S et al., *Oxford Handbook of Gastroenterology and Hepatology*, Oxford University Press, 2012, Section 3, An A to Z, Giardiasis.

33. D. Yellow fever

The clues here are the lack of vaccination history, travel to central America, and jaundice with bleeding which has commenced around ten days after a flu-like illness. Yellow fever is transmitted by the *Haemagogus* mosquito and has an incubation of 3–6 days. Classically, patients recover from a severe flu-like illness, only to fall ill again, with jaundice, bleeding, and mid-zone liver necrosis. Supportive therapy only is possible, and mortality is up to 40%. It is endemic in ten countries across South America and 30 across sub-Saharan Africa. A vaccine is available and mandated when travelling to endemic countries. Diagnosis is clinical, but ELISA and PCR are now available.

Eddleston M, Davidson R, *Oxford Handbook of Tropical Medicine*, Oxford University Press, 2005.

34. E. Weil's disease

A farmer working in the countryside with ditches and ponds might be exposed to rat urine and therefore contact Leptospirosis ictohaemorrhagica (Weil's disease). Characteristically, such patients develop suffused conjunctiva, haemorrhagic manifestations, a dry cough, jaundice, and renal failure. Treatment in severe cases is recommended with penicillin G (1.5 million units six-hourly for one week) or, in milder cases, doxycycline 100 mg b.d. for one week.

Wyatt J et al., *Oxford Handbook of Emergency Medicine*, Fourth Edition, Oxford University Press, 2012, Chapter 5, Infectious diseases, Leptospirosis (Weil's disease).

35. A. A single dose of intramuscular penicillin G benzathine 2.4 mU

Herpetic ulcers are notable for causing pain. This ulcer is painless and rubbery suggesting a chancre, as seen in primary syphilis. The symptoms of syphilis typically present approximately three weeks following exposure. Associated regional lymphadenopathy is common in primary syphilis infection. The treatment of primary syphilis is with intramuscular penicillin G benzathine. Acyclovir is appropriate treatment for herpetic ulcers so is not the correct answer.

Török E et al., *Oxford Handbook of Infectious Diseases and Microbiology*, Oxford University Press, 2009, Chapter 5, Clinical syndromes, Syphilis.

36. D. He has Lyme disease and has no evidence of past or current syphilis

Lyme disease may cause a positive TPPA result but would not be expected to cause a positive IgG or RPR. Infection (TB) or inflammation (lupus) may cause a ly positive RPR and his IgG and TPPA may be positive due to previously treated syphilis infection. If he was previously treated for syphlis then his TPPA and IgG may be positive for that reason. However, if his infection was cleared, the RPR should now be negative. The persistent positive RPR suggests ongoing infection which would need treatment. Yaws is another treponemal infection which is able to cause a positive RPR and TPPA in a patient born in the tropics and is therefore difficult to distinguish from syphilis by serology, though clinically the skin changes may be apparent and it is important to examine the legs of the patient. A new or untreated infection of syphilis would be expected to cause a positive IgG, TPPA, and RPR as seen here.

Tramont EC, Mandell, *Douglas and Bennett's Principles and Practice of Infectious Diseases*, Churchill Livingstone Elsevier, 2010, Treponema pallidum (syphilis), laboratory diagnosis, serological tests, pp. 3044–3048.

37. B. Chlorhexidine 4% bodywash daily from neck to feet and mupirocin nasal ointment for five days followed by a combination of oral doxycycline and rifampicin for five days

This case describes *Staphylococcus aureus* soft tissue infection and colonization. The history of recurrent abscesses and probable close contacts as a military recruit suggests the cause may be a strain of *S. aureus* that produces Panton–Valentine Leukocidin (PVL) toxin. This toxin is produced by less than 2% of *S. aureus*, including MRSA strains. As the nasal swab shows MRSA, the patient is colonized with MRSA. As a result, flucloxacillin or fusidic acid are unlikely to be effective therapies. There appears to be a current active soft tissue infection, which will need a course of oral antibiotics. There is also evidence of nasal colonization, which should be treated topically to prevent future infections. In order to treat the primary infection a course of, for example, doxycylcine and rifampicin is needed. If the organism were resistant to tetracyclines, an alternative regime, such as oral linezolid, may be required. Such cases should be discussed with the local microbiologists. Once the antibiotics for the primary infection are complete the organism should be eradicated using a combination of chlorhexidine 4% bodywash daily from neck to feet and mupirocin nasal ointment for five days.

Health Protection Agency, Guidance on the diagnosis and management of PVL-associated Staphylococcusaureus infections (PVL-SA) in England. http://webarchive.nationalarchives.gov.uk/20140714084352/http://www.hpa.org.uk/webc/HPAwebFile/HPAweb_C/1218699411960

38. A. HIV post-exposure prophylaxis should be started immediately. The donor patient should be tested for HIV, hep B, and hep C, and the duration of prophylaxis can be reviewed with these results

There is a significant risk of HIV if the donor was HIV-positive, and as the donor comes from a high-risk area you would recommend starting HIV prophylaxis immediately whilst awaiting the HIV result from the donor patient. Delays while awaiting donor patient virology results may compromise the efficacy of the post-exposure prophylaxis so the treatment course should be started immediately and can be discontinued if the patient is subsequently found to be HIV-negative. As the doctor is known to have a hepatitis B surface antibody level of about 100 IU, they are likely to be immune and there is no need for a booster immunization against hepatitis B at this time.

http://webarchive.nationalarchives.gov.uk/20130107105354/http://www.dh.gov.uk/prod_consum_dh/groups/dh_digitalassets/@dh/@en/documents/digitalasset/dh_089997.pdf

39. B. Call ITU and administer IV clindamycin, linezolid, and rifampicin

This is a classic description of Panton–Valentine Leukocidin (PVL) necrotizing pneumonia although other forms of pneumonia remain in the differential. Current guidance from the HPA suggests flucloxacillin may worsen outcome and the focus of treatment is on the control of toxin production. Outcome is poor but may be improved through supportive measures such as early ITU care and appropriate antimicrobial therapy. Current recommendations are for the combination of clinamycin, linezolid, and rifampicin. Rifampicin should not be used alone due to the rapid emergence of resistance. Alternative treatment regimes include vancomycin in combination with rifampicin or linezolid.

Health Protection Agency, Guidance on the diagnosis and management of PVL-associated Staphylococcusaureus infections (PVL-SA) in England. http://webarchive.nationalarchives.gov.uk/20140714084352/http://hpa.org.uk/webc/hpawebfile/hpaweb_c/1218699411960

40. E. Colonoscopy would be advised to exclude bowel malignancy

Streptococcus bovis is a Gram-positive coccus commonly found in the alimentary tract of cows, sheep, and other ruminants. It is occasionally encountered in cases of human endocarditis. The most common manifestations of *S. bovis* infection are bacteraemia and infective endocarditis (IE). The organism is usually susceptible to penicillin, and infection generally responds to the same treatment regimens prescribed for infections due to viridans streptococci. In view of the association between *S. bovis* bacteremia or IE with colonic neoplasia, strong recommendations have been put forth that all adult patients with *S. bovis* bacteraemia undergo an aggressive diagnostic evaluation to search for colonic malignancy. The organism is not generally considered to be part of the normal oral flora although bacteria described as *S. bovis* have been identified in cultures of gingiva or throat in small numbers of individuals. Most of these organisms are highly sensitive to penicillin. The bacteriologic cure rate with such treatment is approximately 98%.

Alazmi W et al., The association of *Streptococcus bovis* bacteremia and gastrointestinal diseases: a retrospective analysis, *Digestive Diseases and Sciences* 2006;51(4):732–736.

41. B. Liver abscess

The new murmur is most likely to be a flow murmur in someone who is septic and with a normal echocardiogram. Infective endocarditis is a close second in the differential diagnosis and not excluded by the normal transthoracic echocardiogram, but the patient does not meet Duke's criteria. The pleural effusion is likely to be reactive to the liver abscess and the raised hemidiaphragm secondary to liver enlargement. Pulmonary embolism has been excluded by the CTPA. The low grade uptake of the white cell scan in the right knee is compatible with previous surgery.

Medicalcriteria.com, Duke Criteria for Infective Endocarditis (IE). http://www.medicalcriteria.com/criteria/car_endocarditis.htm

42. B. Oral vancomycin

Clostridium difficile infection causes diarrhoeal illness that could vary in severity. Current guidelines recommend oral metronidazole for initial treatment in patients with mild to moderate disease because it is cheaper than oral vancomycin, and because of concern that overuse of vancomycin may result in the selection of vancomycin-resistant enterococci. Symptoms usually improve within 72 hours and it may take ten days for diarrhoea to stop. If diarrhoea does not improve, patients initially treated with metronidazole may be changed to vancomycin. In severe disease, aggressive treatment with escalating doses of vancomycin, up to 500 mg four times daily, is required. No reliable parenteral treatment for *Clostridium difficile* infection exists. In patients with adynamic ileus (which may reduce the passage of oral preparations to the colon), intravenous metronidazole may be added, but the efficacy of this route of administration is unclear. Intravenous immunoglobulin (400 mg/kg) may be used in selected severe cases although results from case reports and small series have been inconsistent.

Gov.uk, Clostridium difficile infection: how to deal with the problem, Public Health England and Department of Health, 2008. http://www.hpa.org.uk/webc/HPAwebFile/HPAweb_C/1232006607827

43. E. Synovial fluid aspiration and analysis

Septic arthritis is a serious infective disorder with a case fatality of 11%. Delayed or inadequate treatment leads to joint damage. Patients with a short history of a hot, swollen, and tender joint with restriction of movement should be regarded as having septic arthritis until proven otherwise. The synovial fluid must be aspirated immediately, Gram stained and cultured, prior to starting antibiotics. Empirical antibiotic treatment can then be initiated and modified according to the Gram stain results. Cartilage and joint damage is a rapid and irreversible process, so appropriate antibiotics should be commenced as soon as possible and these are mandatory for assured eradication of the infection. Blood and synovial fluid cultures may yield an organism. However, it is often 48 hours before any assured blood culture results become available. Plain radiographs of the affected joint are of no benefit in diagnosing septic arthritis. It is unlikely to show acute changes. CT scans and MRIs are more sensitive for distinguishing osteomyelitis, periarticular abscesses, and identifying joint effusions. There is no role for MRI of the knee in the immediate management of septic arthritis.

Coakley G et al., BSR & BHPR, BOA, RCGP and BSAC guidelines for management of the hot swollen joint in adults, *Rheumatology* 2006;45:1039–1041.

44. E. Shingles

The Health Protection Agency (HPA) is responsible for monitoring the incidence and distribution of some of the important infectious diseases. Conditions that are severe, and those that are vaccinated against, make up a large proportion of this list. It is the doctor's legal responsibility to notify the HPA if they suspect any of the diseases on this list. This list can be found on the link below.

Gov.uk, Notifiable diseases and causative organisms: how to report, Public Health England, 2010. http://www.hpa.org.uk/Topics/InfectiousDiseases/InfectionsAZ/NotificationsOfInfectiousDiseases/ListOfNotifiableDiseases/

45. C. Nevirapine

Nevirapine is an non-nucleoside reverse transcriptase inhibitor (NNRTI). The other options are all nucleoside reverse transcriptase inhibitors (NRTIs). Antiretroviral drugs for treatment of HIV infection fall into three main categories: nucleoside reverse transcriptase inhibitors (NRTIs)—inhibit the enzyme responsible for transcription of viral RNA into DNA which is then integrated into the host genome; non-nucleoside reverse transcriptase inhibitors (NNRTIs)—similar mode of action to NRTIs, but act on different receptors; protease inhibitors (PIs)—inhibit HIV protease, an enzyme which cleaves proteins for assembly of new virions. Most HIV treatment regimens contain a combination of classes of Antiretrovirals. Newer agents target other enzymes involved in the viral replication process (e.g. integrase inhibitors such as raltegravir). (See Table 5.3.)

Török E et al., *Oxford Handbook of Infectious Diseases and Microbiology*, Oxford University Press, 2009, Chapter 2, Antimicrobials, pp. 138–147.

Table 5.3 Summary of commonly used antiretrovirals to treat HIV infection

Class	NRTIs	NNRTIs	PIs
Drug	Tenofovir	Nevirapine	Saquinavir
	Lamivudine	Efavirenz	Lopinavir
	Emtricitabine		Ritonavir
	Stavudine		Atazanavir
	Zidovudine		Fosamprenavir
	Abacavir		Darunavir
	Didanosine		Nelfinavir

46. E. *Streptococcus pneumoniae*

Streptococcus pneumoniae appears as Gram-positive cocci in chains or pairs (diplococcic) on Gram staining. It is alpha haemolytic on blood agar and is differentiated from other streptococci by being optochin-sensitive. It is informally known as 'pneumococcus'. It is the commonest bacterial cause of lobar pneumonia, but can cause other serious infectious (e.g. meningitis). HIV infection is a risk factor for invasive infection with *Streptococcus pneumoniae* with formation of empyema. It is usually sensitive to penicillin but penicillin resistance is recognized, with high rates of resistance in some areas (e.g. Spain).

Török E et al., *Oxford Handbook of Infectious Diseases and Microbiology*, Oxford University Press, 2009, Chapter 4, Systematic microbiology, Streptococcus pneumoniae.

47. C. *Neisseria gonorrhoeae*

Neisseria gonorrhoeae is a Gram-negative diplococcus and is intracellular. It is the causative agent of gonorrhoea, a common sexually transmitted infection that typically presents as urethral discharge. *Candida albicans* would appear as yeast cells with pseudohyphae. *Chlamydia trachomatis* stains poorly with Gram stain and is usually not visible on microscopy. *Staphylococcus aureus* would appear as clustered Gram-positive cocci on Gram staining. It can cause purulent infections but is not sexually transmitted. *Treponema pallidum* is not visible on standard light microscopy and is usually diagnosed by serology. Treponemes can occasionally be visualized by dark field microscopy from a sample taken from a syphilitic chancre.

Török E et al., *Oxford Handbook of Infectious Diseases and Microbiology*, Oxford University Press, 2009, Chapter 4, Systematic microbiology, Neisseria gonorrhoeae.

48. E. Tenofovir

Tenofovir is an NRTI. All the other options are protease inhibitors. Antiretroviral drugs for treatment of HIV infection fall into three main categories: ucleoside reverse transcriptase inhibitors (NRTIs)—inhibit the enzyme responsible for transcription of viral RNA into DNA which is then integrated into the host genome; non-nucleoside reverse transcriptase inhibitors (NNRTIs)—similar mode of action to NRTIs, but act on different receptors; protease inhibitors (PIs)—inhibit HIV protease, an enzyme which cleaves proteins for assembly of new virions. Most HIV treatment regimens contain a combination of classes of Antiretrovirals. Newer agents target other enzymes involved in the viral replication process e.g. integrase inhibitors such as raltegravir. (See Table 5.3.)

Török E et al., *Oxford Handbook of Infectious Diseases and Microbiology*, Oxford University Press, 2009, Chapter 2, Antimicrobials, pp. 138–147.

49. A. *Plasmodium falciparum*

This patient is most likely to have Falciparum malaria. *Plasmodium falciparum* is the commonest form of malaria found in sub-Saharan Africa, and is responsible for the most severe form of the illness, and can lead to cerebral malaria and death if untreated. Most people of West African origin lack the Duffy coat antigen on erythrocytes, which is needed by *Plasmodium vivax* to enter erythrocytes, therefore conferring resistance to Vivax malaria, making vivax less likely in this patient. *Plasmodium ovale* and *Plasmodium vivax* cause a less severe illness than Falciparum malaria, but they can cause relapsing illness many months after infection. This is due to parasites that lie dormant in the liver (hypnozoites) which can reactivate to cause clinical disease. *Plasmodium knowelesi* is found in primates and rarely found in humans. It can occasionally cause fatal disease.

Török E et al., *Oxford Handbook of Infectious Diseases and Microbiology*, Oxford University Press, 2009, Chapter 4, Systematic Microbiology, pp. 562–564.

50. A. Efavirenz

Antiretroviral drugs for treatment of HIV infection fall into three main categories: Nucleoside reverse transcriptase inhibitors (NRTIs)—inhibit the enzyme responsible for transcription of viral RNA into DNA which is then integrated into the host genome; non-nucleoside reverse transcriptase inhibitors (NNRTIs)—similar mode of action to NRTIs, but act on different receptors; protease inhibitors (PIs)—inhibit HIV protease, an enzyme which cleaves proteins for assembly of new virions. Most HIV treatment regimens contain a combination of classes of antiretrovirals. Newer agents target other enzymes involved in the viral replication process (e.g. integrase inhibitors such as raltegravir). (See Table 5.3.)

Török E et al., *Oxford Handbook of Infectious Diseases and Microbiology*, Oxford University Press, 2009, Chapter 2, Antimicrobials, pp. 138–147.

51. A. Typhoid fever

Typhoid fever, otherwise known as Enteric fever, is caused by the Gram-negative bacterium *Salmonella typhi* or *Salmonella paratyphi*. Infection is through the faeco-oral route, usually by ingestion of the organism from contaminated food or water. Poor sanitation, crowding, and lack of hygiene increase the risk of typhoid. The incubation period is 5–21 days. Clinical manifestations are varied; however fever, constipation or diarrhoea, abdominal pain, and chills are the commonest symptoms. Rose spots (pink macules on the trunk) are sometime observed. Patients usually have a neutrophilia, and liver function tests are often abnormal. If left untreated, the illness can progress to severe sepsis, peritonitis, and intestinal perforation. Diagnosis is usually made by isolation of the organism in blood cultures, which are positive in 40–80% of cases. Treatment is with a fourth-generation cephalosporin such as ceftriaxone or azithromycin. Previously, quinolones were commonly used to treat typhoid, but quinolone resistance is increasing and treatment with this class of antimicrobials is no longer reliable. Typhoid is a notifiable disease.

Eddleston M et al., *Oxford Handbook of Tropical Medicine*, Third Edition, Oxford University Press, 2008, Chapter 18, Multi-system diseases and infections, Typhoid and paratyphoid fevers.

52. B. The diagnosis of Karposi's sarcoma confirms the onset of AIDS in patients with HIV

Cancer is responsible for an increasing proportion of deaths amongst patients affected with HIV (currently 25–30%). This is thought to be due primarily to the development of highly active antiretroviral therapy (HAART), fewer deaths from opportunistic infections, and an older population. The effects of chronic immunosuppression may also be contributing. Karposi's sarcoma is a multifocal angioproliferative disorder and is the most common tumour observed in patients with HIV. Although its appearance in a patient with confirmed HIV is AIDS-defining according to current criteria, it can also occur in patients without HIV. Its development is associated with infection with human herpes virus, type 8 (HHV-8). Other AIDS-defining cancers in patients with HIV are primary CNS lymphoma, invasive cervical cancer, and intermediate and high-grade non-Hodgkins lymphoma of B-cell or unknown immunological phenotype. HIV-positive patients with non-Hodgkins lymphoma typically present with advanced disease. Compared to seronegative patients with similar histology, response rates to treatment are less good and the disease tends to follow a more aggressive clinical course. Patients with HIV are also at increased risk of non-AIDS-defining cancers. These are generally associated with higher tumour grade, earlier development of metastases, and a poorer outcome than in the seronegative population.

Cassidy J et al., *Oxford Handbook of Oncology*, Third Edition, Oxford University Press, 2010, Chapter 29, AIDS-related malignancies.

53. C. Untreated, up to 15% of infections with HPV will progress to either cervical intraepithelial neoplasia (CIN) or cervical cancer

Human papilloma virus (HPV) is a small, double-stranded DNA virus that infects squamous epithelial cells of skin and mucous membranes, and is the most frequent sexually acquired infection in the developed world. There are over 90 strains of HPV, although the majority have no known association with malignancy. However, certain strains of HPV are believed to be causative in over 80% of cervical cancers worldwide, as well as being associated with squamous cell carcinomas of the anus, penis, vagina, vulva, and some head and neck cancers. Uterine cancers are typically adenocarcinomas and are not associated with HPV. Unprotected sexual intercourse is the most common cause of genital infection, although any close genital contact with an infected individual places the person at risk. The UK immunization programme began in 2008 and offers a quadrivalent vaccination to girls of secondary school age (12–13 years old). The aim is to immunize girls against the four strains of HPV most commonly associated with malignancy (HPV types 6, 11, 16, and 18) before they are exposed to the HPV virus.

Cassidy J et al., *Oxford Handbook of Oncology,* Third Edition, Oxford University Press, 2010, Chapter 2, Aetiology and epidemiology, Infections.

54. B. *Escherichia coli*

Haemolytic uraemic syndrome (HUS) is classically defined as a triad of microangiopathic haemolytic anaemia, thrombocytopenia, and acute renal failure. Presentations following on from a diarrhoeal illness are typically seen in childhood or early infancy, and are most commonly associated with shiga toxin-producing *Escherichia coli*, or more specifically, *E. coli* serotype O157:H7, which is responsible for 80% of cases of diarrhoea-associated HUS. *E. coli* O157:H7 is found in healthy cattle, and transmission to humans is most frequently in the context of consumption of undercooked meat containing viable bacteria. Treatment is supportive, with strict attention to fluid balance and renal replacement therapy if required. Antibiotics have been shown to increase the risk of HUS in the context of *E. coli O157* infections.

Tan AJ, Hemolytic uremic syndrome in emergency medicine, *eMedicine*, 2010. http://emedicine. medscape.com/article/779218-overview

55. E. Oral vancomycin

Although there is no consensus on what characterizes a 'severe' case of CDAD, this patient has several features commonly used as markers of severity, including fever, high white cell count, and profuse diarrhoea (>6–10 stools in 24 hours). However, she has no colonic dilatation or abdominal symptoms requiring surgical intervention at this point, and is able to tolerate oral fluids and medications. Oral vancomycin has been shown to be superior to metronidazole in the context of severe CDAD, and would be the treatment of choice in this case. Intravenous vancomycin is not used to treat CDAD, as it does not reach the colon, and intracolonic vancomycin is typically used in severe cases of CDAD as an adjunct where other treatments have failed. Oral metronidazole is an option for less severe disease, and intravenous metronidazole could be used if the patient was unable to tolerate any medications orally.

Kelly CP, Lamont JT, Treatment of antibiotic-associated diarrhoea caused by *Clostridium difficile* in adults, *UpToDate*, 2010. http://www.uptodate.com/online/content/topic.do?topicKey=gi_infec/2874&sel ectedTitle=1%7E150&source=search_result

56. C. The production of toxins

Clostridium difficile primarily causes disease through the production of two large clostridial toxins, toxin A and toxin B, which form the target of the ELISA-based assays used in the diagnosis of infection in many microbiology laboratories. Toxin B is essential for disease virulence—several toxin A negative/toxin B positive strains exist that are able to cause disease, but to date no toxin A positive/toxin B negative strains have been isolated. The toxins disrupt the cellular Rho GTPases involved in maintaining the cytoskeleton of enteric epithelial cells, leading to apoptosis and inflammation. The toxins also disrupt the intercellular junctions.

LaMont TJ, Epidemiology, microbiology, and pathophysiology of *Clostridium difficile* infection in adults, *UpToDate*, 2010. http://www.uptodate.com/online/content/topic.do?topicKey=gi_infec/2150&selected Title=3%7E150&source=search_result

57. A. Patients should be isolated in side rooms until they have been diarrhoea-free for at least 48 hours and have passed a formed stool

The nosocomial epidemic of *Clostridium difficile*-associated infection that has taken place in North American and European hospitals has prompted widespread intervention by public health authorities. In the UK, reporting of cases of CDI has become mandatory for patients over the age of 2 years, and routine testing is carried out on diarrhoeal specimens submitted by patients over the age of 65 years. At present there are still around 23000 cases reported annually to the Health Protection Agency in the UK. In 2009, the UK Department of Health and the Health Protection Agency issued guidance on the diagnosis, prevention, and treatment of *Clostridium difficile*-associated infection (CDI), including appropriate infection control measures. All of the above issues are discussed in the document. Alcohol hand rub will kill vegetative forms of the organism, but will not inhibit the spread of spores, and hand washing after each patient contact is recommended. Gloves and aprons should be worn for each patient contact, environmental cleaning should be carried out at least daily, and routine environmental screening is not recommended.

Department of Health and Health Protection Agency, *Clostridium difficile* infection: How to deal with the problem, 2009. http://webarchive.nationalarchives.gov.uk/20140714084352/http://www.hpa.org.uk/web/HPAweb&HPAwebStandard/HPAweb_C/1216105603048

58. A. *Campylobacter jejuni*

This man is presenting with an acute (<14 days) diarrhoeal illness, and has features suggestive of severe and invasive infection (temperature >38.5°C, >6 stools/day, bloody diarrhoea). The commonest bacterial causes of community-acquired diarrhoea in immunocompetent adults are *Campylobacter spp.* (30–40%), non-typhoidal Salmonella (20–30%), Shigella (20%), and enterohaemorrhagic *Escherichia coli* (7%). Whilst this presentation could be consistent with answers A, D, and E, the high fever, incubation period, and relative frequency of *Campylobacter jejuni* as a cause of diarrhoea in this context make it the correct answer.

Gov.uk, Campylobacter: guidance, data and analysis, Public Health England, 2014. http://www.hpa.org.uk/Topics/InfectiousDiseases/InfectionsAZ/Campylobacter/GeneralInformation/campyCampylobacterClinicalinformation/

59. B. GM1 ganglioside

C. jejuni-associated GBS is thought to be caused by antibodies directed against GM1 ganglioside, which is found at high levels in the myelin of peripheral nerves. This is an example of molecular mimicry, where autoantibodies are formed in response to structurally similar epitopes on the surface of the particular 'foreign' immunological target in question. HLA-B27 is a particular human leukocyte antigen haplotype that predisposes individuals infected with *C. jejuni* to the development of post-infectious syndromes, and is associated with a multitude of other immune-mediated disease syndromes, such as reactive arthritis and ankylosing spondylitis. Acetylcholine receptor antibodies are a feature of myasthenia gravis, and NMDA and voltage-gated potassium channel antibodies are found in limbic encephalitides.

Allos BM, Clinical features and treatment of Campylobacter infection, *UpToDate*, 2009. http://www.uptodate.com/online/content/topic.do?topicKey=gi_infec/8685&selectedTitle=1%7E112&source=search_result

60. D. Intravenous artesunate

Parasitaemia >10% is consistent with life-threatening malaria. Randomized controlled studies are difficult to find with this degree of parasitaemia, but both artesunate and exchange transfusion have shown promise in the management of the condition. Out of the two, artesunate is listed here and is therefore the correct answer. It is associated with rapid clearance of parasitaemia.

UK malaria treatment guidelines, *Journal of Infection* 2007;54:111e121

61. B. Intravenous quinine

This patient has severe malaria, as evidenced by a parasitaemia above 5%; life-threatening parasitaemia is defined as above 10%. For life-threatening disease both exchange transfusion and artemesin-based compounds are potential options. In the case of severe malaria, IV quinine is superior to oral quinine, despite the risks of hypoglycaemia which can be managed. Her bloods show evidence of severe haemolytic anaemia, renal failure related to malaria infection and SIADH (low sodium), all recognized in severe falciparum.

gov.uk, Malaria: guidance, data and analysis, Public Health England, 2014. http://www.hpa.org.uk/Topics/InfectiousDiseases/InfectionsAZ/Malaria/Guidelines/mala20guidelinesTreatment/

62. E. Cefixime 400 mg PO

Cefixime 400 mg PO given as a single dose is the most appropriate therapy for gonorrhoea according to guidelines. Ceftriaxone given IM as a single dose is another potential option. Resistance of gonorrhoea to penicillins is now above 10% in the UK, nearly 50% for tetracyclines, and around 15% for quinolones. Of course, the patient should also be screened for other co-existing sexually transmitted diseases, including HIV.

BASHH, National Guideline on the Diagnosis and Treatment of Gonorrhoea in Adults, 2005. http://www.bashh.org/documents/116/116.pdf

63. E. Start cefotaxime 2 g intravenously

Appropriate intravenous antibiotic (e.g. cefotaxime 2 g) should be given without delay. The working diagnosis is meningococcal meningitis. CT scan of the brain is a useful test if the patient's condition deteriorates or the diagnosis remains unconfirmed. Blood cultures should be obtained as soon as possible but this procedure should not take priority over administering appropriate intravenous antibiotic. In the very old or immunocompromised it would be appropriate to add ampicillin 2 g six-hourly to cover Listeria, and acyclovir (10 mg/kg eight-hourly, with dose reduction in renal failure) should also be given if herpes simplex encephalitis is a possibility.

Thompson MJ et al., Clinical recognition of meningococcal disease in children and adolescents, *Lancet* 2006;367:397–403.

64. D. Hepatitis E

Viral hepatitis is one of the most common serious infectious diseases acquired through travel. The most common causes of acute viral hepatitis with jaundice and transaminases elevated to greater than 10x the upper limit of normal are hepatitis A, B, and E. These three viral infections are very difficult to distinguish on clinical grounds. All three present with a non-specific prodromal illness including fever, gastrointestinal upset, and malaise followed by jaundice. This usually resolves spontaneously but in a minority of cases can progress to fulminant liver failure. Hepatitis A and E do not cause chronic infection and are transmitted by the faecal-oral route while hepatitis B frequently causes chronic active hepatitis and is transmitted by blood-to-blood contact, sexually, and vertically. Hepatitis A has traditionally been regarded as the most common cause of acute hepatitis in returning travellers. However, effective vaccination has led to a greatly reduced incidence in recent years and if there is a history of recent hepatitis A vaccination then infection with this virus is extremely unlikely (this is in contrast to the frequently co-administered typhoid vaccine which is of only limited effectiveness and offers no protection against infection by *Salmonella paratyphi*). Hepatitis E has been involved in a number of large outbreaks, particularly in the Indian subcontinent, and has been reported to have become the most frequently identified cause of travel-related acute hepatitis in the UK. Pregnant women appear to be particularly at risk from hepatitis E infection and mortality rates of 20% have been reported among this group. *Entamoeba histolytica* is the protozoan gastrointestinal parasitic cause of amoebic dysentery. It usually presents with bloody diarrhoea and can cause severe illness. It is a cause of liver abscesses but the mild gastrointestinal illness and relatively high AST/ALT in this case make the diagnosis unlikely. Leptospirosis is caused by spirochaetes of the Leptospira family (most commonly *L. icterohaemorrhagiae*). Illness is acquired following contact with water contaminated by rat urine, and ranges in severity from a mild flu-like illness through to multi-organ dysfunction and shock. Hepatitis usually occurs in the context of Weil's disease, a combination of acute renal dysfunction, hepatitis with jaundice, and haemorrhage.

Johnston V et al., Fever in returned travellers presenting in the United Kingdom: recommendations for investigation and initial management, *Journal of Infection* 2009;59:1–18.

65. E. Progressive multifocal

The symptoms and signs point towards the diagnosis of progressive multifocal leucoencephalopathy. The MRI scan of the brain confirms the clinical diagnosis. Intensive antiretroviral chemotherapy is seen as the mainstay of treatment for the condition, although in patients with very low CD4 counts, a paradoxical increase in inflammation may be seen, which can result in a worsening of symptoms.

Longmore M et al., *Oxford Handbook of Clinical Medicine*, Eighth Edition, Oxford University Press, 2010, Chapter 9, Infectious diseases, HIV.

66. C. Schistosomiasis

Schistosomiasis is infection cause by the trematode (fluke) Schistosoma, commonly found in fresh water environments in the tropics. Snails are the intermediate host, which release cercariae. Humans are infected by the cercariae penetrating the skin, which can cause a pruritic rash within 24 hours of infection (Swimmer's Itch). They then migrate to the lungs and liver, settling in the bladder's venous plexus (*Schistosoma haematobium*) or portal venous system (*Schistosoma mansoni*). Eggs are passed out in faeces or urine and hatch in the freshwater, releasing miracidia which infects the snails. Katayama fever is acute schistosomiasis, occurring one or two months after infection, and causing a syndrome of fever, cough, lymphadenopathy, and hepatosplenomegaly. An eosinophilia is usually found in the full blood count. Chronic infection can lead to portal hypertension (*S. mansoni*) or bladder carcinoma (*S. haematobium*). Diagnosis is by visualizing schistosomal eggs in urine or stool, or by serological testing for antibodies. Treatment is with praziquantel.

Doherty JF, Moody AH, Wright SG, Katayama fever: an acute manifestation of schistosomiasis, *British Medical Journal* 1996;313(7064):1071–1072. http://www.ncbi.nlm.nih.gov/pmc/articles/PMC2352353/?tool=pubmed

67. B. Cryptococcal meningitis

Cryptococcal meningitis is caused by the yeast-like organism *Cryptococcus neoformans*. It is ubiquitous in the environment and infection is by inhalation of the organism. Infection is usually asymptomatic in the immunocompetent host but can lead to severe illness in the immunocompromised, particularly those infected with HIV. Cryptococcal meningitis is usually seen in HIV-infected patients with a CD4 count of less than 100 cells per mm³. Presentation is often with severe headache and symptoms of raised intracranial pressure. Focal neurological deficit and papilloedema are often found on examination. Lumbar puncture usually reveals elevated opening pressure. A lymphocytosis, low glucose, and high protein are usually seen in the cerebrospinal fluid (CSF). Diagnosis is confirmed by visualization of the organisms after Indian ink staining. Cryptococcal antigen testing by latex agglutination can be performed on blood or CSF. Treatment is with amphotericin and flucytosine, with long-term fluconazole to prevent relapse.

Török E et al., *Oxford Handbook of Infectious Diseases and Microbiology*, First Edition, Oxford University Press, 2009, Chapter 4, Systematic Microbiology, pp. 527–529.

68. D. Children are affected more than adults

Ascaris lumbricoides is a round worm, which is transmitted via the soil; thus children living in rural conditions are the most highly effected population group. The eggs are ingested and hatch in the small intestine, the larvae then migrate through the wall of the small intestine via the blood stream to the lungs; this is associated with a marked eosinophillia. They mature and work their way up the tracheobronchial tree before returning to the bowel to complete their final maturation and begin egg production. Most infections are asymptomatic, but symptoms are proportional to worm burden and can include abdominal pain, dyspepsia, anaemia, malabsorption, and in the worst cases can cause bowel obstruction, intussusception, or perforation. Ascaris worms do not always migrate as per planned life cycle, and have been known to cause biliary obstruction, pancreatitis, appendicitis, as well as CNS complications due to ectopic migration. Diagnosis is by egg identification in faeces, but occasionally worms may be seen on abdominal X-rays or barium studies. Treatment is with oral albendazole or mebendazole, not tetracycline antibiotics.

Eddleston M et al., *Oxford Handbook of Tropical Medicine*, Third Edition, Oxford University Press, 2008, Chapter 7, Gastroenterology, Ascariasis.

69. C. Metronidazole

Giardia lamblia is a protozoan gastrointestinal parasite that is found worldwide, and is typically transmitted via the faecal-oral route, through water, or in food contaminated with water or soil containing cysts excreted from infected individuals. Although a proportion of infected individuals may be asymptomatic (around 15%), many will suffer symptoms including acute watery diarrhoea, chronic diarrhoea with weight loss and malabsorption, abdominal cramps, bloating, and flatulence. Although some people will recover without treatment, treatment shortens the duration of symptoms and reduces the transmission of cysts. Metronidazole is most commonly used; other antibiotics include tinidazole, nitazoxanide, and paromomycin.

Nazer H, Giardiasis, *Medscape*, 2016. http://emedicine.medscape.com/article/176718-overview

70. C. Cryptosporidiosis

The most likely diagnosis is acute cryptosporidiosis, which is an illness caused by *Cryptosporidium spp.*, which are intracellular protozoal parasites. The main infectious species in humans is *Cryptosporidium parvum*. Infection is typically associated with diarrhoea and biliary tract disease, and can occur in both immunocompetent individuals, in which it is a typically self-limited illness, and in those with impaired cellular (particularly T-cell deficiency, such as in HIV with CD4 counts below

100 cells/microlitre) and/or humoral immunity, where symptoms are more severe and frequently more chronic. A major source of infection is contaminated water, and community outbreaks can be caused by contaminated water in swimming pools and other recreational water sources. Diagnosis is made on microscopy, typically after modified acid-fast staining, where the oocysts can be visualized in faecal specimens. In immunocompetent individuals symptoms usually resolve in 10–14 days, and treatment is supportive.

Leder K, Weller PF, Cryptosporidiosis, *UpToDate*, 2010. http://www.uptodate.com/online/content/topic.do?topicKey=parasite/9473&selectedTitle=1%7E63&source=search_result

71. B. *Plasmodium vivax*

This patient is most likely to have vivax malaria. *Plasmodium vivax* causes a less severe illness than falciparum malaria, but it can cause relapsing illness many months after infection. This is due to parasites which lie dormant in the liver (hypnozoites) which can reactivate to cause clinical disease. *Plasmodium falciparum* is the commonest form of malaria found in sub-Saharan Africa, and is responsible for the most severe form of the illness, and can lead to cerebral malaria and death if untreated. *Plasmodium malariae* does not lead to relapsing infection. Relapsing fever is caused by the bacteria of the genus *Borrelia* and can be transmitted by ticks or lice. It causes a severe febrile illness which has a high mortality without prompt treatment. The bacteria can be seen in a blood film and appear as spiral organisms.

Török E et al., *Oxford Handbook of Infectious Diseases and Microbiology*, Oxford University Press, 2009, Chapter 4, Systematic Microbiology, pp. 562–564.

72. C. Severe malaria

Uganda is an endemic area for malaria infection, and in particular the *Plasmodium falciparum* strain, which may be fatal if left untreated. A patient from that area presenting with an unexplained fever should be considered to have malaria until the diagnosis is confirmed or refuted in the laboratory. Bacterial pneumonia is a possibility but the patient had no respiratory symptoms such as a cough and has no focal consolidation on the CXR. The bibasal crackles on examination are likely to be due to the pulmonary oedema seen on CXR and this is a manifestation of malaria. Features suggestive of more severe disease include the low haemoglobin, renal failure, and pulmonary oedema. The thrombocytopenia and elevated bilirubin in the presence of a normal ALT and ALP are typical of malaria infection. If this patient is shown to have *P. falciparum* malaria they should be treated with parenteral therapy initially in view of the severity of their disease.

CDC, Malaria treatment. http://www.cdc.gov/malaria/diagnosis_treatment/treatment.html

73. A. *Plasmodium falciparum*

Chloroquine-resistant *P. falciparum* is a major worldwide problem. Chloroquine cannot be reliably used to treat falciparum malaria except where infection has been acquired in certain parts of South and Central America. The role of chloroquine as malaria prophylaxis has also been curtailed. Treatment of falciparum malaria acquired from parts of the world with chloroquine resistance must be based either on quinine, artesunate (which does not have a licence for use in the UK but is available from tropical medicine centres for use in severe malaria) or one of the oral combination therapies (which are extensively used for non-severe malaria in endemic countries). The mainstay of treatment in the UK is quinine (in combination with another agent). *Plasmodium vivax* has also acquired chloroquine resistance but this is currently localized to South East Asia and has not yet become a worldwide problem. Other types of malaria generally retain sensitivity to chloroquine. Remember that *Plasmodium vivax* and *Plasmodium ovale* remain within the liver as hypnozoites and therefore therapy with primaquine is required to eliminate them also. *Plasmodium knowlesi* has only recently been identified as a cause of disease in humans. It is morphologically similar to *malariae* but more likely to cause severe disease.

Lalloo DG et al., UK malaria treatment guidelines, *Journal of Infection* 2007;54:111–121. http://www. britishinfection.org/drupal/sites/default/files/malariatreatmentBIS07.pdf

74. C. Invasive cervical cancer

The 1993 CDC definition of AIDS remains the most widely used internationally. Patients infected with HIV are divided into stage A, B, and C. Stage A patients are those who are asymptomatic or have symptoms which do not suggest significant immunosuppression (seroconversion symptoms, persistent lymphadenopathy). Opportunistic infections are rare at this stage. Stage B is also called early symptomatic HIV and includes patients with certain conditions associated with a relatively early immunosuppression. These typically include oropharyngeal or recurrent vulval candida, cervical dysplasia, recurrent shingles, and idiopathic thrombocytopaenic purpura. Finally, stage C disease includes patients who have experienced an illness associated with severe immunosuppression. These are mostly opportunistic infections but there are several important exceptions. It is important for non-specialists to recognize stage B and C indicators because the presence of one of these should prompt the offer of an HIV test. While it is not necessary to memorize all AIDS-defining illnesses, it is important to be familiar with the list as there are some relatively common conditions that might otherwise be overlooked. An abbreviated version of the CDC list is shown in Table 5.4. Whilst Listeria meningitis is rare, it is recognized as occurring in the elderly and those with chronic illnesses apart from HIV, and enterovirus meningitis is very common.

CDC, 1993 Revised Classification System for HIV Infection and Expanded Surveillance Case Definition for AIDS Among Adolescents and Adults, *Morbidity and Mortality Weekly Report* 1992;41:RR17. http://www.cdc.gov/mmwr/preview/mmwrhtml/00018871.htm

Table 5.4 Abbreviated list of AIDS-defining illnesses as defined by the CDC

Candida of the lower respiratory tract or oesophagus	*Mycobacterium tuberculosis* infection at any site*
Invasive cervical cancer*	Disseminated infection by non-tuberculous mycobacterium
Invasive cryptococcal disease	*Pneumocystis jirovecii* pneumonia
Cytomegalovirus disease (except when causing a mononucleosis-like illness)	Recurrent pneumonia*
HIV encephalopathy*	Progressive multifocal
Chronic herpes simplex	leukoencephalopathy
Karposi's sarcoma	Recurrent salmonella sepsis*
Burkitt's lymphoma	Cerbral toxoplasmosis
Primary CNS lymphoma*	Wasting syndrome due to HIV*

Items marked with an asterisk are important to note as they are presentations in which underlying HIV is often not suspected.

75. D. Previous hepatitis B infection

This patient is hepatitis B surface antigen negative, implying that there is no evidence of active infection. The presence of hepatitis B surface antibody implies previous exposure either to the virus or its vaccine. The question of whether the patient has been previously infected or vaccinated can be answered by looking at the hepatitis B core antibody. The presence of core antibody implies previous exposure to the virus. Therefore, this patient with positive surface and core antibody has been previously exposed to hepatitis B virus infection. If the surface antibody were negative then previous hepatitis B vaccination would be the correct answer. Patients with positive surface antigen are infected with hepatitis B. Common serological patterns in active infection are shown in Table

5.5. Note the potential difficulty in the diagnosis of acute hepatitis B infection (although in practice it is usually straightforward). However, there is a brief period between loss of surface antigen and appearance of antibody in which both these markers can be absent. This underlines the importance of informing the laboratory that early hepatitis B is being considered, so that core antibody can be checked since the core IgM will be positive in this instance.

Cooke GS et al., Treatment for hepatitis B, *British Medical Journal* 2010;340:87–91. http://www.bmj.com/content/340/bmj.b5429.long

Table 5.5 Hepatitis serology in active infection

Disease State	Surface Ag	Core Ab (IgG)	Core (IgM)	Hep Be Ae	Hep Be Ab	HBV DNA
Carrier	+	+	–	–	+	Low +
Chronic Infection	+	+	–	+	–	High +
Acute Infection	+/–	+/–	+	+/–	–	–/+

76. B. *Escherichia coli*

Travellers' diarrhoea is common in people travelling from resource-rich to resource-poor countries, with an estimated 30–50% of travellers to nations classified as at high risk of developing this syndrome. High-risk areas include most of Asia, the Middle East, Africa, Mexico, and Central and South America. Surveys identify enterotoxigenic *E. coli* (ETEC) as the most frequently encountered pathogen, with enteric viruses such as norovirus and rotavirus, other bacterial species such as *Campylobacter, Shigella* and non-typhoidal *Salmonella*, and protozoal illnesses such as *Giardia* and *Crytosporidia* seen commonly, but less frequently than ETEC. Cholera is rarely seen in travellers, although it should be considered in people who have a known exposure to an outbreak or who have spent more prolonged periods of time in areas with poor sanitation. The majority of episodes of travellers' diarrhoea are self-limiting and rarely require treatment beyond adequate supportive care, which can be done in the community or in hospital, depending on the severity of the illness.

Travellers' diarrhoea, Travel Health Information Sheet, National Travel Health Network and Centre, 2007. http://www.nathnac.org/pro/factsheets/trav_dir.htm

77. B. It is a cause of toxic shock syndrome

Staphylococcus aureus is a Gram-positive coccus which appears as grape-like clusters on microscopy following Gram staining. It is catalase and coagulase-positive. It is commonly carried in the nose without causing symptoms. It is a common cause of skin and soft tissue infections such as cellulitis. It is usually susceptible to flucloxacillin, but MRSA (methicillin-resistant *Staphylcoccus aureus*—which is resistant to flucloxacillin) is an increasing problem. *Staphylococcus aureus* is an uncommon cause of community-acquired pneumonia but can cause severe, cavitating pneumonia. *Staphylococcus aureus* can cause toxic shock syndrome, a severe systemic illness mediated by bacterial toxins, causing symptoms including high fever, haemodynamic instability, a diffuse, desquamating rash (said to resemble sunburn), and multi-organ involvement such as diarrhoea, hepatic inflammation, and renal impairment.

Török E et al., *Oxford Handbook of Infectious Diseases and Microbiology*, First Edition, Oxford University Press, 2009, Chapter 4, Systematic Microbiology, *Staphylococcus aureus.*

78. B. *Neisseria meningitidis*

All of the organisms named can cause meningitis, but outbreaks are usually caused by *Neiserria meningitidis*. Serogroup B is the most prevalent in the United Kingdom, whilst serogroup A is more commonly the cause of major, seasonal epidemics in areas such as the 'meningitis belt' in sub-Saharan Africa. The meningitis vaccine protects against serogroups A,C, Y, and W-135.

Török E et al., *Oxford Handbook of Infectious Diseases and Microbiology*, First Edition, Oxford University Press, 2009, Chapter 4, Systematic microbiology, *Neisseria meningitidis*.

79. A. Acute motor axonal neuropathy (AMAN)

The most likely answer is acute motor axonal neuropathy (AMAN). AMAN is a variant of Guillain–Barré syndrome, an immunologically mediated neuropathy that typically presents with symmetric progressive weakness, often starting in the lower limbs. Paraesthesiae may be a presenting symptom, but objective sensory loss is not a feature. Dysautonomia may occur in up to 70% of cases (e.g. variable blood pressure, tachycardia). There is no fever. *C. jejuni* is the most commonly identified preceding illness in Guillain–Barré syndrome, and typically occurs 1–2 weeks before the onset of neurological symptoms. Data from the General Practice Research Database in the UK has estimated that the relative risk of GBS in patients with *C. jejuni* infection is around 77 times greater than the general population. Even subclinical infection may trigger GBS: the presence of diarrhoea is not a prerequisite. Campylobacter-associated GBS is more likely to be the axonal as opposed to the demyelinating form, which typically manifests in a slower recovery and greater likelihood of neurological deficit.

Allos BM, Clinical features and treatment of Campylobacter infection, *UpToDate*, 2009. http://www.uptodate.com/online/content/topic.do?topicKey=gi_infec/8685&selectedTitle=1%7E112&source=search_result

80. D. *Campylobacter* infection is a trigger for Guillain–Barré syndrome

Campylobacter infection typically requires an infectious dose of between 500–10000 bacteria, and because the organisms are susceptible to gastric acid, fewer bacteria are needed to establish infection in the context of acid suppression (e.g. with proton pump inhibition.) A higher inoculum is associated with a shorter incubation period and more severe symptoms. The incubation period is typically around three days, and symptoms include abdominal pain, which can sometimes mimic appendicitis, fever (which is often as high as 40°C), and diarrhoea, which is bloody in about 15% of patients. Diarrhoea can be profuse. The illness is usually self-limiting in immunocompetent individuals, with the mean duration of diarrhoea being seven days. Antibiotics should only be considered in severely ill patients, those who are immunocompromised (e.g. HIV), pregnant, or at extremes of age. Relapses occur in around 10–15% of patients, and *Campylobacter* infection is a known trigger for Guillain–Barré syndrome. For diarrhoeal illness the most appropriate antibiotic treatment when indicated would be a macrolide, or ciprofloxacin if resistance is not a problem locally. Human-to-human transmission is rare.

Allos BM, Clinical features and treatment of Campylobacter infection, *UpToDate*, 2009. http://www.uptodate.com/online/content/topic.do?topicKey=gi_infec/8685&selectedTitle=1%7E112&source=search_result

81. A. Clindamycin

Antibiotic use is considered the most widely recognized risk factor for CDAD, and all antibiotics are potential contributors to the development of this disease. However, some antibiotics are associated with a greater risk of CDAD, and these include clindamycin, broad-spectrum cephalosporins such as ceftriaxone, broad-spectrum penicillins such as co-amoxiclav, and fluoroquinolones such as ciprofloxacin. Oral vancomycin is commonly used in the treatment of *C. difficile*, and intravenous vancomycin has minimal effect on the gut flora. Metronidazole, vancomycin, trimethoprim, doxycyline, and aminoglycosides such as gentamicin are considered to put patients at a lower risk of developing CDAD and might be preferentially considered for treatment in high-risk situations or in patients with CDAD who need antibiotic treatment for concomitant infections.

Lamont JT, Epidemiology, microbiology, and pathophysiology of *Clostridium difficile* infection in adults, *UpToDate*, 2010. http://www.uptodate.com/online/content/topic.do?topicKey=gi_infec/2150&selected Title=3%7E150&source=search_result

82. E. Whipple's disease

The unifying diagnosis in this case is Whipple's disease. This is a rare disorder caused by infection with *Tropheryma whipplei*, a Gram-positive bacillus, which can colonize healthy individuals and leads to disease in only a small number of cases. Most patients are white males, with a mean age of onset of 49 years. Approximately two-thirds of cases occur in farmers or individuals with occupational exposure to soil and/or animals. In infected individuals, the main symptoms are arthralgia, weight loss, diarrhoea, and abdominal pain. The arthralgia is typically migratory, affecting the large joints, and can precede the onset of other symptoms by many years. Other systems affected include the central nervous system, with dementia manifesting as a feature of late disease, and the respiratory and cardiac systems resulting in pleural effusions, pericarditis, or endocarditis. The diagnostic test of choice involves biopsies of the small bowel with periodic acid-Schiff staining demonstrating PAS-positive material in the lamina propria in conjunction with villous atrophy; the presence of *T. whipplei* can be confirmed with electron microscopy. Molecular diagnosis by PCR can be done at reference laboratories.

Apstein MD, Schneider T, Whipple's disease, *UpToDate,* 2010. http://www.uptodate.com/online/content/topic.do?topicKey=gi_infec/5305&selectedTitle=1%7E55&source=search_result

83. D. Sputum smear for acid-fast bacilli

The patient described above presents with classical symptoms of respiratory tuberculosis, i.e. infection with Mycobacterium tuberculosis (TB) with weight loss, night sweats, and cough. HIV co-infection is a major risk factor for tuberculosis and should increase the clinical suspicion of tuberculosis. Diagnosis of TB can be challenging. Of the above tests, only visualization of acid-fast bacilli in sputum can confirm the diagnosis. Auramine or Ziehl–Neelsen staining can be performed on sputum in an attempt to visualize AFBs. Smear negative tuberculosis is more common in HIV infection, however, and a negative sputum smear does not exclude infection. The gold standard is culture of the organism, but this can take many weeks, limiting its clinical usefulness, particularly in the developing world. Molecular methods such as PCR are available but are limited by cost and lack of sensitivity. Radiological findings such as upper lobe consolidation and calcification can be suggestive but are not in themselves diagnostic. The Mantoux test involves intracutaneous injection of tuberculin and measurement of induration in the skin. The reliability of the test is limited by positives caused by prior BCG vaccination and the high rate of negatives, particularly in HIV-infected individuals who fail to mount an adequate immune response.

Török E et al., *Oxford Handbook of Infectious Diseases and Microbiology*, Oxford University Press, 2009, Chapter 4, Systematic Microbiology, *Mycobacterium tuberculosis.*

84. D. Necrotizing fasciitis

Mycoplasma pneumoniae is a common cause of community-acquired pneumonia. It lacks a rigid cell wall and therefore is not visualized on Gram staining. Serology can be used for diagnosis by measurement of Mycoplasma-specific IgG and IgM, with a rising titre suggestive of infection. Infection can cause lobar pneumonia. Complications include haemolytic anaemia secondary to cold agglutinins, erythema nodosum and multiforme, Guillain–Barré syndrome, meningo-encephalitis, and Stevens–Johnson syndrome. Necrotizing fasciitis, however, is a rapidly progressive infection of the superficial and deep fascia particularly caused by organisms such as Group A *Streptococcus* and anaerobes. It is a surgical emergency with debridement of infected tissue essential for treatment.

Török E et al., *Oxford Handbook of Infectious Diseases and Microbiology*, Oxford University Press, 2009, Chapter 4, Systematic microbiology, Mycoplasma. http://ohinfdis.oxfordmedicine.com/cgi/content/full/1/1/med-9780198569251-div1-221

85. D. Intravenous ceftriaxone 2 g

This student has signs and symptoms that raise concerns of meningococcal septicaemia with meningitis. The presence of septic shock means a lumbar puncture is not the most urgent step, and may be inappropriate in view of the purpura and possible disseminated intravascular coagulation (DIC). In the presence of shock and absence of neurological signs, a CT brain should be delayed until the patient is stabilized. Acyclovir is appropriate treatment for viral encephalitis, which is unlikely to be the diagnosis in the case described here. Ceftriaxone is the current recommended treatment for meningitis or meningococcal sepsis. The appropriate dose of ceftriaxone in severe illness is 2 g.

British Infection Association guidelines for meningitis, 2003. http://www.britishinfection.org/guidelines-resources/published-guidelines/

86. B. Plain abdominal X-ray

Urinary tract infections are relatively common in women. Single infections may be treated empirically without further investigation while a mid-stream urine should be requested in those women with recurrent infection. Only 4% of women in general practice with recurrent bacterial cystitis have abnormalities on further investigation. The presence of *Proteus* on culture raises the possibility of urolithiasis and a plain urinary tract X-ray may in the first instance identify the presence of renal stones. See NICE guidelines for management of urinary tract infections, asymptomatic bacteriuria (especially in pregnancy) and in those with urinary catheters.

Török E et al., *Oxford Handbook of Infectious Diseases and Microbiology*, Oxford University Press, 2009, Chapter 4, Systematic microbiology, *Proteus*.

87. C. Gram-positive cocci forming into clusters

This question not only tests your knowledge of infective endocarditis but also requires you to know the Gram-stain appearances of common micro-organisms. The Gram stain provides vital clinical information at an early stage of processing a clinical sample. It not only provides morphological characteristics but information about the nature of the cell wall of the organism. It can be carried out directly on clinical samples (e.g. CSF or sputum) or on organisms cultured from any site. It is important to be aware of the microscopic appearance of a range of common pathogens. Several important examples are shown in Table 5.6. Although morphology cannot precisely discriminate between streptococci and staphylococci, streptococci usually form into short chains while staphylococci are usually seen in clusters. Endocarditis in intravenous drug users can be caused by a diverse range of organisms. However, *Staphylococcus aureus* is consistently found to be the most common isolate. Other organisms isolated include streptococci, enterococci, Gram-negative rods, and *Candida* (especially *C. parapsilosis*). A significant minority of infections are polymicrobial. The tricuspid valve is most frequently affected.

Gordon R, Lowy F, Bacterial infections in drug users, *New England Journal of Medicine* 2005;353:1945–1954.

Table 5.6 Gram-stain appearances of common micro-organisms

Gram-positive cocci	Gram-negative cocci
Any *Staphylococcus* species including: *Staphylococcus aureus* Any *Streptococcus* species including: *Streptococcus pyogenes* *Streptococcus viridans* *Streptococcus pneumoniae*	*Neisseria sp.* (*meningitidis* and *gonorrhoea*)
Gram-positive rods	**Gram-negative rods**
Clostridium sp. (*botulinum, tetani,* etc.) *Bacillus anthracis* *Listeria monocytogenes*	*Escherichia coli* *Klebsiella pneumonia* *Pseudomonas aeruginosa* *Haemophilus influenza* *Legionella pneumophila*

88. D. Typhoid

The presentation is that of a typical case of enteric fever caused by *Salmonella typhi* or *Salmonella paratyphi*. The lack of travel advice before travel implies that he was not immunized against typhoid prior to his trip. Fever and gastrointestinal symptoms following travel to a high-risk area are typical of enteric fever. It is common to also develop a cough. The blood tests show a normal total leukocyte count but lymphopenia, with a raised ALT and CRP. Malaria needs to be excluded but the normal platelet count and haemoglobin are reassuring that this is less likely to be the cause of the fever.

Török E et al., *Oxford Handbook of Infectious Diseases and Microbiology*, Oxford University Press, 2009, Chapter 5, Clinical syndromes, Enteric fever.

89. A. Continue oral amoxicillin and commence MRSA eradication therapy with mupirocin

The British Thoracic Society recommends that patients with a low CURB-65 score requiring admission to hospital for social reasons are treated with oral amoxicillin as first-line antibiotic therapy. This patient is responding to amoxicillin as assessed by both the resolution of his fever and improvement in inflammatory markers (CRP). *Staphylococcus aureus* frequently contaminates sputum cultures due to colonization of colonization, systemic therapy with antibiotics active against MRSA is not required. Patients with staphylococcal pneumonia are typically severely unwell. Patients with colonization of the throat with MRSA can sometimes be treated with systemic therapy but this is only rarely indicated in particularly difficult patients and decontamination therapy is usually achieved with topical therapy. Of the alternative antibiotic options suggested in the answer stems, piperacillin/tazobactam is a beta-lactamase inhibitor combination with a spectrum of action against Gram-positive and Gram-negative bacteria. However, it does not have activity against MRSA. The other three suggested antibiotic options all do have activity against MRSA and may be indicated for treatment of symptomatic MRSA infection. Fucidic acid and rifampicin in combination is a commonly recommended oral therapy that is effective in non-severe infection only. Vancomycin (by the intravenous route only) is effective against severe MRSA infection and remains the most commonly used antibiotic for this indication. There are clinical trial data suggesting that linezolid is more effective than vancomycin for ventilator-associated pneumonia (VAP) and many authorities suggest the use of this agent for VAP, particularly if severe. Daptomycin, one of the other newer agents with activity against MRSA, should not be used in pneumonia as it is inactivated by surfactant and likely to be ineffective. In a patient of this age, the isolated MRSA is likely to be healthcare-associated. However, there has been much recent interest in the increasing prevalence of community-acquired MRSA infection, which has been associated with outbreaks of foliculitis (most famously affecting North American sports teams). There have been infrequent cases of severe, necrotizing pneumonias associated with these organisms, which often express the Panton–Valentine leukocidin exotoxin—although the role of this toxin in pathogenesis is disputed. Patients present with severe, usually bilateral, pneumonia with haemoptysis and cavity formation; mortality is high. Community-acquired MRSA remains uncommon in the UK but is common in North America and many other parts of the world.

Coia JE et al., Guidelines for the control and prevention of meticillin-resistant *Staphylococcus aureus* (MRSA) in healthcare facilities, *Journal of Hospital Infection* 2006;63S:S1–44.

90. A. Amoxicillin

Gram-positive rods that exhibit tumbling motility are Listeria monocytogenes. Listeria infection is relatively uncommon in the United Kingdom but there is an association between pregnancy and infection. Invasive infection during pregnancy usually presents with bacteraemia and placental infection whereas meningoencephalitis is the most common presenting feature in older and immunocompromised patients who make up the majority of cases. Listeria is unusual in that it is sensitive to penicillins such as amoxicillin but resistant to cephalosporins and therefore is not covered by the usual UK empirical treatment for meningitis based on a third-generation cephalosporin. Gentamicin is frequently used in combination with amoxicillin in CNS infection but is contraindicated in pregnancy. Pregnancy requires careful consideration of antibiotic therapy as several commonly prescribed antibiotics are contraindicated. Beta-lactams are generally considered to be safe, although a randomized trial of empirical antibiotic therapy for premature rupture of membranes found an association between co-amoxiclav and necrotizing enterocolitis in neonates and this has led to some authorities suggesting that this antibiotic be avoided in late pregnancy. Macrolides are also generally considered safe. However, gentamicin and other aminoglycosides have been associated with hearing impairment in infants while ciprofloxacin was associated with arthropathy in animal models. Folate antagonists such as trimethoprim and co-trimoxazole should be avoided due to the risk of neural tube defects. Tetracyclines are also contraindicated due to problems with skeletal development.

Longmore M et al., *Oxford Handbook of Clinical Medicine*, Eighth Edition, Oxford University Press, 2010, Chapter 9, Infectious diseases, Susceptibilities to antibiotics.

91. E. Oral clarithromycin

The British Thoracic Society (BTS) guidelines for the management of community-acquired pneumonia suggest that all patients with community-acquired pneumonia are assessed using the CURB-65 severity score. This assessment gives one point for each of the five criteria that can be applied to the patient. The criteria are: new confusion, urea greater than 7 mmol/l, respiratory rate greater than 30, systolic blood pressure less than 90 mmHg or diastolic blood pressure less than 60 mmHg, and age greater than 65. Patients with CURB-65 scores of 0 or 1 are generally considered to have non-severe pneumonia and may be candidates for outpatient therapy. Patients with scores of 3 or more are considered to have severe pneumonia with a high risk of complications and death. These patients require aggressive management. The patient described above has a CURB-65 score of 0 and as such has non-severe pneumonia and is likely to be a candidate for outpatient therapy. The BTS guidelines suggest amoxicillin (preferred), clarithromycin, or doxycycline monotherapy for non-severe community-acquired pneumonia managed in the community. Ciprofloxacin is not as effective as other choices against *Streptococcus pneumonia* and is therefore not recommended. If the patient had more severe community-acquired pneumonia, requiring admission to hospital, then combination oral therapy with amoxicillin and clarithromycin in moderate severity (e.g. CURB-65 = 2) or intravenous co-amoxiclav with clarithromycin in high severity (e.g. CURB-65 = 3 or more) are indicated.

Lim WS et al., Guidelines for the management of community acquired pneumonia in adults: update 2009, *Thorax* 2009;64(Suppl III):iii1–iii55.

92. E. Schistosoma mansoni

The combination of fever, splenomegaly, and eosinophilia is the classic presentation of Katayama fever, the acute presentation of schistosomiasis. Given that this patient has just returned from an area with a high incidence of schistosomiasis infection, this is the most likely cause. Malaria is the most important cause of fever in a returning traveller from endemic areas and must be excluded. However, eosinophilia is uncommon in malaria. Eosinophilia is also uncommon in melioidosis (caused by *Burkholderia pseudomallei*), an infection common in Australia and South East Asia. It can cause pneumonia and complicated skin and soft tissue infection which can recur many years after the patient has left an endemic area. Dengue fever can cause fever and rash but is an unusual cause of eosinophilia. Helminth infections are an important cause of peripheral eosinophilia and these also must be considered. Non-infectious causes of eosinophilia, such as asthma and Hodgkin's lymphoma, must also be considered.

Gryseels B et al., Human schistosomiasis, *Lancet* 2006;368:1106–1118.

93. A. Elevated LDH

LDH is typically raised in cases of *Pneumocystis jirovecii* pneumonia, the most likely diagnosis here. It is not however specific or sensitive. Chest X-ray may be normal, although perihilar infiltration/ fluffy shadowing is often seen. Transfer factor is reduced due to pulmonary infiltrates. Pneumocystis pneumonia is an AIDS-defining illness; as such CD4 count is universally reduced. The organism is not identified on routine culture, and specialist staining, usually with silver stains, is required.

Chapman S et al., *Oxford Handbook of Respiratory Medicine*, Second Edition, Oxford University Press, 2009, Chapter 41, Respiratory infection: fungal, Pneumocystis pneumonia (PCP): diagnosis.

94. E. Typhoid (enteric fever)

Typhoid, also known as enteric fever, is not caused by *Rickettsia* but by *Salmonella typhi* or *paratyphi*. Typhoid is a systemic illness with clinical features including abdominal pain with diarrhoea or constipation, fever, often lymphadenopathy, and sometimes a rash resembling 'rose spots'.

Török E et al., *Oxford Handbook of Infectious Diseases and Microbiology*, Oxford University Press, 2009, Chapter 4, Systematic microbiology, Rickettsial diseases.

95. B. It may be auto-inoculated from non-genital to genital sites

HPV virus is one genus of a group of double-stranded DNA viruses. Examination of genital warts (condylomata acuminate) and common skin warts (verrucae vulgares) showed both types of lesions contain morphologically identical virus particles (although much reduced in genital lesions), but they are revealed through immune electron microscopy to be antigenically distinct. Although most cross-sectional studies have shown that the prevalence of type-specific serum antibodies is higher in women than men, the reason is unclear, but may reflect the difference in the numbers of sexual partners between the sexes. Sometimes ano-genital warts are caused by HPV types associated with common skin warts (types 1, 2, or 4), most likely acquired through auto-inoculation.

McMillan A et al., *Sexually Transmissible Infections in Clinical Practice*, Elsevier, 2002, Chapter 5, Human papillomavirus infection.

96. C. Three

BHIVA recommends therapy-naive patients start ART containing 2 NRTIs and one of the following 3 classes of drugs, a ritonavir(r)-boosted protease inhibitor (PI/r), an NNRTI (non-nucleoside reverse transcriptase inhibitor), or an integrase inhibitor (INI).

BHIVA, BHIVA guidelines for the treatment of HIV-1-positive adults with antiretroviral therapy 2012, *HIV Medicine* 13:1–85.

97. A. Doxycycline

Mononeuritis, coupled with arthralgia and relative bradycardia, and exposure to a tick bite, is suggestive of Lyme disease. Doxycycline is the treatment of choice, with amoxicillin the default alternative. In the event that both are unsuitable, then BD cefuroxime is an option. If cellulitis is also suspected, then co-amoxiclav or cefuroxime combined with flucloxacillin are used. Thankfully, although Lyme carditis and mononeuritis can be associated with significant morbidity, they resolve in over 90% of cases.

Johnson C et al, *Oxford Handbook of Expedition and Wilderness Medicine*, Oxford University Press, 2008, Chapter 14, Infectious diseases.

98. A. Check VZV IgG

Most labs can process samples for VZV IgG within 48 hours. If the result shows no evidence of previous chicken pox infection, then this patient is at significant risk of severe disease. VZV IgG can be given at any time up to 10 days post-exposure to an infected person, and is effective at preventing or modifying the severity of an episode in the immunocompromised patient. This can also be supplemented by oral acyclovir. Live attenuated *varicella zoster* vaccinations are available, although they are not indicated for post-exposure prophylaxis.

Ramrakha P et al, *Oxford Handbook of Acute Medicine*, Third Edition, Oxford University Press, 2010, Chaper 7, Infections diseases.

99. A. Metronidazole

Both metronidazole and oral vancomycin are potential options for the treatment of *C. difficile*. Vancomycin may be marginally better due to changes in the luminal concentration of metronidazole meaning that it may be less effective towards the end of a course of therapy. Metronidazole can be given both orally and intravenously, but works better orally. Vancomycin is not absorbed when given orally, and therefore creates a high concentration in the colon. Vancomycin does not work if given intravenously for treatment of *C. difficile* because it is not excreted in the colon. Teicoplanin and rifampicin may be options for resistant disease. Ciprofloxacin is well recognized as a cause of *C. difficile*.

Wiffen P et al, *Oxford Handbook of Clinical Pharmacy*, Second Edition, Oxford University Press, 2012, Therapy-related issues: infections.

100. A. Schistosomiasis

The fact that this man may have been working in a village in Zambia is indicative of possible *Schistosomiasis* infection, through exposure to local water courses. This fits with dysuria, haematuria, proteinuria, and anaemia because of chronic blood loss. The eosinophilia is also suggestive of parasitic infection. Afternoon urine specimens are the optimal way to confirm the diagnosis, with praziquantel the treatment of choice. We are given no history of unprotected sexual intercourse; as such, gonorrhoea is much less likely. *Proteus* urinary tract infection over the longer term is associated with urinary stone formation. With respect to IgA nephropathy, we would have expected a clear history of respiratory tract infection, and in minimal change disease there is predominantly proteinuria.

Pattman R et al, *Oxford Handbook of Genitourinary Medicine, HIV, and Sexual Health*, Second Edition, Oxford University Press, 2010, Chapter 17, Tropical genital and sexually acquired infections,

101. A. Permethrin

This patient's rash, and the position of his most severe symptoms, itching occuring between the web spaces, is most consistent with a diagnosis of scabies. As such, permethrin is the most appropriate first-line therapy. Screening for sexually transmitted diseases is indicated, although at this stage antibiotics are not unless any infection is proven. Hydrocortisone is not indicated whilst there is ongoing parasitic infection.

Pattman R et al, *Oxford Handbook of Genitourinary Medicine, HIV, and Sexual Health*, Second Edition, Oxford University Press, 2010.

102. C. Infection with high-risk HPV type

In women it is correlated with older age (peak age group at which diagnosis made in Scottish clinics was 20–24 years), infection with multiple types of HPV, and infection with high-risk HPV types. Whether infection with one type of HPV confers immunity against either infection with other types or re-infection with the same type is uncertain. Smoking tobacco may also be a risk factor for the development of genital warts in women. A study by Feldman et al. found that current smokers were 5.2 times more likely to develop warts than non-smokers. The reasons are uncertain.

McMillan A et al., *Sexually Transmissible Infections in Clinical Practice*, Elsevier, 2002, Chapter 5, Human papillomavirus infection, p. 78.

103. A. Patients with chronic infection should start treatment when CD4 lymphocyte count is ≤ 350 cells/μl

BHIVA (British HIV Association) guidelines recommend that patients with chronic infection start ART (antiretroviral therapy) if the CD4 cell count is ≤ 350 cells/μl or close to this threshold. Late diagnosis has considerable impact on longevity, with up to 15 years of reduced life expectancy if ART is started later than the current BHIVA guidelines recommend. ART is usually started for the health benefit of the individual, but in certain circumstances it may be beneficial to start ART to primarily reduce the risk of onward sexual transmission of HIV. Treatment does not always start as soon as diagnosis is established but depends on CD4 count, co-morbidity, and stage of pregnancy.

Williams I et al., BHIVA guidelines for the treatment of HIV-1-positive adults with antiretroviral therapy 2012, *HIV Medicine* 2012;13(Suppl. 2):7–11. http://www.bhiva.org/documents/Guidelines/Treatment/2012/hiv1029_2.pdf

104. B. 16

HPV types 16, 18, 31, and 45 are commonly associated with ano-genital carcinomas. Types 2 and 27 are associated with common or mosaic skin warts and type 11 with laryngeal papillomata.

McMillan A et al., *Sexually Transmissible Infections in Clinical Practice*, Elsevier, 2002, Chapter 5, Human papillomavirus infection, p. 72, Table 5.1.

105. A. 6 and 11

Types 3 and 10 are commonly associated with flat warts, types 27 & 2 with common or mosaic warts and types 13 & 32 with focal epithelial hyperplasia.

McMillan A et al., *Sexually Transmissible Infections in Clinical Practice*, Elsevier, 2002, Chapter 5, Human papillomavirus infection, p. 72, Table 5.1.

1. **Regarding diabetic retinopathy, which is true?**
    A. It can cause glaucoma
    B. It is the commonest cause of blindness in the United Kingdom in 30–60-year-olds
    C. Certain forms can be treated with photocoagulation
    D. It can cause rubeosis iridis
    E. There is thinning of the basement membrane of the capillaries

2. **Which of the following abnormalities would one expect to find in a patient with Arnold Chiari malformation?**
    A. Transient visual loss
    B. Third nerve palsy
    C. Sixth nerve palsy
    D. Downbeat nystagmus
    E. Inferior altitudinal field loss in one or both eyes

3. **A patient presents to hospital with a right superior quadrantanopia with no pupillary disturbance. The site of the lesion is:**
    A. Left temporal lobe
    B. Left parietal lobe
    C. Left lateral geniculate nucleus
    D. Optic chiasm
    E. Left optic nerve

4. **A patient presents to hospital with a left inferior homonymous quadrantanopia with no pupillary disturbance. The site of the lesion is:**
    A. Right parietal lobe
    B. Right lateral geniculate nucleus
    C. Optic chiasm
    D. Right temporal lobe
    E. Left optic nerve

5. A 71-year-old woman is admitted to hospital for a routine right total hip replacement. You are asked to see her because she is hallucinating that there is a woman in nineteenth-century clothing at the end of her bed, and she has asked the nurses on a number of occasions to remove the woman. She has a past history of poor vision because of bilateral glaucoma, but there is no other history of note. Her BP is 145/70, pulse is 75 and regular, her hip replacement scar looks clean, chest and abdominal examination are normal. Investigations: haemoglobin 10.1 g/dl (11.5–16.5), white cell count 7.0 x 1(4–11), platelets 212 x 10⁹/l (150–400), serum sodium 136 mmol/l (135–146), serum potassium 4.2 mmol/L (3.5–5), creatinine 99 micromol/l (79–118). What is the most likely diagnosis?

A. Alzheimer's disease
B. Charles Bonnet syndrome
C. Post-operative confusion
D. Urinary sepsis
E. Pick's disease

6. A 35-year-old Caucasian British male develops photophobia and blurred vision. He has a long history of low back pain, and developed mouth ulcers four days ago. He is otherwise fit and well. On examination he has a hypopyon. The most likely of this is:

A. Behçet's disease
B. Syphilis
C. Rheumatoid arthritis
D. Ankylosing spondylitis
E. Sarcoidosis

7. A 28-year-old man with a history of ulcerative colitis which is managed with mesalazine presents with an acutely painful, watering red left eye. Visual acuity is reduced in the left eye; there is direct and consensual photophobia. The eye seems cloudy on examination and you can't see the optic disc clearly. Which of the following is the most likely diagnosis?

A. Posterior uveitis
B. Conjunctivitis
C. Anterior uveitis
D. Acute closed-angle glaucoma
E. Scleritis

8. **A patient has developed retinal damage due to their medication. They have a long history of an arrhythmia, TB, and a connective tissue disease but have always had normal renal function. They have taken all of the drugs listed below. Which of these is most likely to cause retinal toxicity when taken in normal doses?**

   A. Hydroxychloroquine
   B. Cyclophosphamide
   C. Ethambutol
   D. Chloroquine
   E. Digoxin

9. **Bilateral swollen optic discs in the presence of spontaneous retinal venous pulsations are most likely to be seen with?**

   A. Optic disc drusen
   B. Migraine
   C. Multiple sclerosis-associated optic neuritis
   D. Untreated idiopathic intracranial hypertension
   E. Brain tumour

10. **A 32-year-old Caucasian woman with limited adduction of the right eye and nystagmus on abduction in the left eye is likely to have:**

    A. Phenytoin overdose
    B. Arnold Chiari malformation
    C. Thyroid eye disease
    D. Multiple sclerosis
    E. Progressive supra nuclear gaze palsy

11. **Proliferative diabetic retinopathy is best treated by:**

    A. Tight blood sugar control
    B. Tight blood pressure control
    C. Intravitreal lucentis injections
    D. Panretinal photocoagulation laser
    E. Macular grid laser

12. **A 32-year-old woman has multiple cotton wool spots noticed on routine fundoscopy. Which of the following blood tests is least helpful in determining the likely cause?**

    A. Lipid profile
    B. Anti-nuclear antibody
    C. Glucose
    D. Full blood count
    E. HIV test

13. **Which of these best describes the function of the rods in the eye?**

  A. Accommodation for near vision
  B. Depth perception
  C. Colour vision
  D. Image discrimination
  E. Vision in dim light

14. **A 67-year-old woman who has type 2 diabetes mellitus and a previous anterior MI presents to the A and E with sudden, painless central vision loss affecting her right eye. On examination her BP is 185/105, pulse is 80 (atrial fibrillation). Vision on the left is 6/18; it is reduced to count fingers only on the right-hand side. Examination of the retina on the right reveals a pale retina with a cherry red spot in the area of the macula. Which of the following is the most likely diagnosis?**

  A. Branch retinal vein occlusion
  B. Central retinal vein occlusion
  C. Central retinal artery occlusion
  D. Branch retinal artery occlusion
  E. Macular degeneration

15. **A 51-year-old woman with a 40-year history of type 1 diabetes comes to the emergency department complaining of sudden painless loss of vision in her left eye. She has a history of proliferative retinopathy which has required bilateral laser therapy in the last two years. You cannot clearly see the retina and she has lost the red reflex. Which of the following is the most likely diagnosis?**

  A. Central retinal vein occlusion
  B. Central retinal artery occlusion
  C. Ischaemic optic neuritis
  D. Vitreous haemorrhage
  E. CMV retinitis

16. **A 34-year-old woman presents to the emergency department with progressive loss of vision in her left eye. She says over the past 36 hours her colour vision has deteriorated and now she can only see blurred objects out of that eye. There is an afferent pupillary defect on the left, although the disc itself looks normal. Her BP is 122/72, pulse is 74 and regular, and there are no other abnormal features. Which of the following is the most appropriate intervention?**

  A. IV methylprednisolone
  B. IV ganciclovir
  C. Oral aciclovir
  D. Oral prednisolone
  E. IV heparin

17. **A 29-year-old man with a history of ankylosing spondylitis presents with bilateral eye pain, blurred vision, and photophobia. On examination there is bilateral pupil constriction and circumcorneal redness. Slit lamp examination reveals cells in the anterior chamber. Which of the following is the treatment of choice?**

    A. Prednisolone and cyclopentolate eye drops
    B. Oral prednisolone
    C. Prednisolone and atropine eye drops
    D. Prednisolone and timolol eye drops
    E. Timolol and cyclopentolate eye drops

18. **A 54-year-old woman who has a history of type 2 diabetes and hypertension presents to the emergency department with visual loss affecting her right eye. She says that the loss has been painless, and she went from acceptable vision to count fingers only over a period of around 12 hours. Ophthalmoscopy reveals dilated tortuous retinal vessels, cotton wool spots, and retinal haemorrhages in all four quadrants. Which of the following complications gives most cause for concern, around three months after this event?**

    A. Neovascular glaucoma
    B. Vitreous haemorrhage
    C. Central retinal artery occlusion
    D. Optic neuritis
    E. Branch retinal vein occlusion

1. E. There is thinning of the basement membrane of the capillaries

All of the options are true except option E because diabetic retinopathy involves thickening of the basement membrane of the capillaries. Rubeosis iridis is a medical condition of the iris of the eye in which new abnormal blood vessels are found on the surface of the iris.

Collier J et al., *Oxford Handbook of Clinical Specialties*, Eighth Edition, Oxford University Press, 2009, Chapter 5, Ophthalmology, The eye in diabetes mellitus.

2. D. Downbeat nystagmus

Foramen magnum lesions cause downbeat nystagmus, and Arnold Chiari malformation is the condition most likely to cause downbeat nystagmus.

Jackson TL, *Moorfields Manual of Ophthalmology*, Elsevier, 2008, Chapter 4, Neuro-ophthalmology.

3. A. Left temporal lobe

The lesion site for a quadrantanopia can be memorized by the mnenomic PITS: Parietal Inferior, Temporal Superior. Lesions distal to the lateral geniculate nucleus will tend to have pupillary involvement.

Lueck CJ, Loss of vision, *Practical Neurology* 2010;10:315–325.

4. A. Right parietal lobe

The lesion site for a quadrantanopia can be memorized by the mnenomic PITS: Parietal Inferior, Temporal Superior. Lesions distal to the lateral geniculate nucleus will tend to have pupillary involvement.

Lueck CJ, Loss of vision, *Practical Neurology* 2010;10:315–325.

5. B. Charles Bonnet syndrome

Charles Bonnet syndrome occurs in patients with severe visual loss where they may suffer visual hallucinations related to people or objects that are not really there. Recognized associated conditions include age-related macular degeneration, cataract, glaucoma, and diabetic eye disease. Hallucinations may be complex, for instance, seeing a person in the room, or landscape, or just involve repeating patterns. Management involves reassurance, helping patients understand that their poor vision is driving the hallucinations, and making sure the room is well lit and any unusual items are removed from the room. SSRIs have been shown in one study to help with resolution of hallucinations. They become effective slightly more quickly than when used for the treatment of depression, with resolution in one study with venlafexine after only four days.

Lang UE, Charles Bonnet Syndrome: successful treatment of visual hallucinations due to vision loss with selective serotonin reuptake inhibitors, *Journal of Psychopharmacology* 2007;21:553–555. http://jop.sagepub.com/content/21/5/553.short

6. D. Ankylosing spondylitis

This man has uveitis causing a hypopyon. Most anterior uveitis is idiopathic but by far the commonest association with anterior uveitis in the UK is ankylosing spondylitis, particularly in young men with low back pain and a hypopyon. Mouth ulcers are common and are an incidental finding here. Genital ulcers or particularly severe and persistent mouth ulcers might make one consider Behçet's or syphilis. Rheumatoid arthritis is uncommon in young men and does not cause uveitis (juvenile idiopathic arthritis does though). Sarcoidosis can cause anterior uveitis but low back pain and mouth ulcers are not typical features and it is more common in Afro-Carribean patients.

Hakim A et al., *Oxford Handbook of Rheumatology*, Third Edition, Oxford University Press, 2011, Chapter 8, The spondyloarthropathies.

7. C. Anterior uveitis

The history of ulcerative colitis raises the possibility of uveitis, and the combination of conjunctival injection, pain, direct and consensual photophobia supports the diagnosis. The reason that the optic disc isn ot easily visualized is almost certainly due to the presence of cells in the anterior chamber. Cycloplegics such as cyclopentalate, and steroid eye drops are the mainstay of therapy. Azathioprine may be of value in steroid-resistant uveitis. The condition should of course be managed with input from a specialist opthalmologist.

Denniston AKO, Murray PI, *Oxford Handbook of Ophthalmology*, Second Edition, Oxford University Press, 2009, Chapter 11, Uveitis.

8. D. Chloroquine

Chloroquine is now rarely used for connective tissue diseases as long-term use carries a significant risk of retinal toxicity. Patients develop a bull's eye maculopathy and irreversible loss of vision with excessive cumulative dosing. Hydroxychloroquine appears much safer with long-term use, although there is still a small risk particularly after more than six years of treatment or with abnormally high doses. Ethambutol causes an optic neuropathy rather than a retinopathy. Digoxin overdose affects colour vision causing an orange tint to the patient's vision. Cyclophosphamide is a toxic drug but is not a likely cause of a retinopathy.

The Royal College of Ophthalmologists, Hydroxychloroquine and Ocular Toxicity, 2009. https://www.rcophth.ac.uk/2009-sci-010-ocular-toxicity/

9. A. Optic disc drusen

Optic disc drusen are calcific deposits in the optic nerve head which cause the disc to appear swollen. Spontaneous venous pulsations show that the intracranial pressure is not raised although absent pulsations do not necessarily mean the intracranial pressure is raised. Migraine does not cause optic disc swelling, and headache in the presence of optic disc swelling is a worrying finding. Optic neuritis can cause optic disc swelling from direct inflammation of the nerve in one-third of cases but is very unlikely to be bilateral. Both brain tumour and idiopathic intracranial hypertension cause raised intracranial pressure and therefore retinal venous pulsations would not be expected to be present.

Denniston AKO, Murray PI, *Oxford Handbook of Ophthalmology*, Second Edition, Oxford University Press, 2009, Chapter 16, Neuro-ophthalmology, Pseudopapilloedema, Table 16.10.

10. D. Multiple sclerosis

This is a description of internuclear ophthalmoplegia which is usually caused by demyelination affecting the medial longitudinal fasciculus connecting the sixth and third nerve nuclei. Phenytoin overdose may cause nystagmus but not limited adduction. Thyroid eye disease may cause limited adduction but not nystagmus. Progressive supra nuclear gaze palsy causes symmetrical reduction in eye movements, particularly affecting vertical eye movements, and is associated with poor balance and dementia. It affects older patients.

Jackson TL, *Moorfields Manual of Ophthalmology*, Elsevier, 2008, Chapter 14, Neuro-ophthalmology.

11. D. Panretinal photocoagulation laser

Patients with proliferative diabetic retinopathy require urgent panretinal photocoagulation laser (within two weeks). Tightening blood sugar control and blood pressure control in the short term can actually make the retinopathy worse although there is long-term benefit. Macular grid laser is only appropriate for diabetic macular oedema (maculopathy), not for proliferative disease. Lucentis is used for age-related macular oedema and recent trials show it is also effective for diabetic maculopathy but it has not yet been shown to be effective for proliferative disease (December 2010).

Ockrim Z, Yorston D, Managing diabetic retinopathy, *British Medical Journal* 2010;341:c5400.

12. A. Lipid profile

Abnormal lipids are unlikely to cause cotton wool spots; the fundal appearance is typically normal with hyperlipidaemia. Cotton wool spots occur with HIV retinopathy, severe anaemia, systemic lupus erythematosis (signifying a flare-up of the condition), and diabetes.

Jackson TL, *Moorfields Manual of Ophthalmology*, Mosby, 2008.

13. E. Vision in dim light

Cones are involved in colour vision and depth perception. Rods are involved in perception of objects in dim light.

Collier J et al., *Oxford Handbook of Clinical Specialties*, Eighth Edition, Oxford University Press, 2009, Chapter 5, Ophthalmology, Blindness and partial sight.

14. C. Central retinal artery occlusion

Central retinal artery (CRA) occlusion is associated with a pale retina apart from the cherry red spot in the area of the macula—cherry red because of preserved blood supply from intact choroid vessels. Immediate referral is recommended as some blood flow and hence vision may be restored. Treatments including ocular massage, acetazolamide, and locally delivered TPA have all been attempted with variable success.

Denniston AKO, Murray PI, *Oxford Handbook of Ophthalmology*, Second Edition, Oxford University Press, 2009, Chapter 13, Medical retina.

15. D. Vitreous haemorrhage

The sudden painless loss of vision, coupled with loss of the red reflex and obscured retina, fits best with vitreous haemorrhage. It is quite possible this has occurred as a result of neovascularisation leading to the formation of fragile vessels which have a greater propensity to bleed. Where a large haemorrhage has occured, a B-scan ultrasound is employed to determine the site of the bleed. Haemorrhage may take up to three months to resolve.

Collier J et al., *Oxford Handbook of Clinical Specialties*, Eighth Edition, Oxford University Press, 2009, Chapter 5, Opthalmology.

16. A. IV methylprednisolone

The clinical picture and findings on eye examination are consistent with optic neuritis. Initial therapy of choice for optic neuritis is IV methylprednisolone, for 72 hours, followed by oral prednisolone to complete a two-week course of corticosteroid treatment. Recovery is usual over 2–6 weeks, although 40–80% of individuals develop multiple sclerosis in subsequent years. The appearance of the retina does not support an infective cause such as CMV retinitis underlying the visual loss seen here.

Collier J et al., *Oxford Handbook of Clinical Specialties*, Eighth Edition, Oxford University Press, 2009, Chapter 5, Opthalmology.

17. A. Prednisolone and cyclopentolate eye drops

The diagnosis here is anterior uveitis, which occurs more frequently in patients who have seronegative arthritides or inflammatory bowel disease. It is thought to be related to HLA-B27 positivity. The aims of therapy are to prevent damage from prolonged inflammation (because this causes disruption to the flow of aqueous inside the eye, with glaucoma occurring ± adhesions between iris and lens). Drug therapies include steroids, eg 0.5–1% prednisolone drops every two hours, to reduce inflammation (hence pain, redness, and exudate), and to prevent adhesions between lens and iris (synechiae), the pupil is kept dilated with cyclopentolate 0.5% 1–2 drops/8h. Early referral to the ophthalmologist is also very important.

Collier J et al., *Oxford Handbook of Clinical Specialties*, Eighth Edition, Oxford University Press, 2009, Chapter 5, Opthalmology.

18. A. Neovascular glaucoma

The diagnosis here is central retinal vein occlusion, the long-term outcome of which is variable, with possible improvement for six months to one year. The main problems are macular oedema and neovascular glaucoma secondary to iris neovascularization. In ischaemic central retinal vein occlusion, 60% develop neovascular glaucoma (called '100 days glaucoma' as it develops within this time after the occlusion). There is no validated treatment for post-occlusion macular oedema. Neovascular glaucoma requires aggressive panretinal laser photocoagulation. Vitreous haemorrhage is not a major concern after central retinal vein occlusion, being seen most commonly in proliferative retinopathy in patients with diabetes mellitus. Central retinal artery occlusion is most associated with embolic phenomena, and optic neuritis may be ischaemic or inflammatory in origin.

Collier J et al., *Oxford Handbook of Clinical Specialties*, Eighth Edition, Oxford University Press, 2009, Chapter 5, Opthalmology.

INDEX

Note: Page numbers in *q* refer to Question and *a* refer to Answer. References to figures, tables, and boxes are indicated by 'f', 't', and 'b' following the page number, for example 14*af* refers to a figure on page 14.